Cannabis and Cannabinoid-Based Medicines in Cancer Care

Claude Cyr • Mellar P. Davis • Danial Schecter
Paul Daeninck

Cannabis and Cannabinoid-Based Medicines in Cancer Care

A Comprehensive Guide to Medical Management

Springer

Claude Cyr
McGill University
Department of Family Medicine
Montreal, QC, Canada

Danial Schecter
Royal Victoria Regional
Health Centre
Barrie, ON, Canada

Mellar P. Davis
Palliative Care Research
Geisinger Health System
Danville, PA
USA

Paul Daeninck
CancerCare Manitoba, Winnipeg
Regional Palliative Care Program
Max Rady College of Medicine
University of Manitoba
Winnipeg, MB, Canada

ISBN 978-3-030-89917-2 ISBN 978-3-030-89918-9 (eBook)
https://doi.org/10.1007/978-3-030-89918-9

This Springer imprint is published by the registered company Springer Nature Switzerland AG
The registered company address is: Gewerbestrasse 11, 6330 Cham, Switzerland

This book is dedicated to the frontline medical cannabis pioneers in Chile, Peru, Jamaica, Malawi, South Africa, the UK, France, and elsewhere, working towards the decriminalization of an act of compassion, and because they remind me of my father's undying quest to make things right in the world.

Preface

Is cannabis medicine?

Although several synthetic and natural cannabinoid extracts are indeed officially categorized as approved pharmaceuticals, this textbook will focus on all compounds that exhibit clinically significant interactions with the endocannabinoid system in cancer care, including the aforementioned approved medications as well as the more commonly used, and non-approved, natural cannabis products. For the vast majority of cancer patients who presently consider phytocannabinoids to be a valuable adjunct to their treatment regimen, we cannot yet provide them with a definitive answer since the science of using whole plant medicine is complex and will continue to be challenged as novel synthetic cannabinoids or combinations of isolated cannabinoids take on a larger role in future clinical trials. It is the hope that the following chapters will encourage clinicians to make this clear distinction and permit them to remain critical of the limited available data on the use of non-approved cannabis-derived products in any clinical setting.

Though we may be facing the final days of prohibition, the study of cannabis in randomized clinical trials, considered the gold standard to determine efficacy, remains an extremely difficult endeavor for researchers everywhere, even in Canada where comprehensive frameworks for the use of medical and recreational cannabis have been enacted. Unfortunately, many bureaucratic roadblocks continue to thwart researchers, and clinical studies using natural cannabis-based medicines will require protracted efforts in order to provide an acceptable level of evidence of safety and efficacy. This will be further compounded by the inherent diversity of cannabinoids, their complex pharmacodynamic interactions, and the multiple clinical applications for which preclinical trials have suggested possible benefits. The Byzantine system of forestalling research happens to persist in an age where social media has produced a crisis of confidence in many fields of knowledge, from climate science to medicine. The recent discovery of the endocannabinoid system (ECS) could not have arrived at a more perilous time.

Many scientific and government-sanctioned authorities naively believed that their judicious analysis of the science and sage guidance through the impenetrable complexity of the natural world would withstand the democratization and dissemination of information which has increased exponentially in social media. Instead of retaining their status as the most trusted resource, they have in fact met a series of humbling defeats in the forum of public opinion. The medical profession has certainly not been spared, and the increasing availability of cannabis products resulting from the successive breakdown of legal barriers has created a rapidly evolving and mostly unregulated landscape with plenty of flashy promises and little guidance from health authorities. While the reasons for the apparent drop in confidence are still being scrutinized by the *actual* experts in our historically respected medical associations, vulnerable patients are being lured by many *self-proclaimed* experts advancing questionable interpretations from much of the preclinical literature, and claiming that cannabis should be regarded as an adjunct and even alternative treatment to standard cancer care. In an age where obvious facts are considered by some as merely diverging opinions, it's no surprise that the sudden reappearance of an "ancient medicine," victim of a prolonged and senseless prohibition, and often regarded as natural and safe, can become a tempting alternative for desperate and misinformed cancer patients.

To quote Margaret Haney: "With a federally illegal drug legalised in individual states, scientists constrained, and federal agencies somewhat silent, clinicians have none of the data that guide their decisions for medications… In this scientific vacuum, a billion-dollar industry has swept in without evidence but with an obvious conflict of interest and with little regulation of quality control, advertising, or product labeling… The legalization of cannabis and the use of terms such as" medicinal" cannabis or 'medical marijuana' and 'recreational' has provided the public a false sense of safety and legitimacy for its use." This is indeed a sobering statement, and although western medical cannabis literature spans back nearly 200 hundred years and includes hundreds of case reports and expert opinions, these clearly provide an insufficient level of evidence in the age of properly conducted randomized controlled trials.

The vast influence of cannabinoids on multiple organ systems has been rapidly evolving in preclinical models and observational studies over the last few decades. However, these results are considered preliminary and have been the target of many critiques which essentially point to the cold fact that the current level of evidence is insufficient in order to receive an official stamp of approval from medical regulatory authorities. This is further complicated by the fact that cannabis contains over a hundred metabolically active compounds interacting with dozens of molecular targets in multiple organ systems and disease states. Furthermore, trials to date have for the most part used unstandardized cannabis products and derivatives, examined different delivery methods and populations, and used different designs, analysis, outcome measures, and timeframes.

Thus, conclusions drawn from comparing presently available cannabis trials remain weak, contradictory, and largely inconsistent, and we must be reminded that the evidence from replicability is far stronger than the results from a single study with a significant P value, according to Steven N Goodman. The high rate of non-replicability from cannabis research findings has led many stakeholders to rely on "real-world" observational studies and surveys, or claiming conclusive research findings solely on the basis of a single study assessed by formal statistical significance, typically using a P-value of less than 0.05. This convenient perspective is nonetheless considered a failed strategy, according to several authors (Sterne, Davey Smith, Wacholder, and Rish), and has created an unsettled debate. On one hand, discarding observational studies when the evidence from randomized trials is available is to miss an opportunity for exploring similarities and differences. Conversely, favoring observational studies while abandoning the results of randomized trials is considered poor science.

The Thalidomide fiasco of the early 1960s was a defining moment in medical history. The pharmaceutical industry, emboldened by a series of near miraculous discoveries, felt that safety concerns were a hindrance to scientific progress, and also their shareholders' enthusiasm. Many unscrupulous clinicians agreed to turn a blind eye to egregious ethics violations and welcomed the opportunity to be the figureheads for an industry that had lost its moral compass. In some ways, the erosion in public trust which it produced has never completely healed. The western medical establishment, whose purpose is to ensure guidance for safe and effective treatments, struggled to regain its credibility as a benevolent institution. The enactment of evidence-based standards has indeed greatly improved the roadmap for more accountability in future drug development but remains constantly challenged. The intoxicating financial incentives following patent approval still require a watchful eye from trusted and independent authorities, and continued slip ups are not uncommon.

While high-quality randomized controlled trials using medical cannabis can also fall prey to clever design readjustments and statistical manipulations, they also mostly remain financially out of reach since the debate over the intellectual property of cannabis genomics remains unresolved.

This of course has left many clinicians wondering which course of action to take: Should we wait for medical authorities to give the green light, or should we dive in, learn what we can from the art and science that is presently available, and counsel our patients on a safe exploration of this unique set of compounds? One could argue that, since many patients have decided to forgo the evidence and embark in this process with or without their physicians' consent, the answer to this dilemma is self-evident.

Thus, the authors aim not only to provide an overview of the current state of the evidence but also propose a more flexible perspective to justify the clinical use of cannabis and cannabinoids in cancer care. By focusing on principles of compassion and safe integration, this allows for a more pragmatic approach to the introduction and monitoring of these compounds in select cancer patients.

Montreal, QC, Canada Claude Cyr
Danville, PA, USA Mellar P. Davis

Acknowledgments

The writing of this textbook could not have been possible without the unwavering love and support from our better halves. Dr. Daeninck would like to thank his wife Monica, who has shown steadfast support through his career and their shared endeavors. Dr Davis would like to acknowledge the support of his wife Deborah and his children; Luke, Amanda, Meghan, Jessamyn, Emelin and Lilian in all his endeavors. In my case, I would like to show my grateful appreciation to my wonderful family: my love Andreanne, my daughter Emma, and son Théo. You make life a truer, brighter, and nobler experience, respectively.

Many many thanks to my co-authors and co-editors for their dedication to scrupulous research and our shared cautious optimism for cannabinoid-based medicine. Thanks as well to Drs. Connor Prosty, Samuel Qizilbash, and Christian Dabrowski for their valued feedback on the early drafts.

A very special thanks to the man who can process anything and find a solution, my friend and fellow crime fighter Sean Robert Senechal. A loving thanks as well to my siblings, true beings one and all: my sisters Anne, embracing the cause, Julie, forever carrying the family's heart, and of course that shining beacon of reason, my amazing brother Pierre.

Thanks as well to a long list of immensely sympathetic individuals, ranging from my longtime colleague Samer Daher to my rockin' neighbors Fuzz and Mat, Liz, Elise, Sophie (x2), Stuart, Martin P. et T., Dan, Mo, Eric, and my truly gifted clinical, research, and teaching colleagues. A very special thanks to Steph Sherer and Kevin Jones of Americans for Safe Access for their generous insights on the present challenges facing not only patients in search of safe and standardized products but also the majority of clinicians who struggle to find reliable information in order to properly integrate cannabis in their armamentarium.

A very very special thanks to all the movers and shakers who initially got the ball rolling, the visionary politicians and lawmakers Trudeau (*père et fils*), Jean Chrétien, and the Supreme Court of Canada who showed their courage at the turn of the millennium and finally started asking the burning question: "what's all the big fuss about?" Thanks of course to those who are pushing the ball forward, the many friends and colleagues living and working in The Magical Land of Oz, otherwise known as the Canadian cannabis industry. May you flourish and honor good science.

A final word of thanks to my extended family and lovely bunch of eccentric friends who drifted in and out of my parent's funhouse during our halcyon days, when Time was truly golden in the mercy of his means. Starting with the members of the Gambolputty(sp?) Dadaist collective: my goombella Marcey-kins "Full-Goose Bozo" Saint-Peter, Donny "The D is for America," Randy Rhodes, the brothers Danny "Snapper-organs" and Brigadier-General Maurice "knit the bomb" Piranha, Roger "Drum" Tree-Spirit, Phillip "Manhandling is not assault" Scolder, the spirited Sir Paul "Punmeister," and all the other endearing metalheads, Potato Queens, spirit mediums, hippies, and poets (living and dead) who transformed a quiet New Brunswick town into a joyous Fellini movie. You will forever march in the fields of praise.

Montreal, QC, Canada Claude Cyr

About the Book

This textbook aims to address the use of cannabinoids in advanced cancer and palliative care patients and provide the necessary guidance which will allow clinicians to safely introduce these compounds even in frail patients. The proposed recommendations are meant to be used in this specific clinical context only and should not be inferred as being applicable to any other clinical setting. Pending further evidence, the authors believe that access to cannabinoids should be prioritized in advanced cancer and end-of-life settings. This textbook will further argue that the available evidence strongly suggests that early introduction of these compounds should be considered for most patients facing life-threatening illnesses.

The first three chapters will examine the present state and future directions of cannabinoid science. It may be more suitable for readers having a basic understanding of the endocannabinoid system (ECS) and the expanded *endocannabinoidome* and who wish to explore the most recent preclinical and clinical studies which provide a rationale for present and future clinical uses of these compounds in different cancer care settings. For those needing a more general overview of the ECS, many accredited online resources are available, such as those offered by Americans for Safe Access https://www.safeaccessnow.org/, Society of Cannabis Clinicians https://www.cannabisclinicians.org/, and The Canadian Consortium on the Investigation of Cannabinoids (CCIC) https://ccic.net/, among others.

Chapters 4 and 5 will focus more on the applied science of medical cannabis, and are intended for clinicians seeking practical advice on choosing the appropriate clinical settings where cannabis may provide benefits. The level of text presupposes a firm grasp of the medical lexicon. However, Chaps. 6 and 7, which are dedicated to patient evaluation and treatment initiation, including dosing, administration, and management of adverse effects, may be more accessible to most healthcare providers and caregivers.

The final chapter of this textbook will examine the often-ignored benefits of cannabis psychoactivity. The intention to explore these unique effects will invariably face certain cultural biases that must be challenged if clinicians wish to engage in a genuine and fully compassionate discussion centered on the ease of suffering in cancer patients. Therefore, in an attempt to provide a further rationale to consider the use of CBM and cannabis as part of the standard of care for advanced cancer and palliative patients, the reader may need to confront emotionally charged or preconceived notions regarding the psycholytic and psychedelic experiences encountered with increasing doses of THC.

For readers with an emerging interest but only looking for a brief overview of the evidence so far, the authors have provided a summary of key recommendations and suggestions found in the annex. The list is divided in two parts, beginning with *recommendations* for which a higher degree of evidence has been put forward, while the second part offers *suggestions* addressing issues considered more conjectural and are based mostly on interpretations of preclinical data or empirical clinical experience. And finally, the *2021 Cannabis Index* is provided as an amusing list of recent cannabis science facts.

Terminology Used in this Textbook

A glossary can be found in the annex of the terms used in this textbook pertaining to the products, structures, and characteristics which have arisen from this new branch of science. These include many vernacular expressions as well as their scientific equivalents, several of which have only recently been coined. However, this has led to a multiplication of subtly different terms by different authors aiming to describe similar concepts. Pending a wider consensus over which of these should be generally accepted into the medical lexicon, the authors have chosen what they believe to be the most accurate descriptors. Equivalent or semi-equivalent terms will only be mentioned to point out subtle differences when clinically relevant. Of these, three important terms will be quickly mentioned here, since they will be frequently encountered in the textbook:

1. **Endocannabinoid System (ECS)** versus *Endocannabinoidome (eCBome)*. The term “endocannabinoid system (ECS)” refers to the original and basic physiological concepts described earlier. The “endocannabinoidome (eCBome)” may in fact be a more appropriate term since it encompasses the far-reaching effects of this multi organ system. However, the authors have chosen to mostly use the more widely known term “endocannabinoid system (ECS)” when referring to both the original canonical receptors and enzymes or the larger system of molecular targets and ligands. The term “endocannabinoidome” will be discussed in more detail in the first chapter, and will only be further mentioned in order to point out a clinically relevant difference between these two related concepts in the following chapters.
2. **Cannabinoid-Based Medicines (CBM)** versus *Cannabis-Based Medicines or Endocannabinoid System Modulators*. With few exceptions, most presently available products fall under the category of “cannabinoid-based medicines (CBM),” which includes natural and synthetic pharmaceuticals. Although the term “endocannabinoid system modulators” may eventually be regarded as the

general umbrella definition which includes CBM and all compounds that interact either directly or indirectly with the receptors, ion channels, enzymes, and transporter proteins associated with the ECS and the endocannabinoidome, it will not be used in this textbook, unless clinically relevant.

3. **Medical Cannabis** versus *Medical Marij(h)uana/Cannabis/Cannabis for Therapeutic Purposes.* The term "medical cannabis" will be the preferred designation for products specifically derived from the natural cannabis plant and when used for therapeutic purposes.

Contents

1 Overview of the Endocannabinoid System and Endocannabinoidome 1
1.1 Introduction 2
1.2 Terminology 4
1.3 The Canonical Cannabinoid Receptors: CB1 and CB2 5
1.4 Heterodimers and Membrane Influences on Canonical Cannabinoid Signaling 7
1.5 Constitutive Activation of Canonical Receptors 8
1.6 Allosteric Modulation 8
1.7 Canonical Cannabinoid Receptor Locations 9
1.8 Neurophysiology of Canonical Receptor Activation 10
1.9 Orphan Receptors 11
1.10 Endocannabinoid Ion Channels: Transient Receptor Potential Channels 12
1.11 Interactions Between the Endocannabinoid and Endogenous Opioid Systems 13
1.12 N-Methyl-D-aspartate Receptors and Cannabinoids 14
1.13 Cannabinoid Ligands 14
1.14 Synthesis and Catabolism of Anandamide (AEA) 15
1.15 Synthesis and Catabolism of 2-Arachidonoyl Glycerol (2-AG) 16
1.16 Tetrahydrocannabinol 18
1.17 Tetrahydrocannabinol and the Eicosanoid System 19
1.18 Intracellular Binding Proteins 20
1.19 Phytocannabinoids and P-Glycoprotein and Multidrug Transports 20
1.20 N-Acylethanolamines 21
1.21 Conclusion 23
References 24

2 **Cannabinoid-Based Medicine: Pharmacology and Drug Interactions** . . . 41
2.1 Introduction . . . 42
2.2 Terminology . . . 43
2.3 Endocannabinoids and Drug Interactions . . . 43
2.4 Endocannabinoids, Cyclooxygenase, and Drug Interactions . . . 44
2.5 Endocannabinoids and Glucocorticoids . . . 45
2.6 Endocannabinoids and Opioids . . . 46
2.7 Clinical and Animal Studies of Cannabinoid Opioid Interactions . . . 46
2.8 Endocannabinoids, Anxiety and Depression . . . 48
2.8.1 Endocannabinoid "Tone": Beyond the Theory . . . 49
2.9 Endocannabinoids and Post-traumatic Stress Disorder . . . 50
2.10 Endocannabinoid System Disruptions and Potential Impact on Treatment with Antipsychotics . . . 51
2.11 The use of Phytoannabinoids as Antipsychotics . . . 53
2.12 Omega-3 Fatty Acids and effects on the Endocannabinoid System . . . 54
2.13 Phytocannabinoid Pharmacokinetics: THC . . . 55
2.14 Phytocannabinoid Pharmacokinetics: CBD . . . 57
2.15 Cannabidiol and Efflux Pumps . . . 59
2.16 Pharmacokinetics of Approved Cannabinoids . . . 60
2.17 Pharmacokinetic Cannabis-Drug Interactions . . . 60
2.18 Pharmacokinetic Cannabis-Drug Interactions: Relevant Examples . . . 62
2.18.1 Corticosteroids . . . 62
2.18.2 Nonsteroidal Anti-inflammatory Drugs . . . 63
2.18.3 Opioids . . . 63
2.18.4 Antidepressants . . . 63
2.18.5 Janus Kinase Inhibitors . . . 63
2.18.6 Antipsychotics . . . 64
2.18.7 Anticonvulsants . . . 64
2.18.8 Benzodiazepines . . . 64
2.18.9 Ethanol . . . 65
2.18.10 Anticoagulants . . . 65
2.18.11 Antiplatelet Medications . . . 65
2.18.12 HIV Medications . . . 65
2.18.13 Theophylline . . . 66
2.18.14 Chemotherapy . . . 66
2.19 Conclusion . . . 66
References . . . 66

3 **Future Therapeutic Potential of Synthetic Cannabinoids and Endocannabinoid System Modulators** . . . 91
3.1 Introduction . . . 91
3.2 Terminology . . . 93
3.3 Part 1: Synthetic Cannabinoids . . . 93

3.3.1 Synthetic Cannabinoid Use in the Community 93
3.3.2 Pharmacology 94
3.3.3 Conclusion 100
3.4 Part 2: Palmitoylethanolamide (PEA) and the Role of Future Endocannabinoid Modulators in Cancer Care 100
3.4.1 Pharmacodynamics 101
3.4.2 Pharmacokinetics 101
3.4.3 Safety 103
3.5 Conclusion 105
References (Synthetic Cannabinoids) 106

4 Cannabinoid-Based Medicines as Cancer Therapy 117
4.1 Introduction 117
4.2 Terminology 118
4.3 Antineoplastic Activity of Different Cannabis Formulations 119
4.4 Cannabinoids and Graft Versus Host Disease 122
4.5 Cannabinoids and Immune Checkpoint Inhibitors 123
4.6 Using High-Dose Cannabinoids to Treat Cancer (Phoenix Tears/Rick Simpson Oil) 124
4.7 Hail Mary Pass 124
4.8 Conclusion 124
References 125

5 Cannabinoid-Based Medicines and Cancer Symptom Management 129
5.1 Introduction 129
5.2 Terminology 132
5.3 Chemotherapy-Induced Nausea and Vomiting 133
5.4 Appetite Stimulation 136
5.5 Pain 137
5.6 Sleep 140
5.7 Drug-Sparing Effects 141
5.8 Topical Applications for Wound Healing and Analgesia 142
5.9 Multimodal Symptom Treatment in Advanced Cancer 143
5.10 Conclusion 144
References 145

6 Patient Evaluation: Precautions and Managing Expectations 153
6.1 Introduction 154
6.2 Terminology 155
6.3 General Considerations 155
6.4 Risks of Cannabis Use 157
6.5 Potential Increased Cancer Risk with Cannabis Use 159
6.6 Contraindications and Precautions 160
6.7 Managing Physician Expectations 162
6.8 Managing Patient Expectations 163
6.9 Patient Evaluation 164

6.10 The Initial Interview: Key Clinical Questions and Commentary... 165
6.11 Detailed Medical History... 168
6.11.1 Neurological Effects and Driving Performance... 168
6.11.2 Cardiovascular Effects... 170
6.11.3 Pulmonary Effects... 171
6.11.4 Gastrointestinal Effects... 172
6.11.5 Immune System Modulatory Effects... 173
6.12 Detailed Psychiatric History... 173
6.12.1 Screening for Clinical High Risk for Psychosis (CHR)... 174
6.12.2 Possible Protective Effects of CBD in THC-Induced Psychotic-Like Symptoms... 175
6.12.3 Anxiety and Depression... 176
6.12.4 Bipolar Disease... 176
6.12.5 Post-traumatic Stress Disorder... 176
6.12.6 Addiction Issues... 177
6.12.7 Tolerance... 177
6.12.8 Use of Cannabis in Mild Cognitive Impairment or Dementia... 177
6.13 Dealing with Trauma-Sensitive Patients... 178
6.14 Medication History... 179
6.15 Cannabis History... 180
6.16 Conclusion... 181
References... 183

7 Choosing a Product, Route of Administration, Initial Dosage, Titration, Monitoring and Management of Adverse Effects... 191
7.1 Introduction... 192
7.2 Terminology... 193
7.3 General Considerations... 194
7.4 Review of the Principal Active Ingredients of Cannabis... 196
7.4.1 CBD... 197
7.4.2 THC... 197
7.4.3 THCA, CBDA, and Other Secondary Cannabinoids... 198
7.5 Overview of the Main Routes of Administration of Cannabis Products... 198
7.5.1 Oral Ingestion... 199
7.5.2 Oromucosal Ingestion... 201
7.5.3 Inhalation... 201
7.5.4 Topical and Transdermal... 204
7.5.5 Intra-rectal and Vaginal (Suppositories)... 205
7.6 Considering the Initial Use of Approved Pharmaceutical Cannabinoids... 205
7.7 Choosing a Cannabis Formulation... 206
7.7.1 Word of Caution on Product Labeling... 207
7.7.2 Regarding the Therapeutic Dose of THC... 208
7.7.3 Regarding the Protective Effects of CBD on THC Psychoactivity... 208

7.8 Cannabinoid Metabolism: Clinical Considerations Between Inhaled and Oral Routes of Administration 209
7.9 Treatment Selection According to Symptom or Clinical Setting. 209
7.10 Precise Dosing Recommendations. 217
7.10.1 Initial CBD Dosing 217
7.10.2 Initial THC Dosing 217
7.10.3 Considering Microgram THC Dosing 218
7.10.4 Proposed Dosing Protocols from Consensus Groups 218
7.10.5 Considering the Toxic Psychosis Threshold of THC...... 221
7.10.6 Considering the Use of High-Potency Extracts (Rick Simpson Oil, RSO, Phoenix Tears) 222
7.11 Dealing with Hospitalized Patients Already Taking Cannabinoid-Based Medicines 223
7.12 Estimating the Dose of THC in Unsupervised Patients.......... 223
7.13 Patient Monitoring, Record Keeping, and Follow-Up Visits...... 224
7.13.1 Reporting Cannabis Side Effects..................... 225
7.14 Overview of Cannabis Use Disorder and Cannabis Withdrawal Syndrome 226
7.15 Conclusion 227
7.16 Chapter Summary 228
References.. 228

8 Psychoactive Effects of Cannabinoid-Based Medicines: Exploration and Inquiry. 235
8.1 Introduction 236
8.2 Terminology.. 240
8.3 Cannabis Psychoactivity: Current Challenges................. 241
8.3.1 The Complicated Social, Cultural, and Spiritual History of Cannabis Psychoactivity.................. 241
8.3.2 The Evidence Remains Mostly Anecdotal.............. 243
8.3.3 Our Understanding of the Neurocognitive Effects of THC Has Only Just Begun 243
8.3.4 Management Guidelines for Cannabis Psychoactivity Are Not Available. 244
8.3.5 Cannabis Psychoactivity Is Common in Medical Cannabis Patients................................ 244
8.3.6 Avoiding Psychoactivity Is Possible, but Difficult... for Now 245
8.3.7 Precise Dosing Guidelines Are Only Beginning to Emerge.. 245
8.3.8 Prior Experience with Cannabis May Influence Tolerance to Psychoactivity and Even Psychotic-Like Reactions 246
8.4 Basic Precautions.. 247
8.4.1 Introducing Cannabis Early in the Course of Life-Limiting Illnesses............................. 247

8.4.2 Preventing Involuntary Intoxications 248
8.4.3 Low Initial THC Dosing: The Cornerstone of Harm Reduction 249
8.4.4 Route of Administration: Oral Versus Inhaled 249
8.5 Preparing Patients for Cannabis Psychoactivity 250
8.5.1 Set and Setting 251
8.5.2 Integration 252
8.5.3 Trauma Sensitivity 252
8.6 Dealing with an Involuntary Intoxication (Bad Trip) 253
8.7 Overview of the Specific Neurocognitive Effects Associated with Cannabis Psychoactivity 255
8.7.1 Slowed Down Perception of Time 255
8.7.2 Metacognition: Thinking About Thinking 257
8.7.3 Metacognition Versus Mind Wandering. 258
8.7.4 Metacognition Versus Insight. 259
8.7.5 Introspective and Mystical/Spiritual Reflections 260
8.7.6 Reduced Working Memory and Divided Attention 261
8.7.7 Heightened Sense of Awareness and Nonspecific Amplification: The Effects of THC on the Triad Network – Default Mode, Salience, and Central Executive 263
8.7.8 Aversive Memory Extinction 270
8.8 Other Benefits of Cannabis Use in End of Life Situations 271
8.8.1 Cannabis and Creativity 271
8.8.2 Higher-Order Problem-Solving 271
8.8.3 Delaying Palliative Sedation 272
8.8.4 Coping with Forced Confinement 273
8.9 Conclusion 274
References. 274

Summary of Recommendations 283

Cannabis in Cancer Index 2021 287

Patient Evaluation and Monitoring Checklist 289

Clinical High Risk for Psychosis Checklist 295

Trauma Sensitive Screening 297

Glossary of Terms 299

Index 305

List of Figures

Fig. 1.1 CBD cannabidiol, Abn CBD abnormal-CBD, THCV tetrahydrocannabivarin, CBG cannabigerolic acid, CBDV cannabidivarin, THC tetrahydrocannabinol, PLC phospholipase C, Lyso-PLD lysophospholipase D, NAPE-PLD N-acyl phosphatidylethanolamine-specific phospholipase D, DAG-lipase diacylglycerol lipase, MAGL monoacylglycerol lipase, PPAR peroxisome proliferator-activated receptors 3
Fig. 4.1 Schematic representation of the main signaling cascades highlighting the downstream CB receptor activation by cannabinoids which impact all the hallmark processes of cancer such as proliferation, apoptosis, migration, invasion, angiogenesis and EMT (epithelial-mesenchymal transition). (Reference: Das et al. [13]. (Springer publication)). 119
Fig. 5.1 Longitudinal study of >1600 Tilray patients at 20 medical clinics in 5 provinces, the largest Canadian national longitudinal cannabis study to date. This preliminary data is based on 573 patients enrolled before December 1, 2017 143
Fig. 6.1 End of life trajectories. (Adapted from Lunney et al. (2002)) 156
Fig. 7.1 Health Canada approved dried cannabis inhaler devices. (**a**) Volcano Medic™ shown with filling chamber and balloon, (**b**) Volcano Medic 2™, (**c**) Mighty Medic™ shown with filling chamber tool set, (**d**) Syqe™ medical cannabis inhaler device, shown with prefilled replacement cartridge containing dried cannabis. 203
Fig. 8.1 This is an open-access article distributed under the terms of the Creative Commons Attribution License (CC-BY). The use, distribution, or reproduction in other forums is permitted, provided the original author(s) or licensor is credited and that the original publication in this journal is cited, in accordance with accepted academic practice. No use, distribution, or reproduc-

tion is permitted which does not comply with these terms. *Schematic figure of the triple network model consisting of the default mode network (DMN), salience network (SN), and central executive network (CEN).* According to this model, the anterior insula (belonging to the salience network) activates the CEN and deactivates the DMN in response to the salient stimuli. Legend: *ACC* anterior cingulate cortex, *DLPFC* dorsolateral prefrontal cortex, *PPC* posterior parietal cortex, *mPFC* medial prefrontal cortex, *PPC* posterior cingulate cortex, *INS* anterior insula [91]. In healthy humans, the SN efficiently allocates attentional resources to either the DMN or CEN. This anticorrelation (i.e., negative relationship) is necessary for optimal functioning 262
Fig. 8.2 This is an open-access article distributed under the terms of the Creative Commons CC-BY license, which permits unrestricted use, distribution, and reproduction in any medium, provided the original work is properly cited. *The distribution of CB1Rs across the human brain.* Regions with high CB1R concentration include the amygdala (not in view) and substantia nigra (related to salience network), cerebellum, cingulate gyrus, dorsal motor nucleus of the vagus, entorhinal cortex, globus pallidus, hippocampal formation, middle frontal gyrus, and Wernicke's area. Regions with medium CB1R concentration include the auditory cortex (right), caudate nucleus, mediodorsal nucleus of the thalamus, motor cortex, occipitotemporal gyrus, putamen, somatosensory cortex, and visual cortex. Montreal Neurological Institute coordinates (x, y, z) are shown above [18] 266
Fig. 8.3 Illness trajectories in palliative care. (Adapted from: Murray et al. [89]) 272

List of Tables

Table 2.1 Summary of cannabinoid drug interactions 60
Table 2.2 CBD ICD50 [22] 61
Table 2.3 THC IC50 [22] 61
Table 3.1 Synthetic cannabinoid class and metabolizing enzymes 97
Table 3.2 Clinical toxicity noted in PEA trials 104
Table 4.1 Preclinical evidence of cannabinoid antitumor activity 120
Table 4.2 Effects of THC and CBD on specific cancer cell lines. 121
Table 5.1 Adapted from the Consensus-Based Recommendations for Titrating Cannabinoids and Tapering of Opioids [94] 142
Table 6.1 Major adverse effects associated with cannabis use 158
Table 6.2 Likelihood of acute psychotic-like reactions/anxiety attacks with cannabis use. 159
Table 6.3 Medical cannabis contraindications 161
Table 6.4 Medical cannabis precautions 162
Table 6.5 Secondary causes of psychosis (adapted from Matskevich and Keshavan 2019) 175
Table 7.1 Characteristics of frequently used routes of administration for medical cannabis 199
Table 7.2 Dried cannabis blending instructions for reducing THC concentration using high-potency strains and high-CBD strains (containing less than 1% THC). 204
Table 7.3 Cannabis formulations based on THC and CBD content 207
Table 7.4 Disclaimer: The initial introduction of CBD has not yet been demonstrated clinically for these purposes. The following recommendations are based on preclinical evidence, observational data, and clinical experience 219
Table 7.5 Adapted from: Sihota et al., "Consensus-Based Recommendations for Titrating Cannabinoids and Tapering Opioids for Chronic Pain Control", 2020. Disclaimer: The

initial introduction of CBD has not yet been demonstrated clinically for these purposes. These recommendations are based on preclinical evidence, observational data, and clinical experience. 220
Table 7.6 Cannabis dose-related side effects 225
Table 7.7 Cannabis use disorder (DSM-V) 227
Table 8.1 Clinical indications for palliative sedation 271

Contributors

Claude Cyr McGill University, Department of Family Medicine, Montreal, QC, Canada

Paul Daeninck CancerCare Manitoba, Winnipeg Regional Palliative Care Program, Max Rady College of Medicine, University of Manitoba, Winnipeg, MB, Canada

Mellar P. Davis Palliative Care Research, Geisinger Health System, Danville, PA, USA

Rachel Rudney University of Manitoba Max Rady College of Medicine, Winnipeg, MB, Canada

Danial Schecter Royal Victoria Regional Health Centre, Barrie, ON, Canada

Chapter 1
Overview of the Endocannabinoid System and Endocannabinoidome

Contents

1.1 Introduction 2
1.2 Terminology 4
1.3 The Canonical Cannabinoid Receptors: CB1 and CB2 5
1.4 Heterodimers and Membrane Influences on Canonical Cannabinoid Signaling 7
1.5 Constitutive Activation of Canonical Receptors 8
1.6 Allosteric Modulation 8
1.7 Canonical Cannabinoid Receptor Locations 9
1.8 Neurophysiology of Canonical Receptor Activation 10
1.9 Orphan Receptors 11
1.10 Endocannabinoid Ion Channels: Transient Receptor Potential Channels 12
1.11 Interactions Between the Endocannabinoid and Endogenous Opioid Systems 13
1.12 N-Methyl-D-aspartate Receptors and Cannabinoids 14
1.13 Cannabinoid Ligands 14
1.14 Synthesis and Catabolism of Anandamide (AEA) 15
1.15 Synthesis and Catabolism of 2-Arachidonoyl Glycerol (2-AG) 16
1.16 Tetrahydrocannabinol 18
1.17 Tetrahydrocannabinol and the Eicosanoid System 19
1.18 Intracellular Binding Proteins 20
1.19 Phytocannabinoids and P-Glycoprotein and Multidrug Transports 20
1.20 N-Acylethanolamines 21
1.21 Conclusion 23
References 24

C. Cyr et al., *Cannabis and Cannabinoid-Based Medicines in Cancer Care*,
https://doi.org/10.1007/978-3-030-89918-9_1

1.1 Introduction

At the turn of the millennium, the simple elegance of the endocannabinoid system (ECS) was initially thought to be involved in modulating neurotransmitter release in the central nervous system and several immune-related functions, though the latter have only recently begun to reveal their clinical relevance. We are now realizing that we have only breached the surface of a much wider system with far-reaching physiological effects. Over the last decade, the ECS has blossomed into a vast multiorgan network comprising dozens of molecular targets and an exponential number of cannabinoid/receptor interactions. Ligands in this system have been found to be so promiscuous, they make a Texas brothel look like a Catholic convent. Emerging research on the interactions between this extended endocannabinoid system and other pharmacologicals related to symptom control and disease modifying effects is rapidly providing new clinical insights.

This chapter offers a glimpse into the vast world of the extended endocannabinoid system, which some suggest should be referred to as the *endocannabinoidome* [180]. This may be a more appropriate description which puts into question whether the role of endocannabinoids should even be called a system in the first place, since it is involved with regulating nearly every other biological system in one way or another.

Those for whom this chapter will be their first ever encounter with the endocannabinoidome might find the potential pharmacological implications in cancer care overwhelming at first. Although the basic functions of the endocannabinoidome will be covered in this chapter, those who wish to know more about the basic science of the original endocannabinoid system (ECS) and the expanded endocannabinoidome can easily find many reliable online resources. Americans for Safe Access, for example, is a non-profit patient advocacy group which offers accredited advanced level CME for medical professionals as well as regional medical cannabis practice policies and scientific ethics information.

The canonical endocannabinoid system was originally considered to contain two receptors which are 7-transmembrane G-protein-coupled receptors (CB1 and CB2) and two ligands, anandamide (AEA) and 2-arachidonoylglycerol (2-AG). Both CB1 and CB2 receptors have a 7-transmembrane structure with an extracellular N-terminal beginning and C-terminal intracellular tail which activates both G-proteins and beta-arrestin. Ligand binding to the extracellular core within the transmembrane helix alters the intracellular domain conformation allowing for G-protein interactions and/or beta-arrestin-1 or 2 binding to the intracellular C-terminus within the cell. Five enzymes are responsible for biosynthesis of these ligands: N-acyl phosphatidylethanolamine phospholipase D (NAPE-PD) for synthesis of AEA, diacylglycerol lipase-alpha and diacylglycerol lipase-beta (DAGLs) for synthesis of 2-AG, and fatty acid amide hydrolase (FAAH) for catabolism of AEA, and monoacylglycerol lipase (MAGL) for 2-AG catabolism [72].

This original conception turned out to be too simplistic, however. There are now 23 components which have been attributed to the endocannabinoidome, including 7 receptors and 3 enzymes which are membrane bound, 4 enzymes and 3 transporters found in the cytoplasm (FAAH is on the endoplasmic reticulum) and a nuclear transcription factor and peroxisome proliferator activating receptor-alpha (PPAR) which directly interact with endocannabinoids [175]. Also, a set of Transient Receptor Potential Vanilloid channels (TRPVs) are now considered endocannabinoid ion channels [240] (Fig. 1.1).

Arachidonic acid plays a central role in the endocannabinoidome. It is a substrate used in AEA and 2-AG synthesis and is also recycled during catabolism. It also acts as a shared substrate for the eicosanoid system (which produces prostaglandins, leukotrienes, as well as other eicosanoids). Thus, both AEA and 2-AG are indirect sources of prostaglandins by way of cyclooxygenase 2 (COX2) [3, 100, 134, 146, 150].

Anandamide (AEA) and 2-arachidonoylglycerol (2-AG) are also chemically distinct. Anandamide (AEA) belongs to the N-acylethanolamine (NAE) family of biologically active fatty acids which do not contain an arachidonoyl group. Other non-arachidonoyl containing NAEs have been shown to interact with the endocannabinoid system, including palmitoylethanolamide (PEA) and oleoylethanolamine (OEA). These two compounds do not directly interact with CB1 and CB2, but rather indirectly activate both receptors by competing for intracellular endocannabinoid binding proteins (fatty acid binding proteins or FABPs) and anandamide's catabolic

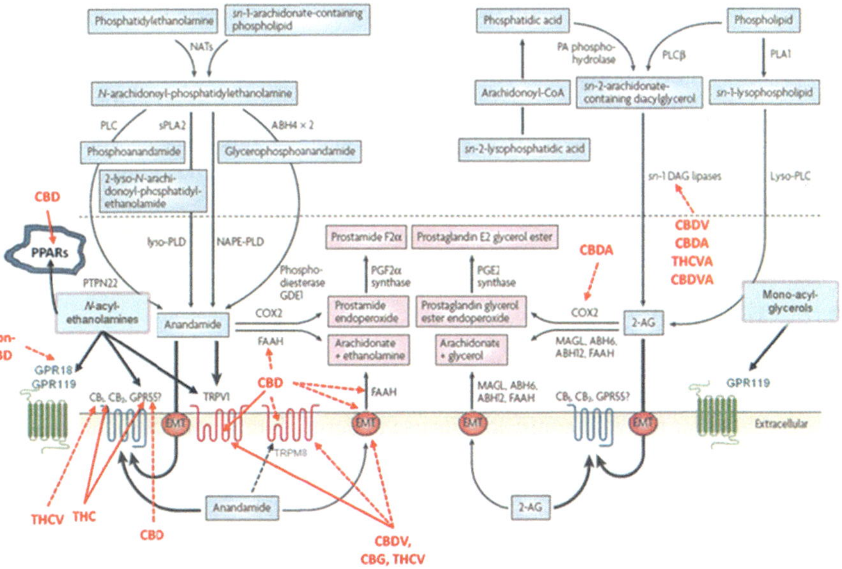

Fig. 1.1 CBD cannabidiol, Abn CBD abnormal-CBD, THCV tetrahydrocannabivarin, CBG cannabigerolic acid, CBDV cannabidivarin, THC tetrahydrocannabinol, PLC phospholipase C, Lyso-PLD lysophospholipase D, NAPE-PLD N-acyl phosphatidylethanolamine-specific phospholipase D, DAG-lipase diacylglycerol lipase, MAGL monoacylglycerol lipase, PPAR peroxisome proliferator-activated receptors

enzyme FAAH. These NAEs also activate the endocannabinoid "orphan receptors" PPAR alpha and positively modulate TRPV1 [62].

The complexity of the endocannabinoidome doesn't stop with direct and indirect CB1 and CB2 receptor binding, however. Multiple orphan receptors have been shown to be the targets for endocannabinoids, phytocannabinoids, and NAEs [157, 235]. Conversely, ligands within this system have been shown to have a large number of other "promiscuous" targets. Furthermore, two separate ligands may complement downstream signaling or reduce side effects by interactions within the endocannabinoidome, a phenomenon described as the "entourage" effect. As an example, cannabidiol (CBD) is postulated to be a negative allosteric modulator at CB1 and has been shown to reduce the psychotomimetic effects of 9-delta-tetrahydrocannabinol (THC), an agonist at CB1 [194]. A central characteristic of the endocannabinoidome is the heterogeneity from gene to intracellular signaling that occurs with multiple endocannabinoid ligands acting on multiple receptors and ion channels simultaneously. Lack of specificity of ligand to receptor response and measured effect and alterations that occur with disease which modify responses means that off-target effects will always be experienced whether positive or negative and dose response may be relatively unpredictable [293].

The endocannabinoidome has been shown to regulate a multitude of biological functions including fertility, sexuality, energy metabolism, cardiovascular function, inflammation, mood, and cognition [22, 124, 143]. In addition, the endocannabinoidome plays an intrinsic role on memory, stress processing, and reward pathways involved in addiction [84]. Alterations in the system are associated with a wide range of diseases: obesity, Parkinson's disease, Alzheimer's dementia, multiple sclerosis, Huntington's chorea, amyotrophic lateral sclerosis, schizophrenia, depression, atherosclerosis, cancer, inflammatory bowel disease, liver steatosis and fibrosis, and infertility [40, 114, 139, 190, 202, 247, 263]. Understanding these alterations in the endocannabinoidome system may allow for future disease modifying or palliative interventions.

1.2 Terminology

The term "endocannabinoidome" is still not widely used by clinicians and researchers, and in order to avoid confusion, its use to describe the *expanded* endocannabinoid system (ECS) will be restricted to this chapter. In the following chapters, the more commonly used term "endocannabinoid system (ECS)" will be used to describe most concepts relating to both the more specific canonical receptors and enzymes and the larger system of molecular targets and ligands. The "endocannabinoidome" will only be mentioned in order to point out a clinically relevant difference between these two related concepts.

1.3 The Canonical Cannabinoid Receptors: CB1 and CB2

Both the CB1 and CB2 recpetor belong to the G-protein-coupled receptor (GPCR) family. There are roughly 750 different types of G-protein-coupled receptors (GPCRs) in the human genome, approximately 350 of which are involved in known physiological functions. These range from detecting hormones, growth factors, neurotransmitters, and other endogenous ligands, as well as sight and smell perception via the olfactory and photoreceptors. However, another 150 are considered orphan receptors with no known ligands or function. GPCRs are important drug targets, and approximately 34% of all FDA-approved drugs target 108 members of this family [109]. The CB1 receptor was initially discovered in 1988 and subsequently cloned based on responsiveness to THC, hence the name cannabinoid receptor [69]. It is also the most abundant GPCR receptor in the brain [115]. The CB2 receptor was isolated 5 years later from differentiated myeloid cells [199]. The two receptors share 44% amino acid homology, and both AEA and 2-AG act as ligands to CB1 and CB2. While 2-AG is a full agonist for CB1, AEA is considered a partial agonist. Paradoxically the extracellular portion of CB2 bound by an antagonist shares conformity with an agonist-bound CB1 receptor. As a result, receptor activity cannot be directly determined by receptor conformational changes alone [162].

CB1 is largely expressed on presynaptic membranes in the central nervous system (CNS), while CB2 is mostly expressed on peripheral immune cells. However, CB2 is also found in small numbers on postsynaptic membranes where it has been shown to hyperpolarize postsynaptic neurons [293]. CB1 receptors far outnumber CB2 in the CNS, with a 100-fold greater expression. CB2 receptors found in the CNS have also been shown to be inducible and upregulate in pathological states such as addiction, anxiety, neuroinflammation, and epilepsy, suggesting that CB2 receptor function in the CNS is involved in modulating disease states. Hence, it is possible that the CB2 receptor may become an important target for neuroprotection in neuropsychiatric disorders and neurodegenerative diseases.

The CB1 receptor gene is located on chromosome 6q14-15 and CB2 on 1p36 [119, 218]. Polymorphisms are described with both receptors and associated with certain disease predispositions. For example, certain CB2 receptor polymorphisms exhibit a reduced efficacy with 2-AG binding as compared with wild-type receptors. On the other hand, certain CB2 polymorphisms exhibit greater constitutional (ligand independent) activity than wild-type receptors [37]. CB2 polymorphisms are also associated with a wide range of psychiatric disorders, addiction, obesity, thrombocytopenia in children, and osteoporosis [52, 83, 117, 130, 132, 151, 179, 192, 223, 271, 291, 292].

CB1 receptor polymorphisms include mRNA splice variants of the four exons. This genetic variation derived from the CB1 gene has demonstrated altered ligand binding affinities and G-protein activation [245, 260].

G-protein-coupled receptors (GPCRs), including CB1 and CB2, have a complex 7-transmembrane structure with an extracellular N-terminal beginning site and a C-terminal intracellular tail where activated G-proteins enable intracellular signaling. Hence, GPCRs are much more than simple on/off switches and have been shown to exhibit a strong influence from internal and external factors which influence downstream effects after receptor activation.

G-protein activation is the necessary first step in transmitting signals from external stimuli into the cell interior. CB1 and CB2 G-protein binding involved in neurotransmitter signaling has been extensively studied. These types of GPCRs are known as pertussis toxin (PTX)-sensitive G-proteins. Pertussis toxin is a unique pharmacological probe used for the study of neuronal signal transduction pathways mediated by this type of G-protein receptor [121]. Receptor binding produces conformational receptor changes which cause the formation of a heterotrimeric complex (G-alpha-G-beta/gamma). Downstream signaling results in inhibition of adenylyl cyclase and cyclic AMP production which in turn downregulates protein kinase A intracellular signaling. G-beta/gamma stimulates phosphatidylinositol 3-kinase which downstream leads to phosphorylation of mitogen-activated protein kinases (MAPKs) [170]. G-proteins activate inward-rectifying potassium channels and inhibit N-type and P/Q type voltage-gated calcium channels resulting in hyperpolarization of presynaptic neurons. The end result of this complex cascade is inhibition of neurotransmitter release [1].

Other downstream signaling include effects on adapter protein AP-3, G-protein-coupled receptor-associated sorting protein, factors associated with neutral sphingomyelinases, and cannabinoid receptor-interacting protein 1a (CRIP-1a) [123, 281].

Receptor deactivation of GPCRs is also influenced by several factors. In order to switch off the response or adapt to a persistent stimulus, the activated receptors need to become desensitized. This is achieved by a two-step process, beginning with phosphorylation of the activated receptor by G-protein receptor kinases (GRKs), which are enzymes that function in concert with beta-arrestins to regulate G-protein receptor activation [42]. Activation of G-protein-coupled receptor kinases (GRKs) cause phosphorylation of C-terminus serine and threonine which facilitates beta-arrestin binding and desensitize the receptor to further G-protein activation [268]. Secondly, phosphorylation of the intracellular C-terminus increases the affinity for beta-arrestin binding which then produces GPCR decoupling and further reduced signaling [1, 167]. Beta-arrestin-mediated decoupling of GPCRs is thus considered an important mechanism involved in receptor desensitization [172].

Furthermore, different agonists have been shown to produce varying effects on the upregulation of GRKs and beta-arrestin in different regions of the brain. Thus, differences in downstream signaling of GPCRs are location-dependent within the central nervous system (CNS), and this effect has also been observed with THC [161, 208].

Cannabinoid receptor-interacting protein 1a (CRIP-1a) has also been shown to modulate GPCR signaling [19]. This protein, which is located on the distal C-terminal, interacts to *prevent* beta-arrestin binding which, in turn, blocks desensitization and internalization of the receptor [17].

Orthosteric ligands (ligands which bind to the *active* receptor site such as AEA, 2-AG, THC, and the synthetic agonists WIN 55,2122, CP55,940) activate various subtypes of G-proteins (G i/o, Gs, Gq11). These various G-proteins have different downstream signaling resulting in ligand-dependent functional selective signaling. Various ligands also differ in the ability to signal through beta-arrestins [155].

In summary, different orthosteric agonists cause different conformational changes in the receptor which result in functional selectivity of downward signaling leading to different cellular responses depending on location within the CNS. This is altered by disease and neuron membrane lipid content [170].

1.4 Heterodimers and Membrane Influences on Canonical Cannabinoid Signaling

Most GPCRs exist as homodimers (formed by two identical proteins). However, it has been shown that GPCRs may dimerize with other types of GPCRs and form a heterodimer. This in turn creates a physical interaction between the two receptors, where activation of one receptor influences the other [13]. Heterodimers of CBI/CB2 have been described with distinctly different signaling compared to their respective monomers. Thus, THC bound to the CB1 monomer has biased signaling toward MAPK activation and does not activate G-proteins at CB2 but is less functionally selective when bound to CB1/CB2 heterodimers [203]. However, reduced THC activity on CB1/CB2 heterodimers may be partly reversed by cannabidiol (CBD). CBD does not strongly bind to either CB1 or CB2 and is considered a negative allosteric modulator of CB1, thereby reducing certain THC-mediated effects. However, when CBD binds to both sites on CB1/CB2 heterodimers, it may in fact increase functionality of THC and anandamide (AEA) [204].

Dimer formation on cell surfaces is dependent on cholesterol content of the membrane [213]. Cholesterol content plays a greater role in CB1 signaling than on CB2. Cholesterol promotes dimerization and contributes to the inactivation of CB1 [213]. Membrane cholesterol content differs regionally within the CNS and content changes with disease such that cannabinoid responses and the heterodimer formation also differs with disease [108, 203, 205]. Increased heterodimer formation also influences drug responses. For example, upregulation of dimers within the striatum in a rat Parkinson's disease model causes dyskinetic responses to levodopa [204].

Heterodimers can also form between canonical CB1and CB2 cannabinoid receptors and other orphan G-protein-coupled receptors. For example, CB1 forms dimers with GPR-55, and THC may activate or inactivate GPR-55 through binding to CB1 within this heterodimer [10, 138, 185, 259]. Heterodimers between CB1 and non-cannabinoid receptors may lead to simultaneous benefits and side effects related to THC. THC memory deficits, anxiolysis, hallucinations, and social impairments may result from activation of 5HT2a receptors which dimerize with CB1, whereas analgesia, anxiogenic reactions, hypo locomotor, and hypothermia may be independent of this dimer [286]. THC binding to the CB1/5HT2A dimer changes the type of G-protein interactions and produces effects resembling those which occur with LSD [105].

1.5 Constitutive Activation of Canonical Receptors

A receptor which is capable of producing a biological response in the absence of a bound ligand is said to display "constitutive activity," which may be blocked by an inverse agonist. Cannabinoid receptors are known to display such constitutive activity. They are considered to be spontaneously active and produce cellular responses without binding ligands. As such, this activation is not reversed by a neutral antagonist but by an inverse agonist [89, 225, 226]. CB1 second transmembrane domain stabilizes the receptor in both an inactive and active state [209]. Constitutively activated CB1 is continuously removed from the plasma membrane by endocytosis in the somatodendritic areas of the neuron but not in axons.

Constitutive activity of receptors may have clinical relevance. Blocking constitutive activity with an inverse agonist increases CB1 plasma membrane expression [158]. Furthermore, CB2 "spontaneous" constitutive activity, which regulates pro-apoptotic brain cortical JNK (c-Jun NH2-terminal kinase) activity, is abolished over time by an inverse agonist which reduces JNK activity [248]. CBD, a partial agonist and an inverse agonist at CB2, may also modulate constitutive activity which may explain its effect on reducing experimental brain injuries [38, 152, 222].

1.6 Allosteric Modulation

Allosteric modulators are compounds that bind to a receptor and change that receptor's response to a specific stimulus. As mentioned above, allosteric modulators change the G-protein coupling and orthosteric signaling. Downstream signaling may be intensified with a positive modulator and weakened by a negative modulator. Signaling bias may change with an allosteric modulator and influence receptor expression and trafficking [170]. CBD, an allosteric modulator at CB1, reduces THC psychotomimetic effects [231, 277]. CBD also reduces the efficacy of 2-AG and THC to phosphorylate extracellular receptor kinase (ERK1/2) and recruit beta-arrestin to the C-terminus [154]. Allosteric modulators at CB1 receptors have been used to treat CNS and peripheral nerve disorders and simultaneously avoid adverse effects associated with orthosteric agonists [154].

There is a feedback loop between neurosteroids and CB1 agonists which can serve to illustrate this. On one hand, THC upregulates pregnenolone. Pregnenolone, however, is a negative allosteric modulator of CB1 and, in conjunction with CRIP1a, decreases CB1 stimulated phosphorylation of ERK1/2 and reduces beta-arrestin interactions with CB1 [283].

Ligands may also demonstrate allosteric modulation depending on drug concentrations. For example, fenofibrate at low concentrations acts as a partial agonist at CB1 but at high concentrations is a negative allosteric modulator to the ligand CP 55, 940 G-protein, and beta-arrestin recruitment [232].

There is as much enthusiasm toward developing allosteric modulators, as much as there is in developing cannabis orthosteric ligands. Modulators have the advantage of reducing the untoward side effects of long-term cannabis therapy and thus increase cannabis safety or specificity. There is also a wider variation of allosteric binding sites relative to orthosteric binding sites and a greater potential for receptor subtype selectivity than with orthosteric cannabis ligands. Another reason for enthusiasm is that allosteric modulators are without intrinsic receptor activity and hence are selective only for regions where endogenous cannabinoids are present and functioning. Hopefully this would reduce off-target toxicities [170].

1.7 Canonical Cannabinoid Receptor Locations

CB1 is one of the most abundant receptors in the brain. It is highly expressed in the basal ganglia nuclei, hippocampus, cortex, and cerebellum [101]. Distribution within the CNS correlates with motor function, cognition, memory, and analgesia. Receptors are largely located in presynaptic terminals in central and peripheral neurons and are classically known to inhibit neurotransmitter release, with the exception of disinhibition which occurs through activation of CB1 receptors located on gamma aminobutyric acid (GABA) inhibitory interneurons [59, 75, 275, 301].

Although much has been written on CB1 receptor inhibition of neurotransmitter release, disinhibition via gamma aminobutyric acid (GABA) inhibitory interneurons may be a further mechanism by which cannabinoids increase appetite and reduce pain. In fact, CB1 receptors are found in greater density on GABAergic than glutaminergic neurons, which may contribute to disinhibition [141, 142].

Both astrocytes and microglia are invested in and have a functional relationship with synapses. Both express CB1 receptors and are influenced by cannabinoid interactions with glia as well as directly via CB1 receptor activation [217]. CB1 is sparsely expressed within the brain stem respiratory nuclei such that cannabinoids usually have not been associated with respiratory depression [178]. However, CB1 is highly expressed within the ventral striatum which accounts for the rewarding or "drug liking" effects and in the cerebellar parallel climbing fibers and basket cells which influences coordination [186, 272, 279]. CB1 is also found within multiple extra-neural sites: adrenal gland, heart, lung, prostate, uterus, testes, thymus, and bone marrow [28, 94].

There are several differences between CB2 and CB1 receptors. As mentioned, CB2 receptor expression in the CNS is 100-fold less than that of CB1 receptors [196, 302]. As opposed to CB1, they are mainly expressed on postsynaptic membranes. CB2 immunoreactivity is found within rat glial and neuronal tissues in a number of brain regions: the olfactory tubercle, cerebral cortex, striatum, thalamic nuclei, hippocampus, amygdala, substantia nigra, and periaqueductal gray, among other sites [104]. Activation of CB2 receptors does cause activation of neurons as demonstrated by the lack of fos protein expression [201].

However, high CB2 receptor density has generally been found in the immune system. It is more highly expressed in spleen, lymph nodes, and thymus than CB1 and is intimately involved in immunomodulation. Descending order of expression is B lymphocytes >> natural killer cells >> monocytes >> polymorphonuclear leukocytes >> CD8+ T lymphocytes >> CD4+ lymphocytes [94].

CB2 is also highly inducible and increased expression usually reflects an underlying disease process [131, 182, 287]. Increased expression of CB2 in the case of neuroinflammation (a hallmark of neuropathic pain) is due in part to migration of inflammatory cells into the CNS [169]. During experimental cerebral ischemia, targeting upregulated CB2 receptors has been found to be a promising approach to treating neuropathic pain. In a cerebral ischemia/reperfusion injury model, inhibition of CB_1 receptor activation has been shown to have protective effects, while inhibition of CB_2 receptor is detrimental. The greatest degree of neuroprotection was shown to occur with combined CB_1 antagonist and CB_2 agonist [304]. Targeting CB2 receptors with an agonist reduced experimental taxane-induced neuropathy [294]. In this model, paclitaxel induced the expression of CB2 receptors in microglia.

1.8 Neurophysiology of Canonical Receptor Activation

Endocannabinoids are produced in postsynaptic neurons upon depolarization and diffuse across the synapse to bind to presynaptic CB1 receptors [137]. There are three forms of synaptic responses that then occur [137, 149, 215]:

1. Depolarization-induced suppression of inhibition or depolarization-induced suppression of excitation
2. Metabotropic-induced suppression of inhibition or metabotropic suppression of excitation through dimers with the glutaminergic receptor mGlu5
3. Endocannabinoid-mediated long-term depression

GPCRs are also known as metabotropic receptors, which are activated by nonionic ligands (as opposed to ionotropic receptors) and are defined by their ability to initiate a number of metabolic steps to modulate cell activity. Thus, endocannabinoids modulate many neurotransmitters by several mechanisms, including cholinergic traffic by depolarization-induced suppression of inhibition or excitation of M1 and M3 receptor, orexin via orexin A receptors, cholecystokinin through CCKa receptors, and adrenergic traffic via alpha1 receptors [137]. However, CB1 receptor activity on GABAergic and glutamatergic synapses has received the most attention to date. Hence, depolarization-induced suppression of inhibition (GABA) and depolarization-induced suppression of excitation (glutamate) are the most commonly known CB1 receptor functions in the CNS and are responsible for modulating nearly every physiological and cognitive function in the CNS. Depolarization-induced suppression of inhibition occurs when release of

GABA, an inhibitory neurotransmitter, is blocked by CB1 receptor agonism. Conversely, depolarization-induced suppression of excitation occurs when release of the excitatory neurotransmitter glutamate is suppressed. Inhibitory synapses (GABA) are more sensitive to CB1-mediated depolarization-induced suppression than excitatory synapses (glutamate), however. Furthermore, THC causes tonic inhibition of inhibitory synapses which modulates the balance between GABAergic and glutamatergic neurotransmission [113].

The endocannabinoid system is also intimately involved in neuroplasticity which can be influenced by long-term synaptic depression. Plasticity is a universal property of neuronal activity and is involved in the refinement of brain connectivity during development and throughout adult life [47]. Long-term synaptic depression produced by THC by way of CB1 activation can modulate synaptic plasticity and can be either homosynaptic (requiring presynaptic activation) or heterosynaptic (independent of presynaptic activation). Long-term depression from sustained low frequency depolarization has been described with glutaminergic synapses in the dorsal and ventral striatum [98], which may be a mechanism behind the rewarding effects of cannabis. Heterosynaptic long-term depression has been described in the hippocampus as well [44].

Glutamate released by activation of Schaffer collaterals activates group I metabotropic glutamate receptors at CA1 pyramidal cells, which causes persistent reduction of GABA release mediated by endocannabinoids and hence are considered heterosynaptic [44]. This function is mediated by endocannabinoids through heterosynaptic pathways [44]. Heterosynaptic long-term depression of inhibitory interneurons is important to dendritic development and in maturing cortical circuits. Thus, early life THC exposure may cause subtle developmental abnormalities by altering this process and later predispose individuals to psychiatric disease as adults [171].

1.9 Orphan Receptors

By definition, an orphan receptor lacks a specific ligand. In the last few decades, several of these orphan receptors have been shown to interact with endocannabinoids. These receptors are GPR3, GPR6, GPR12, GPR18, GPR55, and GPR119. However, this is not an exhaustive list.

Orphan receptors such as GPR55 have a low-sequence amino acid identity with CB1 receptors (13%) and CB2 receptors (14%) and are widely expressed in the brain. GPR55 co-localizes with CB1 and CB2 receptors in dimers. Lysophosphatidylinositol, which is considered an endogenous cannabinoid neurotransmitter, is considered a possible ligand of GPR55 [112, 144]. THC, AEA, and 2-AG also bind to GPR55, while several other CB1 and CB2 receptor ligands are also allosteric modulators of GPR55 [194, 207, 244]. GPR55 activity is implicated in various processes such as cancer, pain, metabolic disorders, vascular function, bone physiology, and motor coordination [195].

GPR18 has low-sequence amino acid identity with CB1 receptors (13%) and CB2 receptors (8%) and is expressed in lymphoid tissue. N-Arachidonoyl glycine, a carboxylic metabolite of anandamide, is thought to be its ligand; however several other ligands bind to GPR18 [187, 188]. Resolvin D2, a polyunsaturated fatty acid metabolite which is involved in promoting normal cellular function following post-injury inflammation, is also an agonist at GPR18 [45].

GPR3, GPR6, and GPR12 were first described in the 1990s and are found in the brain and reproductive tract.

GPR12 was cloned from mouse DNA in 1993, and the human receptor has a 35% transmembrane sequence identity and 60% overall identity with CB1 and CB2 receptors [77, 156]. GPR12 receptors are involved in fertility, metabolic disorders, cell survival including cancer cell migration, and invasion [156]. Certain cannabis derivatives such as cannabidiol are inverse agonists for this receptor [24]. Sphingosine-1-phosphatide and sphingomyelin phosphatidylcholine are also thought to be ligands [128]. Downstream signaling is distinctly different from CB1 and CB2 receptors. These receptors select for Gs rather than Gi/o proteins, activate rather than inhibit adenylyl cyclase, and are functionally selective for beta-arrestin interactions [156, 276]. These receptors may determine some of the biologic effects of cannabidiol (CBD), since THC does not interact with either GPR3, GPR6, or GPR12.

GPR3 modulates amyloid production, and silencing GPR3 receptors has been shown to reduce CNS amyloid [278]. GPR3 receptor agonists may also reduce neuropathic pain, anxiety, and caloric intake and improve fertility [156] and may also reduce the rewarding effects of cocaine [195].

GPR6 receptor agonists have demonstrated protective effects in Alzheimer's disease in animal models but may worsen Parkinson's disease in a different model. GPR6 receptors have also been shown to be important in learning [156].

1.10 Endocannabinoid Ion Channels: Transient Receptor Potential Channels

Transient receptor potential (TRP) channels are membrane-associated proteins involved in the transduction of chemical and physical stimuli. Six of 28 known TRP channels are labeled as "ionotropic cannabinoid receptors": TRPV1, TRPV2, TRPV3, TRPV4, TRPA1, and TRPM8 [66]. These channels modulate ion entry, which influences the temperature sensation, pressure, pH, smell, taste, vision, and pain [198]. TRP channels are primarily found on somatosensory neurons, dorsal root ganglia, blood vessels, and gastrointestinal tract and have been shown to have many interactions with several cannabinoids.

AEA and 2-AG bind, activate, and then desensitize multiple TRPs [67]. Endogenous cannabinoids activate the ankyrin channel, TRPA1, and are antagonists at the melastatin receptor, TRPM8. AEA was the first recognized endogenous TRPV1 agonist and is a TRPA1 agonist and TRPM8 antagonist [198]. THC and CBD activate and then desensitize TRPV1 and TRPV2. CBD and tetrahydrocannabivarin (THCV) activate TRPV3 with high efficacy (50–70%) and potency. Cannabichromene

(CBC), a minor phytocannabinoid, reduces TRPV1, TRPV3, and TRPV4 mRNA in the jejunum and TRPV3 and TRPV4 mRNA in the ileum in mice with experimental colitis [66, 67]. Desensitization of these receptors by cannabinoids has been proposed to be a prime mechanism to explain cannabis analgesia [66].

1.11 Interactions Between the Endocannabinoid and Endogenous Opioid Systems

There is an intimate and complex interaction between the endocannabinoid and the endogenous opioid system, which may explain why there is a growing popularity of using cannabis in pain management and as an "opioid sparing" agent. Interactions between both systems can be direct in the form of heterodimer modulation of endogenous opioid release and upregulation of production of endogenous opioids or via shared downstream signaling leading to analgesic tolerance or improved nociception [181, 256].

To illustrate this complexity, one study demonstrated that THC caused a time-related increase in proenkephalin (endogenous opioid polypeptide hormone) gene expression and mu-opioid receptor activation of G-proteins, but also a time-related decrease in CB1 receptor gene expression and reduction in CB1 receptor activation of G-proteins [54]. In a number of animal models, THC analgesia effect is mediated in part through delta and kappa opioid receptors [50].

Interactions between systems appear to be largely supraspinal. Intracerebral ventricular injections of the CB1 receptor neutral antagonist AM251 completely reverse the central antinociception of morphine in a dose-dependent fashion, and this interaction was specific for mu receptor agonists [219]. There have been animal studies which have demonstrated both antinociceptive synergy and tolerance with cannabinoid/morphine combinations as well [35, 50, 57, 285].Cannabinoid receptor antagonists have also been shown to blunt opioid withdrawal and opioid physical dependence in animal models [242].

The endocannabinoid/opioid interaction may also play a role in addiction, since the endocannabinoid system synergistically interacts with opioid receptors in the nucleus accumbens increasing the rewarding effects of both drugs [289]. Cannabinoid receptor blockers have been shown to reduce dopamine release within the nucleus accumbens and heroin self-administration in animals [87, 193].

In individuals with chronic low back pain, low endogenous opioid and endocannabinoid levels have been found and may predict morphine responses to continuous pain, whereas high endocannabinoid and low endogenous opioids predicts morphine responses to evoked pain and also morphine rewarding effects [25]. The interactions may not only be related to pain but also metabolism. Individuals who are obese and <30 years have lower methylation of both the mu-opioid receptor (MOR) gene and CB1 receptor gene with increased expression of both in circulating mononuclear cells. Incidentally, this epigenetic phenomenon may be a biomarker of early obesity [233], since these epigenetic changes reflect events occurring in the hypothalamus in areas governing appetite.

1.12 N-Methyl-D-aspartate Receptors and Cannabinoids

The NMDA receptor is a glutamate and ion channel receptor activated by glutamate and glycine and which has received much attention as a result of recent ketamine trials in mental health. Both direct and indirect interactions between the endocannabinoid system and NMDA receptors have also been found. On one hand, the activation of the CB1 receptor modulates NMDA receptor activity. Preventing glutamate overactivity and downregulating the expression of glutamate receptors results in effects which are similar to ketamine and lead to both analgesic and psychotomimetic effects [133, 166, 241]. Activation of CB1 receptors also directly stimulates release of calcium from intracellular stores. This rise in cytosolic calcium inhibits the NMDA-mediated calcium influx [166]. Furthermore, the endocannabinoid system interacts in an indirect fashion with these receptors via Sigma-1 receptor activation. Sigma-1 receptors on endoplasmic reticulum influence mitochondrial calcium flux. Activation of sigma-1 receptors causes migration of receptors to the plasma membrane resulting in activation of NMDA receptors and dampening of mu receptor G-protein signaling [61]. Activation of Sigma-1 receptors is also associated with seizure activity [284]. This may explain the analgesic and anti-seizure effects of cannabidiol (CBD) which blocks Sigma-1 receptors and eventually dampens NMDA receptor activity [237]. A recent study has suggested that ketamine analgesia may be dependent on endocannabinoid release [220]. This complex interaction may also play a role in certain mental health conditions. CB1 receptor agonists negatively regulate NMDA receptors, provoking dysregulation of dopamine in striatal nuclei and prefrontal cortex which is a hallmark of psychosis [97]. Finally, endocannabinoids may modulate NMDA receptor activity through Dimer formation. CB1 receptors form dimers with NMDA receptors through interactions with the NR1 subunit of NMDA receptors [249].

1.13 Cannabinoid Ligands

The complexity and promiscuity of endocannabinoids and phytocannabinoids are quite remarkable. CBD, for example, has a very low affinity for CB1 and CB2 receptors and is potentially an inverse agonist at CB1 receptors. However, it also binds to several orphan receptors, including GPR3, GPR6, and GPR12 as previously outlined. It also acts as an agonist for serotonin receptors 5HT1A and 5HT3A; blocks receptor GPR55 and TRPM8 [110, 140, 250, 295]; allosterically modulates mu-opioid receptors (MOR) and delta-opioid receptors (DOR); activates PPAR-alpha; activates and desensitizes TRPV1, TRPV2, and TRPA1; is a glycine receptor agonist at alpha1, alpha2, and alpha3; and is a sigma1 receptor blocker [36, 154, 227, 239, 243, 244]. These many targets and promiscuous nature of CBD may explain the multiple benefits seen in anxiety, analgesia, anti-seizure activity, etc. However, this may also mean that off-target adverse effects are inevitable.

1.14 Synthesis and Catabolism of Anandamide (AEA)

The two principal endocannabinoid signaling molecules, anandamide (AEA) and 2-AG, share certain metabolic commonalities. Both are mainly synthesized on demand, have a very short half-life (approximately 15 minutes), and are dependent on arachidonic acid for their synthesis. Furthermore, the classical concept that endocannabinoids are only produced upon depolarization and not stored in vesicles is not completely true. Endocannabinoids are in part stored in intracellular organelles called adiposomes [214].

There are two steps in synthesizing AEA which have been described involving two membrane-bound enzymes though this may be a bit simplistic. A calcium-dependent N-acyltransferase (NAT) then N-acyl phosphatidylethanolamine-specific phospholipase D (NAPE-PLD) releases AEA from postsynaptic membranes. There is an alternative route involving glycerol phosphodiesterases (GDE 1,4,7) and then alpha/beta hydrolases domain containing protein 4 (ABHD4) which then generates AEA [88, 127, 216]. NAT activity is the rate-limiting step to AEA production [264]. AEA is then catabolized by membrane-bound enzymes NAPE-PLD and fatty acid amide hydrolase (FAAH). FAAH activity is allosterically modified by various hormones (pregnenolone, estradiol, cortisone, progesterone, testosterone). Binding of these compounds to the allosteric site increases enzyme activity and affinity for AEA, thus reducing AEA levels [246].

Membrane lipid composition, and cholesterol in particular, can also modulate FAAH enzyme activity. Cholesterol content is further altered in many disease states; thus, AEA production changes depending on disease activity [60]. Further mechanisms can also modulate AEA activity. For example, AEA diffuses readily through lipid membranes but requires transporters through the cytosol to get to the endoplasmic reticulum to reach FAAH [46, 177]. AEA thus binds to two protein transporters, fatty acid binding proteins (FABPs) and heat shock protein 70 (HSP70) [80]. The function of these proteins may be altered by other compounds, thus modulating endocannabinoid activity. For example, palmitoylethanolamide (PEA), a non-arachidonic acid containing compound, has been shown to increase AEA levels as an entourage effect by competing with AEA at its binding site on FAAH and inhibiting its expression [71, 90]. In this case, it may be more appropriate to define PAE as an endocannanabinoid system modulator. Furthermore, both AEA and 2-AG can also be transported through membranes through microvesicles rather than directly released [92, 93]. This may be important in presynaptic GABA and dopaminergic signaling.

Both AEA and 2-AG are major sources of arachidonic acid and are metabolized by cyclooxygenase 2 (COX-2), lipoxygenases, and mixed function oxidases (P450 enzymes). There are regional metabolizing enzyme and transporter differences within the CNS which lead to regional differences in signaling [174, 177]. As a result, arachidonic acid derived from AEA is metabolized into prostaglandins (PGE2) which is associated with pronociceptive signaling and regional inflammation [146]. Eicosanoid endocannabinoids will be discussed later.

1.15 Synthesis and Catabolism of 2-Arachidonoyl Glycerol (2-AG)

Synthesis of 2-AG largely occurs in postsynaptic membranes [280]. The first step in the synthesis of 2-AG involves phospholipase C activation with subsequent release of diacylglycerol from membranes which then is metabolized to 2-AG by membrane bound diacylglycerol lipase (DAGL) [12, 197, 228]. DAGL is rate limiting to 2-AG production. This enzyme is dynamically expressed through endocytosis and is also dependent on protein kinase C. Diminished expression of DAGL reduces 2-AG production by 60–80% [95, 306]. DAGL is also more active in microglia than in postsynaptic neurons [299].

Like anandamide, 2-AG is largely made "on demand" [173], with the exception of sperm where 2-AG levels are kept constant and inhibit the calcium channel CATsper [191].

2-AG catabolism is carried out by several different pathways. The main route is by way of monoacylglycerol lipase (MAGL), which is responsible for 85% of 2-AG catabolism [16]. However, other enzymatic pathways have been shown to play a role, including ABHD2, ABHD6, and ABHD12 but also COX-2 and lipoxygenases [73, 91, 163, 183, 206]. Both MAGL and other secondary catabolic enzymes may hold interesting therapeutic potential.

The functional details of 2-AG's main catabolic enzyme MAGL have been studied extensively. MAGL is attached to cellular membranes such that the active enzyme site faces the cytosol. As opposed to its anabolic enzyme DAGL, expression of MAGL is greater in neurons than microglia and largely located in presynaptic membranes [43, 122, 280].

The therapeutic applications which may be derived by increasing 2-AG levels with the use of MAGL inhibitors have generated much interest, particularly as potential analgesics. Although preliminary research in mice with MAGL inhibitors has been associated with adverse effects such as hypothermia, hypomobility, and catalepsy [168], there is reason to believe that manipulating this enzymatic pathway might provide certain therapeutic advantages. Preclinical data suggests that chronic reductions in MAGL desensitize and reduce the expression of CB1 receptors. Furthermore, MAGL-deficient mice do not develop hypothermia, hypomobility, or catalepsy with high 2-AG levels [257]. Intermittent MAGL inhibitors or low affinity/efficacy inhibitors maintain CB1 expression while increasing 2-AG signaling through CB1 receptors [274]. Another advantage to low efficacy blockers is reduction in prostaglandin production resulting in analgesia and reduced neuroinflammation. This is because 2-AG levels are 100- to 1000-fold higher than AEA and are the major source of arachidonic acid. Blocking MAGL activity reduces PGE2 and PGD2 levels which are key molecules in the neuroinflammatory cascade [211, 273].

In sperm, the catabolic enzyme ABHD2 plays a more important role. It is a progesterone-dependent hydrolase which catabolizes 2-AG and has been proposed as a potential target to explain the association between progesterone and male infertility [9, 14, 51, 160].

Although FAAH and MAGL are considered the main enzymes responsible for endocannabinoid catabolism, secondary arachidonic enzymatic pathways can come into play if these are blocked [91]. Like anandamide (AEA), 2-AG can also be metabolized by COX2 and lipoxygenases, which are the main enzymes families involved in the production of eicosanoids (prostaglandins, leukotrienes, hydroperoxides, etc.). Endocannabinoid synthesis and catabolism modulate the availability of arachidonic acid and its availability to form inflammatory metabolites.

2-AG has the same affinity for COX2 as arachidonic acid, and, in fact, COX2 plays an important role in terminating 2-AG signaling [145]. 2-AG is also involved in a feedback loop reducing COX2 expression through interactions with CB1 receptors and PPAR alpha [303]. Arachidonic acid derived from 2-AG catabolism is also used to generate glyceryl ester PGE2 via COX-2 which plays a major role in pain, immunomodulation, neuroinflammation, and synaptic plasticity [106, 251–253]. Thus, the analgesic effect of COX2 inhibitors may be explained in part by enhanced 2-AG availability.

Eiocosanoids are a class of signaling molecules, mostly derived from arachidonic acid, and include a multitude of important players in endocrine systems. Examples include leucotrienes, thromboxanes and prostaglandines, among others. After COX 1 and 2, lipoxygenases are the second enzyme family involved in eicos anoid production. Of the six known human lipoxygenases, several are also involved in 2-AG metabolism and endocannabinoid system modulation. For example, 12-lipoxygenase (LOX) efficiently oxygenates 2-AG. Another lipoxygenase, 15-LOX-2, also oxygenates 2-AG and is a source of the hydroperoxide 15(S)-hydroperoxyeicosatetraenoic (HETE-G) acid glyceryl ester. 15-HETE-G is a peroxisome proliferator-activated receptor alpha (PPAR alpha) agonist [147] and is also involved in inflammation. Hydroperoxides generated from arachidonic acid by 5-LOX inhibit FAAH, thereby increasing AEA levels [176]. Arachidonic acid-derived HETE is associated with certain types of colon polyps [8].

2-AG-derived arachidonic acid is metabolized to leukotriene B (4) which then binds to leukotriene B (4) receptor 1 [48]. 2-AG, in turn, rapidly induces robust biosynthesis of leukotrienes in leukocytes resulting in myeloperoxidase release, kinase activation, and calcium mobilization. Thus, 2-AG contributes to inflammation and tumor formation through LOX and leukotriene transformation.

Transport of 2-AG to metabolic sites requires a carrier. As such, 2-AG shares this commonality with anandamide and is also bound by the same carrier, thus leading to competition between the two endocannabinoids [15]. The transporter is bidirectional and leads to release of 2-AG from the cell. This common carrier appears to be FABP5 [46, 254]. 2-AG, like AEA, can be ferried across synaptic membranes by microvesicles [92, 93].

2-AG is also promiscuous in regard to receptors and ion channels and produces a wide range of physiological effects. 2-AG binds to GABAa receptors and potentiates receptor activation at low concentrations [261]. It also activates PPAR alpha which reduces interleukin-2 and COX-2 expression [76]. 2-AG is also an allosteric modulator of adenosine A3 receptors which reduces inflammation [99]. TRPV1 is activated then desensitized by 2-AG which is a mechanism involved in long-term synaptic depression [300]. 2-AG induces phosphorylation of vasodilator-stimulated phosphoprotein in cerebrovascular endothelial cells which is mediated by TRPV1 receptors [103]. The enzyme monoacylglycerol kinase (MGK) has been shown to metabolize 2-AG to 2-arachidonoyl lysophosphatidic acid (LPA) which is an agonist to GPR55 [305]. Thus, this secondary pathway may be clinically relevant since preclinical evidence suggests that GPR55 modulates anxiety and substance use [2].

1.16 Tetrahydrocannabinol

Tetrahydrocannabinol (THC) is the most common phytocannabinoid in cannabis and is presently in concentrations of 12–20% in recreational cannabis, while strains found in dispensaries have been known to contain up to 25% or more. The influence of THC on the endocannabinoid system is quite wide ranging.

THC activates CB1 which produces psychoactivity, including the "drug liking" effects sought after with street and recreational cannabis [269]. This "drug liking" effect is a result of inhibition of GABAergic neurotransmission within the nucleus accumbens which facilitates dopamine release [96]. Stereoisomers of THC are known to exist and exhibit different receptor affinity. The enantiomer trans-delta-9 THC has greater affinity for CB1 receptors than cis-delta-9 THC, but both have a lower efficacy for both CB1 and CB2 receptors than anandamide AEA [227]. Furthermore, THC has a lower efficacy for G-protein activation than AEA and 2-AG and will act as an antagonist for both CB1 and CB2 where receptor density is sparse. Furthermore, coupling efficiency with cannabinoid receptors is lowered by various disease states [227].

Long-term exposure to THC produces downregulation of CB1 receptors, reducing surface expression of CB1 and increasing expression of CB1 receptor mRNA [238]. This has been associated with increased tolerance to THC' where responses to many adverse and recreational effects may decrease over time. It is unclear if tolerance to the therapeutic effects occurs as well. On the other hand, diseases such as cancer increased expression of CB1 or CB2 receptors [225, 226], although it is unclear what role this may play in THC-induced receptor downregulation.

The activation of CB1 receptors by THC enhances CBD-negative allosteric modulation of the receptor [49]. As a result, cannabis containing CBD and THC is likely to have less psychotomimetic adverse effects, and individuals will tolerate higher doses of THC. Preclinical data has shown that THC-induced analgesia may not require the presence of CB1 receptors [308], suggesting that non-canonical receptor interactions with THC also play a clinically important role.

Though THC has a high affinity for both CB1 and CB2 receptors, it has greater efficacy (receptor activation) at GPR55 receptors, which are not only involved in drug rewarding effects but also anxiety, pain, food intake, fat storage, gut motility, and insulin secretion [164, 227]. THC also modulates conductance through glycine, the serotonin 5HT3a receptor and TRP channels [11, 72, 310]. These interactions may be important contributors to THC-related analgesia and anti-emesis.

1.17 Tetrahydrocannabinol and the Eicosanoid System

The fatty acids linoleic acid and arachidonic acid are metabolized to eicosanoids via cycloxygenases (COX 1 and 2) and lipoxygenases (LOX). Eisocanoids, in turn, are known to play major roles in inflammation, pain response, immunity and cancer growth, among others. There is a complex interaction between THC and the eicosanoid system, which will be briefly reviewed here. Of these, the relationship between THC and COX2 is of particular interest. THC stimulates phospholipase A2 which releases arachidonic acid from membranes. Arachidonic acid is then subjected to cycloxygenase-2 (COX2) or lipoxygenase (LOX) metabolism [290].

THC also increases brain prostaglandin but its metabolite delta 1-tetrahydrocannabinol-7-oic acid (delta 1-THC-7-oic acid) blocks THC stimulated prostaglandin (PG) synthesis [29, 30]. The effect of THC on the increase in PG and PGE2 is not uniform in the brain, however. THC reduces PGE2 in the hypothalamus, which may be the cause of hypothermia in animals exposed to THC [56], and the (-) THC isomer seems to be more potent to produce this effect [29, 30].

Delta 1-THC-7-oic acid has been shown to exhibit antinociceptive effects in animals and blocks THC hyperalgesia [34, 74]. Catalepsy, which is a THC-mediated side effect in rodents, is also blocked by THC-7-oic acid [31].

One of the main metabolites of THC, THC-11-oic acid (THC-COOH), may have interesting clinical properties. It is the main metabolite of THC used for drug testing, since it has a very long half-life, from days to weeks in heavy users [126]. Although it does not have any psychoactive properties, it may have analgesic and anti-inflammatory effects [34]. A synthetic derivative of THC, Ajulemic acid (CT3), is a potent analog of THC-11-oic acid (THC-COOH) and has demonstrated several interesting properties as well, including anti-inflammatory properties resembling NSAIDs. It is non-ulcerogenic in animal models and has no psychotomimetic effects [32, 33, 309]. The anti-inflammatory activity and analgesic effects of THC-11-oic acid (THC-COOH) are in part explained by activation of PPAR-gamma [4], which is a molecular target of ajulemic acid resulting in anti-inflammatory actions [165].

On the other hand, THC activation of CB2 leading to arachidonic acid release by phospholipase A2 leads to an increased production of resolvin eicosanoids which dampen inflammation [27, 41].

Effects of NSAID on THC are also complex. NSAIDS shift arachidonic acid toward endocannabinoid production which may be one mechanism by which NSAIDS reduce pain [258].

Indomethacin effects on THC have been studied in preclinical models. Indomethacin blocks THC-induced PGE2 synthesis and may also block THC psychotomimetic effects [29, 30, 297]. Thus, indomethacin may block the subjective high that cannabis smokers experience [224]. The increase in arachidonic acid produced by THC may also be an important mechanism to addiction relapses [298]. Indomethacin also reduces PGE2 brain levels which do not seem to alter THC analgesia. Indomethacin also blocks THC-induced cerebral arteriolar dilatation likely through altered prostaglandins [78].

COX2 inhibitors have been shown to cause withdrawal behaviors in THC-tolerant animals. However, when diclofenac is started with THC, it seems to prevent

THC withdrawal behaviors [5, 6, 296]. THC sedation is blocked by COX2 antagonists [230]. THC catalepsy in mice is blocked by aspirin, indomethacin, and other COX2 inhibitors [86].

1.18 Intracellular Binding Proteins

Previous sections touched on intracellular binding proteins which help carry endocannabinoids to their catabolic sites. This section will go into a little more depth.

Fatty acid binding proteins (FABPs) are a family of proteins that "solubilize" and transport fatty acids from the extracellular membrane and across the hydrophilic cytosol to intracellular membranes. Both AEA and 2-AG readily cross the cell membrane, but AEA requires FABP to reach its catabolic enzyme FAAH, which governs AEA intracellular levels, and is located on the endoplasmic reticulum. However, 2-AG's catabolic enzyme, MAGL, is bound to the extracellular membrane with the active site facing the cytosol.

There are multiple FABPs that bind AEA and 2-AG in the cell: FABP1 is limited to the liver, while FABP3, FABP5, and FABP7 are found in the CNS [68, 189].

Compounds that bind to FABPs increase AEA and 2-AG levels through competitive inhibition. These include endogenous fatty acid amides belonging to the N-acylethanolamine(NAE) family, such as palmitoylethanolamide (PEA) [68]. PEA is also metabolized by the same enzyme as anandamide, FAAH. Thus, PEA increases AEA signaling through a second mechanism by competing with FAAH. Mice lacking FABP5 and FABP7, which exhibit highest affinities for endocannabinoids, have elevated levels of AEA, PEA, and oleoylethanolamide [135]. Blocking FABPs in animals has been shown to improve endocannabinoid antinociception and reduce anxiety and depression [107].

Both CBD and THC also have affinities for FABPs similar to AEA and 2-AG [79]. Thus, competitive inhibition with FABPs, which increase intracellular AEA levels, may be a further mechanism which explains some of the therapeutic benefits encountered with the use of phytocannabinoids [159]. However, there are important differences between THC and non-THC FABP blockers. THC directly desensitizes CB1 through recruitment of beta-arrestin, whereas AEA does not [23]. FABP1 is particularly important to THC intracellular uptake, elimination, and induced gene expression governing lipid metabolism in the liver [125]. Interestingly, blocking FABP1, which is not found in the CNS, increases brain AEA, 2-AG, and NAT levels [184].

1.19 Phytocannabinoids and P-Glycoprotein and Multidrug Transports

P-Glycoprotein 1 (Pgp or P-gp), also known as multidrug resistance protein 1 (MDR1), is an important cell membrane protein which pumps toxins and drugs out of cells. This ATP-dependent efflux pump has broad substrate specificity and, in oncology, is involved in reduced chemotherapeutic drug efficacy. Many drugs inhibit Pgp, but there are conflicting findings in the literature about efflux protein pumps and interactions with CBD and THC.

In vitro, CBD and THC seem to inhibit P-glycoprotein function and multidrug transporters. THC increases rhodamine (dye) and doxorubicin intracellular levels 2.2- and 2.6-fold, respectively. Both were described as P-glycoprotein substrates [307]. In this regard, both cannabinoids could potentially increase anthramycin tumor kill but also perhaps toxicity. Mice deficient in P-glycoprotein have a 2.17 increase absorption of oral THC. THC oral absorption is improved with an oral P-glycoprotein blocker [18]. THC with prolonged exposure reduces the expression of P-glycoprotein in a T-lymphoblastic cell line but acutely does not block vinblastine (a multidrug transporter substrate) efflux [307]. This has been described in a second study using topotecan and mitoxantrone [120].

On the other hand, THC produces opposite effects with antipsychotics. THC reduces risperidone intracellular accumulation even though risperidone is a P-glycoprotein substrate. The assumption here is that THC actually increases risperidone efflux through P-glycoprotein. In addition, THC has been noted to increase P-glycoprotein expression at multiple sites within the CNS. In this regard THC has been noted to reduce the antipsychotic neurotoxicity in animals [26]. However, additional studies will need to be done to clarify the relationship between phytocannabinoids and efflux pumps.

1.20 N-Acylethanolamines

N-Acylethanolamines (NAEs) are a family of bioactive fatty acid amides, of which anandamide (AEA) is a member. It has been known for a long time that these compounds were found in animal tissues and they are particularly present in the CNS. Their receptors are widely expressed in glial cells and neurons. However, their properties and function have only recently been elucidated, and they are believed to interact with the endocannabinoid system and are involved in the regulation of appetite, mood, reward, sleep, and cognitive functions [34]. They are now considered to be part of the larger endocannabinoidome and could reasonably be described as endocannabinoid system modulators. The most studied NAEs are anandamide (AEA), palmitoylethanolamide (PEA), oleoylethanolamide (OEA), stearoylethanolamide (SEA), and linoleoylethanolamide (LEA).

There is a plethora of basic science studies, clinical trials, systematic reviews, and meta-analyses on palmitoylethanolamide (PEA) [62]. PEA is produced endogenously and is also available as a nutraceutical which does not require a prescription. PEA is produced from membranes on demand with the first step being transfer of palmitic acid to a phospholipid donor through a calcium-dependent N-acyl transferase (NAPE), and then the phosphatidyl group is removed by NAPE phospholipase [234]. Local levels of PEA are governed by a balance of synthesis and catabolism with local AEA levels which compete for FABPs binding and FAAH sites [135, 136, 282]. NAEs such as PEA do not directly activate CB1 or CB2 receptors nor contribute to prostaglandin production as NAEs lack arachidonic acid. PEA stimulates 2-AG biosynthesis through DAGLs [229]. NAEs clinically improve mood and reduce pain, peripheral inflammation, and neuroinflammation [53, 58, 62, 64, 200, 270].

PEA is a positive allosteric TRPV1 modulator which initially increases activation of the ion channel in the presence of AEA [65, 118]. Postsynaptic TRPV1 inhibits GABAergic control within the rostral ventromedial medulla and periaqueductal gray activating OFF neurons which enhances analgesia. TRPV1 activation stimulates glutamate release within the PAG which binds to metabotropic glutamate receptors leading to inhibition of GABA release which facilitates analgesia [70].

PEA is a full agonist at GPR55 and GPR18 [244]. GPR55 acts to potentiate synaptic communication, in an opposite manner to CB_1, and thus is pronociceptive within the dorsal horn and brain stem. GPR55 knockout mice are resistant to mechanical hyperalgesia from Freund's complete adjuvant induced inflammatory pain and partial nerve ligation. GPR55 antagonists are antinociceptive in animal models [111, 288]. GPR55 activation in the PAG reduces nociceptive thresholds. In addition, PEA modulates mesolimbic dopaminergic activity states through the GPR55 receptor. This did not increase morphine rewarding effects but did cause disruption of social interactions, recognition memory, spatial location memory, and reduced fear memory formation in animals [148]. PEA has also been shown to reduce plaque size in early and established atherosclerosis and promotes plaque stability through GPR55 [236]. PEA improves murine experimental colitis, in part through GPR55, by increasing 2-AG which activates CB2, and through PPAR alpha and modulation of TRPV1 channels [21]. PEA also helps to regulate intestinal motility, secretion, inflammation, and cellular proliferation through GPR55 [20].

The complex interaction and biologic effect of PEA through GPR55 receptors requires further exploration. PEA may have a multitude of benefits which are yet unexplored. Furthermore, there have been no psychotomimetic effects noted with PEA in clinical trials [62]. Contrary to animal studies which explored GPR55/PEA interactions and pronociceptive effects, systematic reviews of clinical trials have demonstrated robust analgesia [7, 62, 129].

There has been extensive work done on understanding the interactions between PPAR alpha and PEA, which may be the most important targets for PEA [55]. PEA, once bound to PPAR alpha, causes a dimer to form between the retinoic acid receptor and PPAR alpha which then binds to peroxisome proliferator response elements on DNA [63]. This causes an upregulation of PPAR alpha and downregulation of Nuclear Factor Kappa-B (NF kappa-B) which in turn down-modulates COX-2 and inflammatory cytokines [81, 82]. The PEA-PPAR alpha dimer also upregulates CB2 receptors, adding a further mechanism which dampens inflammatory responses [212]. PPAR alpha increases neurosteroids (allopregnanolone) which alters calcium and potassium channel activation and reinforces GABA signaling. This, in turn, may reduce pain and seizures [255].

PEA has also been shown to interact with mast cells within the CNS. Mast cells are involved with neuroinflammation, neuropathic pain, and cerebral edema from injury and also contribute to demyelination [153]. PEA reduces mast cell-mediated toxicity from brain ischemia [39, 85, 221, 266]. Mast cells have functional CB2 receptors which are negative regulators to mast cell activation. PEA and AEA by way of CB2 bind to the mast cell, but only PEA down-modulates mast cell activation [85]. PEA reduces spinal cord damage from trauma, delays neuron loss from glutamate excitotoxicity, and reduces amyloid deposits, learning deficits and memory loss in animals [116, 265, 267].

Another NAE, oleoylethanolamide (OEA), activates the orphan receptor GPR119, an important modulator of glucagon-like-peptide-1 in the GI tract involved in glycemic control and insulin secretion. OEA is increased in the GI tract with food intake and produces satiety [102, 210]. Oleic canola oil and olive oil consumption in hamsters increases OEA and reduces food intake [262]. OEA influences intestinal motility, inflammation, and cellular proliferation through GPR119 and PPAR alpha and to a lesser extent GPR55 [20].

1.21 Conclusion

The early understanding of the endocannabinoid system has gradually evolved to include complex interactions with multiple non-canonical receptors and ion channels, making its boundaries now harder to define. As advancing research has uncovered the activities which cannabinoids and endocannabinoid system modulators possess, some have suggested the term "endocannabinoidome" to designate the far-reaching influences of this elaborate system, and we have barely scratched the surface. Human clinical trials will require meticulous planning in order to untangle the promiscuous nature of cannabinoid ligand targets which interact at multiple sites resulting in a mixture of both direct and indirect benefits, but also side effects and detriments. Study designs will be further compounded by the fact that disease processes often alter the cannabinoid system as well. Hence, there is a tremendous gap between dispensing phytocannabinoids and knowing what the particular cannabis mixture is actually targeting. Owing to its universal availability, the cannabis plant and its derived products will continue to be studied in human trials. However, future research will undoubtedly explore many natural and synthetic cannabinoid system modulators, either isolated or in combination with other active compounds, though there remain many hurdles in order to effectively develop safe and effective medicinal cannabinoid derivatives.

References

1. Al-Zoubi R, Morales P, Reggio PH. Structural insights into CB1 receptor biased signaling. Int J Mol Sci. 2019;20(8):1837.
2. Alavi MS, Shamsizadeh A, Azhdari-Zarmehri H, Roohbakhsh A. Orphan G protein-coupled receptors: the role in CNS disorders. Biomed Pharmacother. 2018;98:222–32.
3. Alhouayek M, Muccioli GG. COX-2-derived endocannabinoid metabolites as novel inflammatory mediators. Trends Pharmacol Sci. 2014;35(6):284–92.
4. Ambrosio AL, Dias SM, Polikarpov I, Zurier RB, Burstein SH, Garratt RC. Ajulemic acid, a synthetic nonpsychoactive cannabinoid acid, bound to the ligand binding domain of the human peroxisome proliferator-activated receptor gamma. J Biol Chem. 2007;282(25):18625–33.
5. Anggadiredja K, Yamaguchi T, Tanaka H, Shoyama Y, Watanabe S, Yamamoto T. Prostaglandin E2 attenuates SR141716A-precipitated withdrawal in tetrahydrocannabinol-dependent mice. Brain Res. 2003;966(1):47–53.
6. Anggadiredja K, Yamaguchi T, Tanaka H, Shoyama Y, Watanabe S, Yamamoto T. Decrease in prostaglandin level is a prerequisite for the expression of cannabinoid withdrawal: a quasi abstinence approach. Brain Res. 2005;1066(1-2):201–5.
7. Artukoglu BB, Beyer C, Zuloff-Shani A, Brener E, Bloch MH. Efficacy of palmitoylethanolamide for pain: a meta-analysis. Pain Physician. 2017;20(5):353–62.
8. Austin Pickens C, Yin Z, Sordillo LM, Fenton JI. Arachidonic acid-derived hydroxyeicosatetraenoic acids are positively associated with colon polyps in adult males: a cross-sectional study. Sci Rep. 2019;9(1):12033.
9. Baggelaar MP, den Dulk H, Florea BI, Fazio D, Perruzza D, Bernabo N, Raspa M, Janssen APA, Scavizzi F, Barboni B, Overkleeft HS, Maccarrone M, van der Stelt M. ABHD2 inhibitor identified by activity-based protein profiling reduces acrosome reaction. ACS Chem Biol. 2019;14(12):2943.
10. Balenga NA, Martinez-Pinilla E, Kargl J, Schroder R, Peinhaupt M, Platzer W, Balint Z, Zamarbide M, Dopeso-Reyes IG, Ricobaraza A, Perez-Ortiz JM, Kostenis E, Waldhoer M, Heinemann A, Franco R. Heteromerization of GPR55 and cannabinoid CB2 receptors modulates signalling. Br J Pharmacol. 2014;171(23):5387–406.
11. Barann M, Molderings G, Bruss M, Bonisch H, Urban BW, Gothert M. Direct inhibition by cannabinoids of human 5-HT3A receptors: probable involvement of an allosteric modulatory site. Br J Pharmacol. 2002;137(5):589–96.
12. Basavarajappa BS. Critical enzymes involved in endocannabinoid metabolism. Protein Pept Lett. 2007;14(3):237–46.
13. Barnes PJ. Receptor heterodimerization: a new level of cross-talk. J Clin Invest. 2006;116:1210–2.
14. Battista N, Meccariello R, Cobellis G, Fasano S, Di Tommaso M, Pirazzi V, Konje JC, Pierantoni R, Maccarrone M. The role of endocannabinoids in gonadal function and fertility along the evolutionary axis. Mol Cell Endocrinol. 2012;355(1):1–14.
15. Beltramo M, Piomelli D. Carrier-mediated transport and enzymatic hydrolysis of the endogenous cannabinoid 2-arachidonylglycerol. Neuroreport. 2000;11(6):1231–5.
16. Blankman JL, Simon GM, Cravatt BF. A comprehensive profile of brain enzymes that hydrolyze the endocannabinoid 2-arachidonoylglycerol. Chem Biol. 2007;14(12):1347–56.
17. Blume LC, Leone-Kabler S, Luessen DJ, Marrs GS, Lyons E, Bass CE, Chen R, Selley DE, Howlett AC. Cannabinoid receptor interacting protein suppresses agonist-driven CB1 receptor internalization and regulates receptor replenishment in an agonist-biased manner. J Neurochem. 2016;139(3):396–407.
18. Bonhomme-Faivre L, Benyamina A, Reynaud M, Farinotti R, Abbara C. Disposition of Delta tetrahydrocannabinol in CF1 mice deficient in mdr1a P-glycoprotein. Addict Biol. 2008;13(3-4):295–300.
19. Booth WT, Walker NB, Lowther WT, Howlett AC. Cannabinoid receptor interacting protein 1a (CRIP1a): function and structure. Molecules. 2019;24:E3672.

20. Borrelli F, Izzo AA. Role of acylethanolamides in the gastrointestinal tract with special reference to food intake and energy balance. Best Pract Res Clin Endocrinol Metab. 2009;23(1):33–49.
21. Borrelli F, Romano B, Petrosino S, Pagano E, Capasso R, Coppola D, Battista G, Orlando P, Di Marzo V, Izzo AA. Palmitoylethanolamide, a naturally occurring lipid, is an orally effective intestinal anti-inflammatory agent. Br J Pharmacol. 2015;172(1):142–58.
22. Bowles NP, Karatsoreos IN, Li X, Vemuri VK, Wood JA, Li Z, Tamashiro KL, Schwartz GJ, Makriyannis AM, Kunos G, Hillard CJ, McEwen BS, Hill MN. A peripheral endocannabinoid mechanism contributes to glucocorticoid-mediated metabolic syndrome. Proc Natl Acad Sci U S A. 2015;112(1):285–90.
23. Breivogel CS, Lambert JM, Gerfin S, Huffman JW, Razdan RK. Sensitivity to delta9-tetrahydrocannabinol is selectively enhanced in beta-arrestin2 -/- mice. Behav Pharmacol. 2008;19(4):298–307.
24. Brown KJ, Laun AS, Song ZH. Cannabidiol, a novel inverse agonist for GPR12. Biochem Biophys Res Commun. 2017;493(1):451–4.
25. Bruehl S, Burns JW, Morgan A, Koltyn K, Gupta R, Buvanendran A, Edwards D, Chont M, Kingsley PJ, Marnett L, Stone A, Patel S. The association between endogenous opioid function and morphine responsiveness: a moderating role for endocannabinoids. Pain. 2019;160(3):676–87.
26. Brzozowska NI, de Tonnerre EJ, Li KM, Wang XS, Boucher AA, Callaghan PD, Kuligowski M, Wong A, Arnold JC. The differential binding of antipsychotic drugs to the ABC transporter P-glycoprotein predicts cannabinoid-antipsychotic drug interactions. Neuropsychopharmacology. 2017;42(11):2222–31.
27. Buckley CD, Gilroy DW, Serhan CN. Proresolving lipid mediators and mechanisms in the resolution of acute inflammation. Immunity. 2014;40(3):315–27.
28. Bukiya AN, Dopico AM. Cannabinoid interactions with proteins: insights from structural studies. Adv Exp Med Biol. 2019;1162:39–50.
29. Burstein S, Hunter SA, Latham V, Mechoulam R, Melchior DL, Renzulli L, Tefft RE Jr. Prostaglandins and cannabis XV. Comparison of enantiomeric cannabinoids in stimulating prostaglandin synthesis in fibroblasts. Life Sci. 1986a;39(19):1813–23.
30. Burstein S, Hunter SA, Latham V, Renzulli L. Prostaglandins and cannabis--XVI. Antagonism of delta 1-tetrahydrocannabinol action by its metabolites. Biochem Pharmacol. 1986b;35(15):2553–8.
31. Burstein S, Hunter SA, Latham V, Renzulli L. A major metabolite of delta 1-tetrahydrocannabinol reduces its cataleptic effect in mice. Experientia. 1987;43(4):402–3.
32. Burstein SH. Ajulemic acid (CT3): a potent analog of the acid metabolites of THC. Curr Pharm Des. 2000;6(13):1339–45.
33. Burstein SH, Friderichs E, Kogel B, Schneider J, Selve N. Analgesic effects of 1',1' dimethylheptyl-delta8-THC-11-oic acid (CT3) in mice. Life Sci. 1998;63(3):161–8.
34. Burstein SH, Hull K, Hunter SA, Latham V. Cannabinoids and pain responses: a possible role for prostaglandins. FASEB J. 1988;2(14):3022–6.
35. Cadoni C, Pisanu A, Solinas M, Acquas E, Di Chiara G. Behavioural sensitization after repeated exposure to Delta 9-tetrahydrocannabinol and cross-sensitization with morphine. Psychopharmacology (Berl). 2001;158(3):259–66.
36. Campos AC, Guimaraes FS. Involvement of 5HT1A receptors in the anxiolytic-like effects of cannabidiol injected into the dorsolateral periaqueductal gray of rats. Psychopharmacology (Berl). 2008;199(2):223–30.
37. Carrasquer A, Nebane NM, Williams WM, Song ZH. Functional consequences of nonsynonymous single nucleotide polymorphisms in the CB2 cannabinoid receptor. Pharmacogenet Genomics. 2010;20(3):157–66.
38. Ceprian M, Jimenez-Sanchez L, Vargas C, Barata L, Hind W, Martinez-Orgado J. Cannabidiol reduces brain damage and improves functional recovery in a neonatal rat model of arterial ischemic stroke. Neuropharmacology. 2017;116:151–9.

39. Cerrato S, Brazis P, della Valle MF, Miolo A, Puigdemont A. Effects of palmitoylethanolamide on immunologically induced histamine, PGD2 and TNFalpha release from canine skin mast cells. Vet Immunol Immunopathol. 2010;133(1):9–15.
40. Chanda D, Kim YH, Kim DK, Lee MW, Lee SY, Park TS, Koo SH, Lee CH, Choi HS. Activation of cannabinoid receptor type 1 (Cb1r) disrupts hepatic insulin receptor signaling via cyclic AMP-response element-binding protein H (Crebh)-mediated induction of Lipin1 gene. J Biol Chem. 2012;287(45):38041–9.
41. Chang YH, Lee ST, Lin WW. Effects of cannabinoids on LPS-stimulated inflammatory mediator release from macrophages: involvement of eicosanoids. J Cell Biochem. 2001;81(4):715–23.
42. Chaudhary PK, Kim S. The GRKs reactome: role in cell biology and pathology. Int J Mol Sci. 2021;22:3375.
43. Chen Y, Liu X, Vickstrom CR, Liu MJ, Zhao L, Viader A, Cravatt BF, Liu QS. Neuronal and astrocytic monoacylglycerol lipase limit the spread of endocannabinoid signaling in the cerebellum. eNeuro. 2016;3(3):ENEURO.0048-16.2016.
44. Chevaleyre V, Castillo PE. Heterosynaptic LTD of hippocampal GABAergic synapses: a novel role of endocannabinoids in regulating excitability. Neuron. 2003;38(3):461–72.
45. Chiang N, Dalli J, Colas RA, Serhan CN. Identification of resolvin D2 receptor mediating resolution of infections and organ protection. J Exp Med. 2015;212(8):1203–17.
46. Chicca A, Marazzi J, Nicolussi S, Gertsch J. Evidence for bidirectional endocannabinoid transport across cell membranes. J Biol Chem. 2012;287(41):34660–82.
47. Chistiakova M, Bannon NM, Bazhenov M, Volgushev M. Heterosynaptic plasticity: multiple mechanisms and multiple roles. Neuroscientist. 2014;20:483–98.
48. Chouinard F, Lefebvre JS, Navarro P, Bouchard L, Ferland C, Lalancette-Hebert M, Marsolais D, Laviolette M, Flamand N. The endocannabinoid 2-arachidonoyl-glycerol activates human neutrophils: critical role of its hydrolysis and de novo leukotriene B4 biosynthesis. J Immunol. 2011;186(5):3188–96.
49. Chung H, Fierro A, Pessoa-Mahana CD. Cannabidiol binding and negative allosteric modulation at the cannabinoid type 1 receptor in the presence of delta-9-tetrahydrocannabinol: an In Silico study. PLoS One. 2019;14(7):e0220025.
50. Cichewicz DL. Synergistic interactions between cannabinoid and opioid analgesics. Life Sci. 2004;74(11):1317–24.
51. Cobellis G, Ricci G, Cacciola G, Orlando P, Petrosino S, Cascio MG, Bisogno T, De Petrocellis L, Chioccarelli T, Altucci L, Fasano S, Meccariello R, Pierantoni R, Ledent C, Di Marzo V. A gradient of 2-arachidonoylglycerol regulates mouse epididymal sperm cell start-up. Biol Reprod. 2010;82(2):451–8.
52. Col Araz N, Nacak M, Oguzkan Balci S, Benlier N, Araz M, Pehlivan S, Balat A, Aynacioglu AS. Childhood obesity and the role of dopamine D2 receptor and cannabinoid receptor-1 gene polymorphisms. Genet Test Mol Biomarkers. 2012;16(12):1408–12.
53. Coppola M, Mondola R. Is there a role for palmitoylethanolamide in the treatment of depression? Med Hypotheses. 2014;82(5):507–11.
54. Corchero J, Romero J, Berrendero F, Fernandez-Ruiz J, Ramos JA, Fuentes JA, Manzanares J. Time-dependent differences of repeated administration with Delta9-tetrahydrocannabinol in proenkephalin and cannabinoid receptor gene expression and G-protein activation by mu-opioid and CB1-cannabinoid receptors in the caudate-putamen. Brain Res Mol Brain Res. 1999;67(1):148–57.
55. Costa B, Comelli F, Bettoni I, Colleoni M, Giagnoni G. The endogenous fatty acid amide, palmitoylethanolamide, has anti-allodynic and anti-hyperalgesic effects in a murine model of neuropathic pain: involvement of CB(1), TRPV1 and PPARgamma receptors and neurotrophic factors. Pain. 2008;139(3):541–50.
56. Coupar IM, Taylor DA. Alteration in the level of endogenous hypothalamic prostaglandins induced by delta 9-tetrahydrocannabinol in the rat. Br J Pharmacol. 1982;76(1):115–9.

57. Cox ML, Haller VL, Welch SP. Synergy between delta9-tetrahydrocannabinol and morphine in the arthritic rat. Eur J Pharmacol. 2007;567(1-2):125–30.
58. Crupi R, Paterniti I, Ahmad A, Campolo M, Esposito E, Cuzzocrea S. Effects of palmitoylethanolamide and luteolin in an animal model of anxiety/depression. CNS Neurol Disord Drug Targets. 2013;12(7):989–1001.
59. Cruz-Martinez AM, Tejas-Juarez JG, Mancilla-Diaz JM, Floran-Garduno B, Lopez-Alonso VE, Escartin-Perez RE. CB1 receptors in the paraventricular nucleus of the hypothalamus modulate the release of 5-HT and GABA to stimulate food intake in rats. Eur Neuropsychopharmacol. 2018;28(11):1247–59.
60. Dainese E, De Fabritiis G, Sabatucci A, Oddi S, Angelucci CB, Di Pancrazio C, Giorgino T, Stanley N, Del Carlo M, Cravatt BF, Maccarrone M. Membrane lipids are key modulators of the endocannabinoid-hydrolase FAAH. Biochem J. 2014;457(3):463–72.
61. Davis MP. Sigma-1 receptors and animal studies centered on pain and analgesia. Expert Opin Drug Discovery. 2015;10(8):885–900.
62. Davis MP, Behm B, Mehta Z, Fernandez C. The potential benefits of palmitoylethanolamide in palliation: a qualitative systematic review. Am J Hosp Palliat Care. 2019;36(12):1134–54.
63. Daynes RA, Jones DC. Emerging roles of PPARs in inflammation and immunity. Nat Rev Immunol. 2002;2(10):748–59.
64. De Gregorio D, Manchia M, Carpiniello B, Valtorta F, Nobile M, Gobbi G, Comai S. Role of palmitoylethanolamide (PEA) in depression: Translational evidence: special section on "Translational and Neuroscience Studies in Affective Disorders". Section Editor, Maria Nobile MD, PhD. This Section of JAD focuses on the relevance of translational and neuroscience studies in providing a better understanding of the neural basis of affective disorders. The main aim is to briefly summaries relevant research findings in clinical neuroscience with particular regards to specific innovative topics in mood and anxiety disorders. J Affect Disord. 2019;255:S0165-0327(18)31599-4.
65. De Petrocellis L, Di Marzo V. Lipids as regulators of the activity of transient receptor potential type V1 (TRPV1) channels. Life Sci. 2005;77(14):1651–66.
66. De Petrocellis L, Ligresti A, Moriello AS, Allara M, Bisogno T, Petrosino S, Stott CG, Di Marzo V. Effects of cannabinoids and cannabinoid-enriched Cannabis extracts on TRP channels and endocannabinoid metabolic enzymes. Br J Pharmacol. 2011;163(7):1479–94.
67. De Petrocellis L, Orlando P, Moriello AS, Aviello G, Stott C, Izzo AA, Di Marzo V. Cannabinoid actions at TRPV channels: effects on TRPV3 and TRPV4 and their potential relevance to gastrointestinal inflammation. Acta Physiol (Oxf). 2012;204(2):255–66.
68. Deutsch DG. A personal retrospective: elevating anandamide (AEA) by targeting fatty acid amide hydrolase (FAAH) and the fatty acid binding proteins (FABPs). Front Pharmacol. 2016;7:370.
69. Devane WA, Dysarz FA 3rd, Johnson MR, Melvin LS, Howlett AC. Determination and characterization of a cannabinoid receptor in rat brain. Mol Pharmacol. 1988;34(5):605–13.
70. Di Marzo V, De Petrocellis L. Why do cannabinoid receptors have more than one endogenous ligand? Philos Trans R Soc Lond B Biol Sci. 2012;367(1607):3216–28.
71. Di Marzo V, Melck D, Orlando P, Bisogno T, Zagoory O, Bifulco M, Vogel Z, De Petrocellis L. Palmitoylethanolamide inhibits the expression of fatty acid amide hydrolase and enhances the anti-proliferative effect of anandamide in human breast cancer cells. Biochem J. 2001;358(Pt 1):249–55.
72. Di Marzo V, Piscitelli F. The endocannabinoid system and its modulation by phytocannabinoids. Neurotherapeutics. 2015;12(4):692–8.
73. Dinh TP, Freund TF, Piomelli D. A role for monoglyceride lipase in 2-arachidonoylglycerol inactivation. Chem Phys Lipids. 2002;121(1-2):149–58.
74. Doyle SA, Burstein SH, Dewey WL, Welch SP. Further studies on the antinociceptive effects of delta 6-THC-7-oic acid. Agents Actions. 1990;31(1-2):157–63.
75. Drew GM, Lau BK, Vaughan CW. Substance P drives endocannabinoid-mediated disinhibition in a midbrain descending analgesic pathway. J Neurosci. 2009;29(22):7220–9.

76. Du H, Chen X, Zhang J, Chen C. Inhibition of COX-2 expression by endocannabinoid 2-arachidonoylglycerol is mediated via PPAR-gamma. Br J Pharmacol. 2011;163(7):1533–49.
77. Eggerickx D, Denef JF, Labbe O, Hayashi Y, Refetoff S, Vassart G, Parmentier M, Libert F. Molecular cloning of an orphan G-protein-coupled receptor that constitutively activates adenylate cyclase. Biochem J. 1995;309(Pt 3):837–43.
78. Ellis EF, Moore SF, Willoughby KA. Anandamide and delta 9-THC dilation of cerebral arterioles is blocked by indomethacin. Am J Physiol. 1995;269(6 Pt 2):H1859–64.
79. Elmes MW, Kaczocha M, Berger WT, Leung K, Ralph BP, Wang L, Sweeney JM, Miyauchi JT, Tsirka SE, Ojima I, Deutsch DG. Fatty acid-binding proteins (FABPs) are intracellular carriers for Delta9-tetrahydrocannabinol (THC) and cannabidiol (CBD). J Biol Chem. 2015;290(14):8711–21.
80. Elmes MW, Prentis LE, McGoldrick LL, Giuliano CJ, Sweeney JM, Joseph OM, Che J, Carbonetti GS, Studholme K, Deutsch DG, Rizzo RC, Glynn SE, Kaczocha M. FABP1 controls hepatic transport and biotransformation of Delta(9)-THC. Sci Rep. 2019;9(1):7588.
81. Esposito E, Cuzzocrea S. Palmitoylethanolamide is a new possible pharmacological treatment for the inflammation associated with trauma. Mini Rev Med Chem. 2013;13(2):237–55.
82. Esposito G, Capoccia E, Turco F, Palumbo I, Lu J, Steardo A, Cuomo R, Sarnelli G, Steardo L. Palmitoylethanolamide improves colon inflammation through an enteric glia/toll like receptor 4-dependent PPAR-alpha activation. Gut. 2014;63(8):1300–12.
83. Ezzat DA, Hammam AA, El-Malah WM, Khattab RA, Mangoud EM. Role of cannabinoid CB2 receptor gene (CNR2) polymorphism in children with immune thrombocytopenic purpura in Beni-Suef governorate in Egypt. Egypt J Immunol. 2017;24(1):57–66.
84. Ezzili C, Otrubova K, Boger DL. Fatty acid amide signaling molecules. Bioorg Med Chem Lett. 2010;20(20):5959–68.
85. Facci L, Dal Toso R, Romanello S, Buriani A, Skaper SD, Leon A. Mast cells express a peripheral cannabinoid receptor with differential sensitivity to anandamide and palmitoylethanolamide. Proc Natl Acad Sci U S A. 1995;92(8):3376–80.
86. Fairbairn JW, Pickens JT. The oral activity of delta'-tetrahydrocannabinol and its dependence on prostaglandin E2. Br J Pharmacol. 1979;67(3):379–85.
87. Fattore L, Spano S, Cossu G, Deiana S, Fadda P, Fratta W. Cannabinoid CB(1) antagonist SR 141716A attenuates reinstatement of heroin self-administration in heroin-abstinent rats. Neuropharmacology. 2005;48(8):1097–104.
88. Fiskerstrand T, H'Mida-Ben Brahim D, Johansson S, M'Zahem A, Haukanes BI, Drouot N, Zimmermann J, Cole AJ, Vedeler C, Bredrup C, Assoum M, Tazir M, Klockgether T, Hamri A, Steen VM, Boman H, Bindoff LA, Koenig M, Knappskog PM. Mutations in ABHD12 cause the neurodegenerative disease PHARC: an inborn error of endocannabinoid metabolism. Am J Hum Genet. 2010;87(3):410–7.
89. Fong TM. Constitutive activity in cannabinoid receptors. Adv Pharmacol. 2014;70:121–33.
90. Fowler CJ, Jonsson KO, Tiger G. Fatty acid amide hydrolase: biochemistry, pharmacology, and therapeutic possibilities for an enzyme hydrolyzing anandamide, 2-arachidonoylglycerol, palmitoylethanolamide, and oleamide. Biochem Pharmacol. 2001;62(5):517–26.
91. Fowler CJ. The contribution of cyclooxygenase-2 to endocannabinoid metabolism and action. Br J Pharmacol. 2007;152:594–601.
92. Gabrielli M, Battista N, Riganti L, Prada I, Antonucci F, Cantone L, Lombardi M, Matteoli M, Maccarrone M, Verderio C. Active endocannabinoids are secreted on the surface of microglial microvesicles. Springerplus. 2015a;4(Suppl 1):L29.
93. Gabrielli M, Battista N, Riganti L, Prada I, Antonucci F, Cantone L, Matteoli M, Maccarrone M, Verderio C. Active endocannabinoids are secreted on extracellular membrane vesicles. EMBO Rep. 2015b;16(2):213–20.
94. Galiegue S, Mary S, Marchand J, Dussossoy D, Carriere D, Carayon P, Bouaboula M, Shire D, Le Fur G, Casellas P. Expression of central and peripheral cannabinoid receptors in human immune tissues and leukocyte subpopulations. Eur J Biochem. 1995;232(1):54–61.

95. Gao Y, Vasilyev DV, Goncalves MB, Howell FV, Hobbs C, Reisenberg M, Shen R, Zhang MY, Strassle BW, Lu P, Mark L, Piesla MJ, Deng K, Kouranova EV, Ring RH, Whiteside GT, Bates B, Walsh FS, Williams G, Pangalos MN, Samad TA, Doherty P. Loss of retrograde endocannabinoid signaling and reduced adult neurogenesis in diacylglycerol lipase knock-out mice. J Neurosci. 2010;30(6):2017–24.
96. Gardner EL. Endocannabinoid signaling system and brain reward: emphasis on dopamine. Pharmacol Biochem Behav. 2005;81(2):263–84.
97. Gaspar PA, Bustamante ML, Silva H, Aboitiz F. Molecular mechanisms underlying glutamatergic dysfunction in schizophrenia: therapeutic implications. J Neurochem. 2009;111(4):891–900.
98. Gerdeman GL, Ronesi J, Lovinger DM. Postsynaptic endocannabinoid release is critical to long-term depression in the striatum. Nat Neurosci. 2002;5(5):446–51.
99. Gessi S, Merighi S, Varani K, Leung E, Mac Lennan S, Borea PA. The A3 adenosine receptor: an enigmatic player in cell biology. Pharmacol Ther. 2008;117(1):123–40.
100. Glaser ST, Kaczocha M. Cyclooxygenase-2 mediates anandamide metabolism in the mouse brain. J Pharmacol Exp Ther. 2010;335(2):380–8.
101. Glass M, Dragunow M, Faull RL. Cannabinoid receptors in the human brain: a detailed anatomical and quantitative autoradiographic study in the fetal, neonatal and adult human brain. Neuroscience. 1997;77(2):299–318.
102. Godlewski G, Offertaler L, Wagner JA, Kunos G. Receptors for acylethanolamides-GPR55 and GPR119. Prostaglandins Other Lipid Mediat. 2009;89(3-4):105–11.
103. Golech SA, McCarron RM, Chen Y, Bembry J, Lenz F, Mechoulam R, Shohami E, Spatz M. Human brain endothelium: coexpression and function of vanilloid and endocannabinoid receptors. Brain Res Mol Brain Res. 2004;132(1):87–92.
104. Gong JP, Onaivi ES, Ishiguro H, Liu QR, Tagliaferro PA, Brusco A, Uhl GR. Cannabinoid CB2 receptors: immunohistochemical localization in rat brain. Brain Res. 2006;1071(1):10–23.
105. Gonzalez-Maeso J, Yuen T, Ebersole BJ, Wurmbach E, Lira A, Zhou M, Weisstaub N, Hen R, Gingrich JA, Sealfon SC. Transcriptome fingerprints distinguish hallucinogenic and non hallucinogenic 5-hydroxytryptamine 2A receptor agonist effects in mouse somatosensory cortex. J Neurosci. 2003;23(26):8836–43.
106. Guindon J, Hohmann AG. A physiological role for endocannabinoid-derived products of cyclooxygenase-2-mediated oxidative metabolism. Br J Pharmacol. 2008;153(7):1341–3.
107. Hamilton J, Koumas C, Clavin BH, Marion M, Figueiredo A, Gonzalez S, O'Rourke JR, Deutsch D, Kaczocha M, Haj-Dahmane S, Thanos PK. Fatty acid-binding proteins 5 and 7 gene deletion increases sucrose consumption and diminishes forced swim immobility time. Behav Pharmacol. 2018;29(6):503–8.
108. Harayama T, Riezman H. Understanding the diversity of membrane lipid composition. Nat Rev Mol Cell Biol. 2018;19(5):281–96.
109. Hauser AS, Chavali S, Masuho I, Jahn LJ, Martemyanov KA, Gloriam DE, Babu MM. Pharmacogenomics of GPCR drug targets. Cell. 2018;172:41–54.e19.
110. Hayashi T, Tsai SY, Mori T, Fujimoto M, Su TP. Targeting ligand-operated chaperone sigma-1 receptors in the treatment of neuropsychiatric disorders. Expert Opin Ther Targets. 2011;15(5):557–77.
111. Henstridge CM. Off-target cannabinoid effects mediated by GPR55. Pharmacology. 2012;89(3-4):179–87.
112. Henstridge CM, Balenga NA, Ford LA, Ross RA, Waldhoer M, Irving AJ. The GPR55 ligand L-alpha-lysophosphatidylinositol promotes RhoA-dependent Ca2+ signaling and NFAT activation. FASEB J. 2009;23(1):183–93.
113. Hentges ST, Low MJ, Williams JT. Differential regulation of synaptic inputs by constitutively released endocannabinoids and exogenous cannabinoids. J Neurosci. 2005;25(42):9746–51.
114. Hermanson DJ, Marnett LJ. Cannabinoids, endocannabinoids, and cancer. Cancer Metastasis Rev. 2011;30(3-4):599–612.

115. Herkenham M, Lynn AB, Little MD, Johnson MR, Melvin LS, de Costa BR, Rice KC. Cannabinoid receptor localization in brain. PNAS. 1990;87:1932–6.
116. Hind WH, Tufarelli C, Neophytou M, Anderson SI, England TJ, O'Sullivan SE. Endocannabinoids modulate human blood-brain barrier permeability in vitro. Br J Pharmacol. 2015;172(12):3015–27.
117. Ho BC, Wassink TH, Ziebell S, Andreasen NC. Cannabinoid receptor 1 gene polymorphisms and marijuana misuse interactions on white matter and cognitive deficits in schizophrenia. Schizophr Res. 2011;128(1-3):66–75.
118. Ho WS, Barrett DA, Randall MD. 'Entourage' effects of N-palmitoylethanolamide and N-oleoylethanolamide on vasorelaxation to anandamide occur through TRPV1 receptors. Br J Pharmacol. 2008;155(6):837–46.
119. Hoehe MR, Caenazzo L, Martinez MM, Hsieh WT, Modi WS, Gershon ES, Bonner TI. Genetic and physical mapping of the human cannabinoid receptor gene to chromosome 6q14-q15. New Biol. 1991;3(9):880–5.
120. Holland ML, Lau DT, Allen JD, Arnold JC. The multidrug transporter ABCG2 (BCRP) is inhibited by plant-derived cannabinoids. Br J Pharmacol. 2007;152(5):815–24.
121. Holz GG, Turner TJ. Pertussis toxin-sensitive GTP-binding proteins characterized in synaptosomal fractions of embryonic avian cerebral cortex. Comp Biochem Physiol B Biochem Mol Biol. 1998;119:201–11.
122. Horvath E, Woodhams SG, Nyilas R, Henstridge CM, Kano M, Sakimura K, Watanabe M, Katona I. Heterogeneous presynaptic distribution of monoacylglycerol lipase, a multipotent regulator of nociceptive circuits in the mouse spinal cord. Eur J Neurosci. 2014;39(3):419–34.
123. Howlett AC, Blume LC, Dalton GD. CB(1) cannabinoid receptors and their associated proteins. Curr Med Chem. 2010;17(14):1382–93.
124. Hsiao P, Clavijo RI. Adverse effects of cannabis on male reproduction. Eur Urol Focus. 2018;4(3):324–8.
125. Huang H, McIntosh AL, Martin GG, Dangott LJ, Kier AB, Schroeder F. Structural and functional interaction of delta(9)-tetrahydrocannabinol with liver fatty acid binding protein (FABP1). Biochemistry. 2018;57(41):6027–42.
126. Huestis MA, Mitchell JM, Cone EJ. Detection times of marijuana metabolites in urine by immunoassay and GC-MS. J Anal Toxicol. 1995;19:443–9.
127. Hussain Z, Uyama T, Tsuboi K, Ueda N. Mammalian enzymes responsible for the biosynthesis of N-acylethanolamines. Biochim Biophys Acta Mol Cell Biol Lipids. 2017;1862(12):1546–61.
128. Ignatov A, Lintzel J, Hermans-Borgmeyer I, Kreienkamp HJ, Joost P, Thomsen S, Methner A, Schaller HC. Role of the G-protein-coupled receptor GPR12 as high-affinity receptor for sphingosylphosphorylcholine and its expression and function in brain development. J Neurosci. 2003;23(3):907–14.
129. Indraccolo U, Indraccolo SR, Mignini F. Micronized palmitoylethanolamide/trans-polydatin treatment of endometriosis-related pain: a meta-analysis. Ann Ist Super Sanita. 2017;53(2):125–34.
130. Ishiguro H, Carpio O, Horiuchi Y, Shu A, Higuchi S, Schanz N, Benno R, Arinami T, Onaivi ES. A nonsynonymous polymorphism in cannabinoid CB2 receptor gene is associated with eating disorders in humans and food intake is modified in mice by its ligands. Synapse. 2010a;64(1):92–6.
131. Ishiguro H, Horiuchi Y, Ishikawa M, Koga M, Imai K, Suzuki Y, Morikawa M, Inada T, Watanabe Y, Takahashi M, Someya T, Ujike H, Iwata N, Ozaki N, Onaivi ES, Kunugi H, Sasaki T, Itokawa M, Arai M, Niizato K, Iritani S, Naka I, Ohashi J, Kakita A, Takahashi H, Nawa H, Arinami T. Brain cannabinoid CB2 receptor in schizophrenia. Biol Psychiatry. 2010b;67(10):974–82.
132. Jaeger JP, Mattevi VS, Callegari-Jacques SM, Hutz MH. Cannabinoid type-1 receptor gene polymorphisms are associated with central obesity in a Southern Brazilian population. Dis Markers. 2008;25(1):67–74.

133. Javitt DC. Glutamate and schizophrenia: phencyclidine, N-methyl-D-aspartate receptors, and dopamine-glutamate interactions. Int Rev Neurobiol. 2007;78:69–108.
134. Jhaveri MD, Richardson D, Robinson I, Garle MJ, Patel A, Sun Y, Sagar DR, Bennett AJ, Alexander SP, Kendall DA, Barrett DA, Chapman V. Inhibition of fatty acid amide hydrolase and cyclooxygenase-2 increases levels of endocannabinoid related molecules and produces analgesia via peroxisome proliferator-activated receptor-alpha in a model of inflammatory pain. Neuropharmacology. 2008;55(1):85–93.
135. Kaczocha M, Glaser ST, Maher T, Clavin B, Hamilton J, O'Rourke J, Rebecchi M, Puopolo M, Owada Y, Thanos PK. Fatty acid binding protein deletion suppresses inflammatory pain through endocannabinoid/N-acylethanolamine-dependent mechanisms. Mol Pain. 2015;11:52.
136. Kaczocha M, Vivieca S, Sun J, Glaser ST, Deutsch DG. Fatty acid-binding proteins transport N-acylethanolamines to nuclear receptors and are targets of endocannabinoid transport inhibitors. J Biol Chem. 2012;287(5):3415–24.
137. Kano M, Ohno-Shosaku T, Hashimotodani Y, Uchigashima M, Watanabe M. Endocannabinoid-mediated control of synaptic transmission. Physiol Rev. 2009;89(1):309–80.
138. Kapur A, Zhao P, Sharir H, Bai Y, Caron MG, Barak LS, Abood ME. Atypical responsiveness of the orphan receptor GPR55 to cannabinoid ligands. J Biol Chem. 2009;284(43):29817–27.
139. Karasu T, Marczylo TH, Maccarrone M, Konje JC. The role of sex steroid hormones, cytokines and the endocannabinoid system in female fertility. Hum Reprod Update. 2011;17(3):347–61.
140. Kathmann M, Flau K, Redmer A, Trankle C, Schlicker E. Cannabidiol is an allosteric modulator at mu- and delta-opioid receptors. Naunyn Schmiedebergs Arch Pharmacol. 2006;372(5):354–61.
141. Katona I, Rancz EA, Acsady L, Ledent C, Mackie K, Hajos N, Freund TF. Distribution of CB1 cannabinoid receptors in the amygdala and their role in the control of GABAergic transmission. J Neurosci. 2001;21(23):9506–18.
142. Katona I, Sperlagh B, Sik A, Kafalvi A, Vizi ES, Mackie K, Freund TF. Presynaptically located CB1 cannabinoid receptors regulate GABA release from axon terminals of specific hippocampal interneurons. J Neurosci. 1999;19(11):4544–58.
143. Kaur R, Ambwani SR, Singh S. Endocannabinoid system: a multi-facet therapeutic target. Curr Clin Pharmacol. 2016;11(2):110–7.
144. Kihara Y, Maceyka M, Spiegel S, Chun J. Lysophospholipid receptor nomenclature review: IUPHAR Review 8. Br J Pharmacol. 2014;171(15):3575–94.
145. Kim J, Alger BE. Inhibition of cyclooxygenase-2 potentiates retrograde endocannabinoid effects in hippocampus. Nat Neurosci. 2004;7(7):697–8.
146. Kozak KR, Crews BC, Morrow JD, Wang LH, Ma YH, Weinander R, Jakobsson PJ, Marnett LJ. Metabolism of the endocannabinoids, 2-arachidonylglycerol and anandamide, into prostaglandin, thromboxane, and prostacyclin glycerol esters and ethanolamides. J Biol Chem. 2002a;277(47):44877–85.
147. Kozak KR, Gupta RA, Moody JS, Ji C, Boeglin WE, DuBois RN, Brash AR, Marnett LJ. 15-Lipoxygenase metabolism of 2-arachidonylglycerol. Generation of a peroxisome proliferator-activated receptor alpha agonist. J Biol Chem. 2002b;277(26):23278–86.
148. Kramar C, Loureiro M, Renard J, Laviolette SR. Palmitoylethanolamide modulates GPR55 receptor signaling in the ventral Hippocampus to regulate mesolimbic dopamine activity, social interaction, and memory processing. Cannabis Cannabinoid Res. 2017;2(1):8–20.
149. Kreitzer AC, Regehr WG. Retrograde inhibition of presynaptic calcium influx by endogenous cannabinoids at excitatory synapses onto Purkinje cells. Neuron. 2001;29(3):717–27.
150. Kudalkar SN, Kingsley PJ, Marnett LJ. Assay of endocannabinoid oxidation by cyclooxygenase-2. Methods Mol Biol. 2016;1412:205–15.
151. Kuliczkowska Plaksej J, Laczmanski L, Milewicz A, Lenarcik-Kabza A, Trzmiel-Bira A, Zaleska-Dorobisz U, Lwow F, Hirnle L. Cannabinoid receptor 1 gene polymorphisms and nonalcoholic Fatty liver disease in women with polycystic ovary syndrome and in healthy controls. Int J Endocrinol. 2014;2014:232975.

152. Lafuente H, Alvarez FJ, Pazos MR, Alvarez A, Rey-Santano MC, Mielgo V, Murgia-Esteve X, Hilario E, Martinez-Orgado J. Cannabidiol reduces brain damage and improves functional recovery after acute hypoxia-ischemia in newborn pigs. Pediatr Res. 2011;70(3):272–7.
153. Lambracht-Hall M, Dimitriadou V, Theoharides TC. Migration of mast cells in the developing rat brain. Brain Res Dev Brain Res. 1990;56(2):151–9.
154. Laprairie RB, Bagher AM, Kelly ME, Denovan-Wright EM. Cannabidiol is a negative allosteric modulator of the cannabinoid CB1 receptor. Br J Pharmacol. 2015;172(20):4790–805.
155. Laprairie RB, Bagher AM, Kelly ME, Dupre DJ, Denovan-Wright EM. Type 1 cannabinoid receptor ligands display functional selectivity in a cell culture model of striatal medium spiny projection neurons. J Biol Chem. 2014;289(36):24845–62.
156. Laun AS, Shrader SH, Brown KJ, Song ZH. GPR3, GPR6, and GPR12 as novel molecular targets: their biological functions and interaction with cannabidiol. Acta Pharmacol Sin. 2019;40(3):300–8.
157. Laun AS, Song ZH. GPR3 and GPR6, novel molecular targets for cannabidiol. Biochem Biophys Res Commun. 2017;490(1):17–21.
158. Leterrier C, Laine J, Darmon M, Boudin H, Rossier J, Lenkei Z. Constitutive activation drives compartment-selective endocytosis and axonal targeting of type 1 cannabinoid receptors. J Neurosci. 2006;26(12):3141–53.
159. Leweke FM, Piomelli D, Pahlisch F, Muhl D, Gerth CW, Hoyer C, Klosterkotter J, Hellmich M, Koethe D. Cannabidiol enhances anandamide signaling and alleviates psychotic symptoms of schizophrenia. Transl Psychiatry. 2012;2:e94.
160. Lewis SE, Rapino C, Di Tommaso M, Pucci M, Battista N, Paro R, Simon L, Lutton D, Maccarrone M. Differences in the endocannabinoid system of sperm from fertile and infertile men. PLoS One. 2012;7(10):e47704.
161. Li L, Homan KT, Vishnivetskiy SA, Manglik A, Tesmer JJ, Gurevich VV, Gurevich EV. G protein-coupled receptor kinases of the GRK4 protein subfamily phosphorylate inactive G protein-coupled receptors (GPCRs). J Biol Chem. 2015;290(17):10775–90.
162. Li X, Hua T, Vemuri K, Ho JH, Wu Y, Wu L, Popov P, Benchama O, Zvonok N, Locke K, Qu L, Han GW, Iyer MR, Cinar R, Coffey NJ, Wang J, Wu M, Katritch V, Zhao S, Kunos G, Bohn LM, Makriyannis A, Stevens RC, Liu ZJ. Crystal structure of the human cannabinoid receptor CB2. Cell. 2019;176(3):459–467 e413.
163. Ligresti A, Cascio MG, Di Marzo V. Endocannabinoid metabolic pathways and enzymes. Curr Drug Targets CNS Neurol Disord. 2005;4(6):615–23.
164. Liu B, Song S, Jones PM, Persaud SJ. GPR55: from orphan to metabolic regulator? Pharmacol Ther. 2015;145:35–42.
165. Liu J, Li H, Burstein SH, Zurier RB, Chen JD. Activation and binding of peroxisome proliferator-activated receptor gamma by synthetic cannabinoid ajulemic acid. Mol Pharmacol. 2003;63(5):983–92.
166. Liu Q, Bhat M, Bowen WD, Cheng J. Signaling pathways from cannabinoid receptor-1 activation to inhibition of N-methyl-D-aspartic acid mediated calcium influx and neurotoxicity in dorsal root ganglion neurons. J Pharmacol Exp Ther. 2009;331(3):1062–70.
167. Lohse MJ, Benovic JL, Codina J, Caron MG, Lefkowitz RJ. beta-Arrestin: a protein that regulates beta-adrenergic receptor function. Science. 1990;248:1547–50.
168. Long JZ, Li W, Booker L, Burston JJ, Kinsey SG, Schlosburg JE, Pavon FJ, Serrano AM, Selley DE, Parsons LH, Lichtman AH, Cravatt BF. Selective blockade of 2-arachidonoylglycerol hydrolysis produces cannabinoid behavioral effects. Nat Chem Biol. 2009;5(1):37–44.
169. Lou ZY, Zhao CB, Xiao BG. Immunoregulation of experimental autoimmune encephalomyelitis by the selective CB1 receptor antagonist. J Neurosci Res. 2012;90(1):84–95.
170. Lu D, Immadi SS, Wu Z, Kendall DA. Translational potential of allosteric modulators targeting the cannabinoid CB1 receptor. Acta Pharmacol Sin. 2019;40(3):324–35.
171. Lu HC, Mackie K. An introduction to the endogenous cannabinoid system. Biol Psychiatry. 2016;79(7):516–25.

172. Luttrell LM, Lefkowitz RJ. The role of beta-arrestins in the termination and transduction of G-protein-coupled receptor signals. J Cell Sci. 2002;115:455–65.
173. Maccarrone M. Missing pieces to the endocannabinoid puzzle. Trends Mol Med. 2020;26(3):263–72.
174. Maccarrone M, Attina M, Bari M, Cartoni A, Ledent C, Finazzi-Agro A. Anandamide degradation and N-acylethanolamines level in wild-type and CB1 cannabinoid receptor knockout mice of different ages. J Neurochem. 2001;78(2):339–48.
175. Maccarrone M, Bab I, Biro T, Cabral GA, Dey SK, Di Marzo V, Konje JC, Kunos G, Mechoulam R, Pacher P, Sharkey KA, Zimmer A. Endocannabinoid signaling at the periphery: 50 years after THC. Trends Pharmacol Sci. 2015;36(5):277–96.
176. Maccarrone M, Salvati S, Bari M, Finazzi A. Anandamide and 2-arachidonoylglycerol inhibit fatty acid amide hydrolase by activating the lipoxygenase pathway of the arachidonate cascade. Biochem Biophys Res Commun. 2000;278(3):576–83.
177. Maccarrone M, van der Stelt M, Rossi A, Veldink GA, Vliegenthart JF, Agro AF. Anandamide hydrolysis by human cells in culture and brain. J Biol Chem. 1998;273(48):32332–9.
178. Mackie K. Distribution of cannabinoid receptors in the central and peripheral nervous system. Handb Exp Pharmacol. 2005;(168):299–325.
179. Mahmoud Gouda H, Mohamed Kamel NR. Cannabinoid CB2 receptor gene (CNR2) polymorphism is associated with chronic childhood immune thrombocytopenia in Egypt. Blood Coagul Fibrinolysis. 2013;24(3):247–51.
180. Maione S, Costa B, Di Marzo V. Endocannabinoids: a unique opportunity to develop multitarget analgesics. Pain. 2013;154(Suppl 1):S87–93.
181. Manzanares J, Corchero J, Romero J, Fernandez-Ruiz JJ, Ramos JA, Fuentes JA. Pharmacological and biochemical interactions between opioids and cannabinoids. Trends Pharmacol Sci. 1999;20(7):287–94.
182. Maresz K, Carrier EJ, Ponomarev ED, Hillard CJ, Dittel BN. Modulation of the cannabinoid CB2 receptor in microglial cells in response to inflammatory stimuli. J Neurochem. 2005;95(2):437–45.
183. Marrs WR, Blankman JL, Horne EA, Thomazeau A, Lin YH, Coy J, Bodor AL, Muccioli GG, Hu SS, Woodruff G, Fung S, Lafourcade M, Alexander JP, Long JZ, Li W, Xu C, Moller T, Mackie K, Manzoni OJ, Cravatt BF, Stella N. The serine hydrolase ABHD6 controls the accumulation and efficacy of 2-AG at cannabinoid receptors. Nat Neurosci. 2010;13(8):951–7.
184. Martin GG, Chung S, Landrock D, Landrock KK, Huang H, Dangott LJ, Peng X, Kaczocha M, Seeger DR, Murphy EJ, Golovko MY, Kier AB, Schroeder F. FABP-1 gene ablation impacts brain endocannabinoid system in male mice. J Neurochem. 2016;138(3):407–22.
185. Martinez-Pinilla E, Reyes-Resina I, Onatibia-Astibia A, Zamarbide M, Ricobaraza A, Navarro G, Moreno E, Dopeso-Reyes IG, Sierra S, Rico AJ, Roda E, Lanciego JL, Franco R. CB1 and GPR55 receptors are co-expressed and form heteromers in rat and monkey striatum. Exp Neurol. 2014;261:44–52.
186. Matyas F, Watanabe M, Mackie K, Katona I, Freund TF. Molecular architecture of the cannabinoid signaling system in the core of the nucleus accumbens. Ideggyogy Sz. 2007;60(3-4):187–91.
187. McHugh D, Hu SS, Rimmerman N, Juknat A, Vogel Z, Walker JM, Bradshaw HB. N-arachidonoyl glycine, an abundant endogenous lipid, potently drives directed cellular migration through GPR18, the putative abnormal cannabidiol receptor. BMC Neurosci. 2010;11:44.
188. McHugh D, Page J, Dunn E, Bradshaw HB. Delta(9) -Tetrahydrocannabinol and N-arachidonyl glycine are full agonists at GPR18 receptors and induce migration in human endometrial HEC-1B cells. Br J Pharmacol. 2012;165(8):2414–24.
189. McIntosh AL, Huang H, Landrock D, Martin GG, Li S, Kier AB, Schroeder F. Impact of Fabp1 gene ablation on uptake and degradation of endocannabinoids in mouse hepatocytes. Lipids. 2018;53(6):561–80.

190. Mechoulam R, Parker LA. The endocannabinoid system and the brain. Annu Rev Psychol. 2013;64:21–47.
191. Miller MR, Mannowetz N, Iavarone AT, Safavi R, Gracheva EO, Smith JF, Hill RZ, Bautista DM, Kirichok Y, Lishko PV. Unconventional endocannabinoid signaling governs sperm activation via the sex hormone progesterone. Science. 2016;352(6285):555–9.
192. Minocci D, Massei J, Martino A, Milianti M, Piz L, Di Bello D, Sbrana A, Martinotti E, Rossi AM, Nieri P. Genetic association between bipolar disorder and 524A>C (Leu133Ile) polymorphism of CNR2 gene, encoding for CB2 cannabinoid receptor. J Affect Disord. 2011;134(1-3):427–30.
193. Mitchell MR, Berridge KC, Mahler SV. Endocannabinoid-enhanced "liking" in nucleus Accumbens shell Hedonic hotspot requires endogenous opioid signals. Cannabis Cannabinoid Res. 2018;3(1):166–70.
194. Morales P, Goya P, Jagerovic N, Hernandez-Folgado L. Allosteric modulators of the CB1 cannabinoid receptor: a structural update review. Cannabis Cannabinoid Res. 2016;1(1):22–30.
195. Morales P, Reggio PH. An update on non-CB1, non-CB2 cannabinoid related G-protein-coupled receptors. Cannabis Cannabinoid Res. 2017;2(1):265–73.
196. Morgan NH, Stanford IM, Woodhall GL. Functional CB2 type cannabinoid receptors at CNS synapses. Neuropharmacology. 2009;57(4):356–68.
197. Muccioli GG, Xu C, Odah E, Cudaback E, Cisneros JA, Lambert DM, Lopez Rodriguez ML, Bajjalieh S, Stella N. Identification of a novel endocannabinoid-hydrolyzing enzyme expressed by microglial cells. J Neurosci. 2007;27(11):2883–9.
198. Muller C, Morales P, Reggio PH. Cannabinoid ligands targeting TRP channels. Front Mol Neurosci. 2018;11:487.
199. Munro S, Thomas KL, Abu-Shaar M. Molecular characterization of a peripheral receptor for cannabinoids. Nature. 1993;365(6441):61–5.
200. Naccarato M, Pizzuti D, Petrosino S, Simonetto M, Ferigo L, Grandi FC, Pizzolato G, Di Marzo V. Possible Anandamide and Palmitoylethanolamide involvement in human stroke. Lipids Health Dis. 2010;9:47.
201. Nackley AG, Makriyannis A, Hohmann AG. Selective activation of cannabinoid CB(2) receptors suppresses spinal fos protein expression and pain behavior in a rat model of inflammation. Neuroscience. 2003;119(3):747–57.
202. Nasser Y, Bashashati M, Andrews CN. Toward modulation of the endocannabinoid system for treatment of gastrointestinal disease: FAAHster but not "higher". Neurogastroenterol Motil. 2014;26(4):447–54.
203. Navarro G, Borroto-Escuela D, Angelats E, Etayo I, Reyes-Resina I, Pulido-Salgado M, Rodriguez-Perez AI, Canela EI, Saura J, Lanciego JL, Labandeira-Garcia JL, Saura CA, Fuxe K, Franco R. Receptor-heteromer mediated regulation of endocannabinoid signaling in activated microglia. Role of CB1 and CB2 receptors and relevance for Alzheimer's disease and levodopa-induced dyskinesia. Brain Behav Immun. 2018a;67:139–51.
204. Navarro G, Reyes-Resina I, Rivas-Santisteban R, Sanchez de Medina V, Morales P, Casano S, Ferreiro-Vera C, Lillo A, Aguinaga D, Jagerovic N, Nadal X, Franco R. Cannabidiol skews biased agonism at cannabinoid CB1 and CB2 receptors with smaller effect in CB1-CB2 heteroreceptor complexes. Biochem Pharmacol. 2018b;157:148–58.
205. Navarro G, Varani K, Reyes-Resina I, Sanchez de Medina V, Rivas-Santisteban R, Sanchez-Carnerero Callado C, Vincenzi F, Casano S, Ferreiro-Vera C, Canela EI, Borea PA, Nadal X, Franco R. Cannabigerol action at cannabinoid CB1 and CB2 receptors and at CB1-CB2 heteroreceptor complexes. Front Pharmacol. 2018c;9:632.
206. Navia-Paldanius D, Savinainen JR, Laitinen JT. Biochemical and pharmacological characterization of human alpha/beta-hydrolase domain containing 6 (ABHD6) and 12 (ABHD12). J Lipid Res. 2012;53(11):2413–24.
207. Nevalainen T, Irving AJ. GPR55, a lysophosphatidylinositol receptor with cannabinoid sensitivity? Curr Top Med Chem. 2010;10(8):799–813.

208. Nguyen PT, Schmid CL, Raehal KM, Selley DE, Bohn LM, Sim-Selley LJ. beta-arrestin2 regulates cannabinoid CB1 receptor signaling and adaptation in a central nervous system region-dependent manner. Biol Psychiatry. 2012;71(8):714–24.
209. Nie J, Lewis DL. Structural domains of the CB1 cannabinoid receptor that contribute to constitutive activity and G-protein sequestration. J Neurosci. 2001;21(22):8758–64.
210. Nielsen MJ, Petersen G, Astrup A, Hansen HS. Food intake is inhibited by oral oleoylethanolamide. J Lipid Res. 2004;45(6):1027–9.
211. Nomura DK, Morrison BE, Blankman JL, Long JZ, Kinsey SG, Marcondes MC, Ward AM, Hahn YK, Lichtman AH, Conti B, Cravatt BF. Endocannabinoid hydrolysis generates brain prostaglandins that promote neuroinflammation. Science. 2011;334(6057):809–13.
212. O'Sullivan SE. An update on PPAR activation by cannabinoids. Br J Pharmacol. 2016;173(12):1899–910.
213. Oddi S, Dainese E, Fezza F, Lanuti M, Barcaroli D, De Laurenzi V, Centonze D, Maccarrone M. Functional characterization of putative cholesterol binding sequence (CRAC) in human type-1 cannabinoid receptor. J Neurochem. 2011;116(5):858–65.
214. Oddi S, Fezza F, Pasquariello N, De Simone C, Rapino C, Dainese E, Finazzi-Agro A, Maccarrone M. Evidence for the intracellular accumulation of anandamide in adiposomes. Cell Mol Life Sci. 2008;65(5):840–50.
215. Ohno-Shosaku T, Maejima T, Kano M. Endogenous cannabinoids mediate retrograde signals from depolarized postsynaptic neurons to presynaptic terminals. Neuron. 2001;29(3):729–38.
216. Okamoto Y, Morishita J, Tsuboi K, Tonai T, Ueda N. Molecular characterization of a phospholipase D generating anandamide and its congeners. J Biol Chem. 2004;279(7):5298–305.
217. Oliveira da Cruz JF, Robin LM, Drago F, Marsicano G, Metna-Laurent M. Astroglial type-1 cannabinoid receptor (CB1): a new player in the tripartite synapse. Neuroscience. 2016;323:35–42.
218. Onaivi ES, Ishiguro H, Sejal P, Meozzi PA, Myers L, Tagliaferro P, Hope B, Leonard CM, Uhl GR, Brusco A, Gardner E. Methods to study the behavioral effects and expression of CB2 cannabinoid receptor and its gene transcripts in the chronic mild stress model of depression. Methods Mol Med. 2006;123:291–8.
219. Pacheco Dda F, Klein A, Perez AC, Pacheco CM, de Francischi JN, Reis GM, Duarte ID. Central antinociception induced by mu-opioid receptor agonist morphine, but not delta- or kappa-, is mediated by cannabinoid CB1 receptor. Br J Pharmacol. 2009;158(1):225–31.
220. Pacheco DDF, Romero TRL, Duarte IDG. Ketamine induces central antinociception mediated by endogenous cannabinoids and activation of CB1 receptors. Neurosci Lett. 2019;699:140–4.
221. Parrella E, Porrini V, Iorio R, Benarese M, Lanzillotta A, Mota M, Fusco M, Tonin P, Spano P, Pizzi M. PEA and luteolin synergistically reduce mast cell-mediated toxicity and elicit neuroprotection in cell-based models of brain ischemia. Brain Res. 2016;1648(Pt A):409–17.
222. Pazos MR, Cinquina V, Gomez A, Layunta R, Santos M, Fernandez-Ruiz J, Martinez-Orgado J. Cannabidiol administration after hypoxia-ischemia to newborn rats reduces long-term brain injury and restores neurobehavioral function. Neuropharmacology. 2012;63(5):776–83.
223. Peiro AM, Garcia-Gutierrez MS, Planelles B, Femenia T, Mingote C, Jimenez-Trevino L, Martinez-Barrondo S, Garcia-Portilla MP, Saiz PA, Bobes J, Manzanares J. Association of cannabinoid receptor genes (CNR1 and CNR2) polymorphisms and panic disorder. Anxiety Stress Coping. 2020;33:1–10.
224. Perez-Reyes M, Burstein SH, White WR, McDonald SA, Hicks RE. Antagonism of marihuana effects by indomethacin in humans. Life Sci. 1991;48(6):507–15.
225. Pertwee RG. Inverse agonism and neutral antagonism at cannabinoid CB1 receptors. Life Sci. 2005a;76(12):1307–24.
226. Pertwee RG. The therapeutic potential of drugs that target cannabinoid receptors or modulate the tissue levels or actions of endocannabinoids. AAPS J. 2005b;7(3):E625–54.

227. Pertwee RG. The diverse CB1 and CB2 receptor pharmacology of three plant cannabinoids: delta9-tetrahydrocannabinol, cannabidiol and delta9-tetrahydrocannabivarin. Br J Pharmacol. 2008;153(2):199–215.
228. Pertwee RG, Ross RA. Cannabinoid receptors and their ligands. Prostaglandins Leukot Essent Fatty Acids. 2002;66(2-3):101–21.
229. Petrosino S, Schiano Moriello A, Verde R, Allara M, Imperatore R, Ligresti A, Mahmoud AM, Peritore AF, Iannotti FA, Di Marzo V. Palmitoylethanolamide counteracts substance P-induced mast cell activation in vitro by stimulating diacylglycerol lipase activity. J Neuroinflammation. 2019;16(1):274.
230. Pickens JT. Sedative activity of cannabis in relation to its delta'-trans-tetrahydrocannabinol and cannabidiol content. Br J Pharmacol. 1981;72(4):649–56.
231. Price MR, Baillie GL, Thomas A, Stevenson LA, Easson M, Goodwin R, McLean A, McIntosh L, Goodwin G, Walker G, Westwood P, Marrs J, Thomson F, Cowley P, Christopoulos A, Pertwee RG, Ross RA. Allosteric modulation of the cannabinoid CB1 receptor. Mol Pharmacol. 2005;68(5):1484–95.
232. Priestley RS, Nickolls SA, Alexander SP, Kendall DA. A potential role for cannabinoid receptors in the therapeutic action of fenofibrate. FASEB J. 2015;29(4):1446–55.
233. Pucci M, Micioni Di Bonaventura MV, Zaplatic E, Bellia F, Maccarrone M, Cifani C, D'Addario C. Transcriptional regulation of the endocannabinoid system in a rat model of binge-eating behavior reveals a selective modulation of the hypothalamic fatty acid amide hydrolase gene. Int J Eat Disord. 2019;52(1):51–60.
234. Rahman IA, Tsuboi K, Hussain Z, Yamashita R, Okamoto Y, Uyama T, Yamazaki N, Tanaka T, Tokumura A, Ueda N. Calcium-dependent generation of N-acylethanolamines and lysophosphatidic acids by glycerophosphodiesterase GDE7. Biochim Biophys Acta. 2016;1861(12 Pt A):1881–92.
235. Ramirez-Orozco RE, Garcia-Ruiz R, Morales P, Villalon CM, Villafan-Bernal JR, Marichal-Cancino BA. Potential metabolic and behavioural roles of the putative endocannabinoid receptors GPR18, GPR55 and GPR119 in feeding. Curr Neuropharmacol. 2019;17(10):947–60.
236. Rinne P, Guillamat-Prats R, Rami M, Bindila L, Ring L, Lyytikainen LP, Raitoharju E, Oksala N, Lehtimaki T, Weber C, van der Vorst EPC, Steffens S. Palmitoylethanolamide promotes a proresolving macrophage phenotype and attenuates atherosclerotic plaque formation. Arterioscler Thromb Vasc Biol. 2018;38(11):2562–75.
237. Rodriguez-Munoz M, Onetti Y, Cortes-Montero E, Garzon J, Sanchez-Blazquez P. Cannabidiol enhances morphine antinociception, diminishes NMDA-mediated seizures and reduces stroke damage via the sigma 1 receptor. Mol Brain. 2018;11(1):51.
238. Romero J, Garcia-Palomero E, Castro JG, Garcia-Gil L, Ramos JA, Fernandez-Ruiz JJ. Effects of chronic exposure to delta9-tetrahydrocannabinol on cannabinoid receptor binding and mRNA levels in several rat brain regions. Brain Res Mol Brain Res. 1997;46(1-2):100–8.
239. Rong C, Lee Y, Carmona NE, Cha DS, Ragguett RM, Rosenblat JD, Mansur RB, Ho RC, McIntyre RS. Cannabidiol in medical marijuana: research vistas and potential opportunities. Pharmacol Res. 2017;121:213–8.
240. Rosenbaum T, Simon SA. TRPV1 Receptors and Signal Transduction. In: Liedtke WB, Heller S, editors. TRP Ion Channel Function in Sensory Transduction and Cellular Signaling Cascades. Boca Raton; 2007.
241. Roser P, Haussleiter IS, Chong HJ, Maier C, Kawohl W, Norra C, Juckel G. Inhibition of cerebral type 1 cannabinoid receptors is associated with impaired auditory mismatch negativity generation in the ketamine model of schizophrenia. Psychopharmacology (Berl). 2011;218(4):611–20.
242. Rubino T, Massi P, Vigano D, Fuzio D, Parolaro D. Long-term treatment with SR141716A, the CB1 receptor antagonist, influences morphine withdrawal syndrome. Life Sci. 2000;66(22):2213–9.
243. Russo EB, Burnett A, Hall B, Parker KK. Agonistic properties of cannabidiol at 5-HT1a receptors. Neurochem Res. 2005;30(8):1037–43.

244. Ryberg E, Larsson N, Sjogren S, Hjorth S, Hermansson NO, Leonova J, Elebring T, Nilsson K, Drmota T, Greasley PJ. The orphan receptor GPR55 is a novel cannabinoid receptor. Br J Pharmacol. 2007;152(7):1092–101.
245. Ryberg E, Vu HK, Larsson N, Groblewski T, Hjorth S, Elebring T, Sjogren S, Greasley PJ. Identification and characterisation of a novel splice variant of the human CB1 receptor. FEBS Lett. 2005;579(1):259–64.
246. Sabatucci A, Simonetti M, Tortolani D, Angelucci CB, Dainese E, Maccarrone M. Role of steroids on the membrane binding ability of fatty acid amide hydrolase. Cannabis Cannabinoid Res. 2019;4(1):42–50.
247. Saito A, Ballinger MD, Pletnikov MV, Wong DF, Kamiya A. Endocannabinoid system: potential novel targets for treatment of schizophrenia. Neurobiol Dis. 2013;53:10–7.
248. Salort G, Alvaro-Bartolome M, Garcia-Sevilla JA. Regulation of cannabinoid CB2 receptor constitutive activity in vivo: repeated treatments with inverse agonists reverse the acute activation of JNK and associated apoptotic signaling in mouse brain. Psychopharmacology (Berl). 2017;234(6):925–41.
249. Sanchez-Blazquez P, Rodriguez-Munoz M, Vicente-Sanchez A, Garzon J. Cannabinoid receptors couple to NMDA receptors to reduce the production of NO and the mobilization of zinc induced by glutamate. Antioxid Redox Signal. 2013;19(15):1766–82.
250. Sanchez-Fernandez C, Nieto FR, Gonzalez-Cano R, Artacho-Cordon A, Romero L, Montilla-Garcia A, Zamanillo D, Baeyens JM, Entrena JM, Cobos EJ. Potentiation of morphine-induced mechanical antinociception by sigma(1) receptor inhibition: role of peripheral sigma(1) receptors. Neuropharmacology. 2013;70:348–58.
251. Sang N, Chen C. Lipid signaling and synaptic plasticity. Neuroscientist. 2006;12(5):425–34.
252. Sang N, Zhang J, Chen C. PGE2 glycerol ester, a COX-2 oxidative metabolite of 2-arachidonoyl glycerol, modulates inhibitory synaptic transmission in mouse hippocampal neurons. J Physiol. 2006;572(Pt 3):735–45.
253. Sang N, Zhang J, Chen C. COX-2 oxidative metabolite of endocannabinoid 2-AG enhances excitatory glutamatergic synaptic transmission and induces neurotoxicity. J Neurochem. 2007;102(6):1966–77.
254. Sanson B, Wang T, Sun J, Wang L, Kaczocha M, Ojima I, Deutsch D, Li H. Crystallographic study of FABP5 as an intracellular endocannabinoid transporter. Acta Crystallogr D Biol Crystallogr. 2014;70(Pt 2):290–8.
255. Sasso O, Russo R, Vitiello S, Raso GM, D'Agostino G, Iacono A, Rana GL, Vallee M, Cuzzocrea S, Piazza PV, Meli R, Calignano A. Implication of allopregnanolone in the antinociceptive effect of N-palmitoylethanolamide in acute or persistent pain. Pain. 2012;153(1):33–41.
256. Scavone JL, Mackie K, Van Bockstaele EJ. Characterization of cannabinoid-1 receptors in the locus coeruleus: relationship with mu-opioid receptors. Brain Res. 2010;1312:18–31.
257. Schlosburg JE, Blankman JL, Long JZ, Nomura DK, Pan B, Kinsey SG, Nguyen PT, Ramesh D, Booker L, Burston JJ, Thomas EA, Selley DE, Sim-Selley LJ, Liu QS, Lichtman AH, Cravatt BF. Chronic monoacylglycerol lipase blockade causes functional antagonism of the endocannabinoid system. Nat Neurosci. 2010;13(9):1113–9.
258. Seidel K, Hamza M, Ates M, Guhring H. Flurbiprofen inhibits capsaicin induced calcitonin gene related peptide release from rat spinal cord via an endocannabinoid dependent mechanism. Neurosci Lett. 2003;338(2):99–102.
259. Sharir H, Console-Bram L, Mundy C, Popoff SN, Kapur A, Abood ME. The endocannabinoids anandamide and virodhamine modulate the activity of the candidate cannabinoid receptor GPR55. J Neuroimmune Pharmacol. 2012;7(4):856–65.
260. Shire D, Carillon C, Kaghad M, Calandra B, Rinaldi-Carmona M, Le Fur G, Caput D, Ferrara P. An amino-terminal variant of the central cannabinoid receptor resulting from alternative splicing. J Biol Chem. 1995;270(8):3726–31.

261. Sigel E, Baur R, Racz I, Marazzi J, Smart TG, Zimmer A, Gertsch J. The major central endocannabinoid directly acts at GABA(A) receptors. Proc Natl Acad Sci U S A. 2011;108(44):18150–5.
262. Sihag J, Jones PJH. Dietary fatty acid composition impacts plasma fatty acid ethanolamide levels and body composition in golden Syrian hamsters. Food Funct. 2018;9(6):3351–62.
263. Silvestri C, Di Marzo V. The endocannabinoid system in energy homeostasis and the etiopathology of metabolic disorders. Cell Metab. 2013;17(4):475–90.
264. Simon GM, Cravatt BF. Anandamide biosynthesis catalyzed by the phosphodiesterase GDE1 and detection of glycerophospho-N-acyl ethanolamine precursors in mouse brain. J Biol Chem. 2008;283(14):9341–9.
265. Skaper SD. Impact of inflammation on the blood-neural barrier and blood-nerve interface: from review to therapeutic preview. Int Rev Neurobiol. 2017;137:29–45.
266. Skaper SD, Facci L, Giusti P. Glia and mast cells as targets for palmitoylethanolamide, an anti-inflammatory and neuroprotective lipid mediator. Mol Neurobiol. 2013;48(2):340–52.
267. Skaper SD, Facci L, Zusso M, Giusti P. Neuroinflammation, mast cells, and Glia: dangerous Liaisons. Neuroscientist. 2017;23(5):478–98.
268. Smith JS, Rajagopal S. The beta-Arrestins: multifunctional regulators of G protein-coupled receptors. J Biol Chem. 2016;291(17):8969–77.
269. Spiller KJ, Bi GH, He Y, Galaj E, Gardner EL, Xi ZX. Cannabinoid CB1 and CB2 receptor mechanisms underlie cannabis reward and aversion in rats. Br J Pharmacol. 2019;176(9):1268–81.
270. Steels E, Venkatesh R, Steels E, Vitetta G, Vitetta L. A double-blind randomized placebo controlled study assessing safety, tolerability and efficacy of palmitoylethanolamide for symptoms of knee osteoarthritis. Inflammopharmacology. 2019;27(3):475–85.
271. Suarez-Pinilla P, Roiz-Santianez R, Ortiz-Garcia de la Foz V, Guest PC, Ayesa-Arriola R, Cordova-Palomera A, Tordesillas-Gutierrez D, Crespo-Facorro B. Brain structural and clinical changes after first episode psychosis: focus on cannabinoid receptor 1 polymorphisms. Psychiatry Res. 2015;233(2):112–9.
272. Suarez J, Bermudez-Silva FJ, Mackie K, Ledent C, Zimmer A, Cravatt BF, de Fonseca FR. Immunohistochemical description of the endogenous cannabinoid system in the rat cerebellum and functionally related nuclei. J Comp Neurol. 2008;509(4):400–21.
273. Sugiura T, Kishimoto S, Oka S, Gokoh M. Biochemistry, pharmacology and physiology of 2-arachidonoylglycerol, an endogenous cannabinoid receptor ligand. Prog Lipid Res. 2006;45(5):405–46.
274. Sumislawski JJ, Ramikie TS, Patel S. Reversible gating of endocannabinoid plasticity in the amygdala by chronic stress: a potential role for monoacylglycerol lipase inhibition in the prevention of stress-induced behavioral adaptation. Neuropsychopharmacology. 2011;36(13):2750–61.
275. Szabo B, Schlicker E. Effects of cannabinoids on neurotransmission. Handb Exp Pharmacol. 2005;(168):327–65.
276. Tanaka S, Ishii K, Kasai K, Yoon SO, Saeki Y. Neural expression of G protein-coupled receptors GPR3, GPR6, and GPR12 up-regulates cyclic AMP levels and promotes neurite outgrowth. J Biol Chem. 2007;282(14):10506–15.
277. Tham M, Yilmaz O, Alaverdashvili M, Kelly MEM, Denovan-Wright EM, Laprairie RB. Allosteric and orthosteric pharmacology of cannabidiol and cannabidiol-dimethylheptyl at the type 1 and type 2 cannabinoid receptors. Br J Pharmacol. 2019;176(10):1455–69.
278. Thathiah A, Horre K, Snellinx A, Vandewyer E, Huang Y, Ciesielska M, De Kloe G, Munck S, De Strooper B. beta-arrestin 2 regulates Abeta generation and gamma-secretase activity in Alzheimer's disease. Nat Med. 2013;19(1):43–9.
279. Tsou K, Brown S, Sanudo-Pena MC, Mackie K, Walker JM. Immunohistochemical distribution of cannabinoid CB1 receptors in the rat central nervous system. Neuroscience. 1998;83(2):393–411.

280. Tsuboi K, Uyama T, Okamoto Y, Ueda N. Endocannabinoids and related N-acylethanolamines: biological activities and metabolism. Inflamm Regen. 2018;38:28.
281. Turu G, Hunyady L. Signal transduction of the CB1 cannabinoid receptor. J Mol Endocrinol. 2010;44(2):75–85.
282. Ueda N, Tsuboi K, Uyama T. Metabolism of endocannabinoids and related N-acylethanolamines: canonical and alternative pathways. FEBS J. 2013;280(9):1874–94.
283. Vallee M, Vitiello S, Bellocchio L, Hebert-Chatelain E, Monlezun S, Martin-Garcia E, Kasanetz F, Baillie GL, Panin F, Cathala A, Roullot-Lacarriere V, Fabre S, Hurst DP, Lynch DL, Shore DM, Deroche-Gamonet V, Spampinato U, Revest JM, Maldonado R, Reggio PH, Ross RA, Marsicano G, Piazza PV. Pregnenolone can protect the brain from cannabis intoxication. Science. 2014;343(6166):94–8.
284. Vavers E, Svalbe B, Lauberte L, Stonans I, Misane I, Dambrova M, Zvejniece L. The activity of selective sigma-1 receptor ligands in seizure models in vivo. Behav Brain Res. 2017;328:13–8.
285. Vigano D, Rubino T, Parolaro D. Molecular and cellular basis of cannabinoid and opioid interactions. Pharmacol Biochem Behav. 2005;81(2):360–8.
286. Vinals X, Moreno E, Lanfumey L, Cordomi A, Pastor A, de La Torre R, Gasperini P, Navarro G, Howell LA, Pardo L, Lluis C, Canela EI, McCormick PJ, Maldonado R, Robledo P. Cognitive Impairment Induced by Delta9-tetrahydrocannabinol Occurs through Heteromers between Cannabinoid CB1 and Serotonin 5-HT2A Receptors. PLoS Biol. 2015;13(7):e1002194.
287. Viscomi MT, Oddi S, Latini L, Pasquariello N, Florenzano F, Bernardi G, Molinari M, Maccarrone M. Selective CB2 receptor agonism protects central neurons from remote axotomy-induced apoptosis through the PI3K/Akt pathway. J Neurosci. 2009;29(14):4564–70.
288. Wang XF, Galaj E, Bi GH, Zhang C, He Y, Zhan J, Bauman MH, Gardner EL, Xi ZX. Different receptor mechanisms underlying phytocannabinoid- versus synthetic cannabinoid-induced tetrad effects: opposite roles of CB1 /CB2 versus GPR55 receptors. Br J Pharmacol. 2020;177(8):1865–80.
289. Wenzel JM, Cheer JF. Endocannabinoid regulation of reward and reinforcement through interaction with Dopamine and endogenous opioid signaling. Neuropsychopharmacology. 2018;43(1):103–15.
290. White HL, Tansik RL. Effects of delta 9-tetrahydrocannabinol and cannabidiol on phospholipase and other enzymes regulating arachidonate metabolism. Prostaglandins Med. 1980;4(6):409–17.
291. Woo JH, Kim H, Kim JH, Kim JG. Cannabinoid receptor gene polymorphisms and bone mineral density in Korean postmenopausal women. Menopause. 2015;22(5):512–9.
292. Woolmore J, Stone M, Holley S, Jenkinson P, Ike A, Jones P, Fryer A, Strange R, Stephens R, Langdon D, Hawkins C. Polymorphisms of the cannabinoid 1 receptor gene and cognitive impairment in multiple sclerosis. Mult Scler. 2008;14(2):177–82.
293. Wu J. Cannabis, cannabinoid receptors, and endocannabinoid system: yesterday, today, and tomorrow. Acta Pharmacol Sin. 2019;40(3):297–9.
294. Wu J, Hocevar M, Bie B, Foss JF, Naguib M. Cannabinoid type 2 receptor system modulates paclitaxel-induced microglial dysregulation and central sensitization in rats. J Pain. 2019;20(5):501–14.
295. Xiong W, Cui T, Cheng K, Yang F, Chen SR, Willenbring D, Guan Y, Pan HL, Ren K, Xu Y, Zhang L. Cannabinoids suppress inflammatory and neuropathic pain by targeting alpha3 glycine receptors. J Exp Med. 2012;209(6):1121–34.
296. Yamaguchi T, Kubota T, Watanabe S, Yamamoto T. Activation of brain prostanoid EP3 receptors via arachidonic acid cascade during behavioral suppression induced by Delta8-tetrahydrocannabinol. J Neurochem. 2004;88(1):148–54.
297. Yamaguchi T, Shoyama Y, Watanabe S, Yamamoto T. Behavioral suppression induced by cannabinoids is due to activation of the arachidonic acid cascade in rats. Brain Res. 2001;889(1-2):149–54.

298. Yamamoto T, Anggadiredja K, Hiranita T. New perspectives in the studies on endocannabinoid and cannabis: a role for the endocannabinoid-arachidonic acid pathway in drug reward and long-lasting relapse to drug taking. J Pharmacol Sci. 2004;96(4):382–8.
299. Yoshida T, Fukaya M, Uchigashima M, Miura E, Kamiya H, Kano M, Watanabe M. Localization of diacylglycerol lipase-alpha around postsynaptic spine suggests close proximity between production site of an endocannabinoid, 2-arachidonoyl-glycerol, and presynaptic cannabinoid CB1 receptor. J Neurosci. 2006;26(18):4740–51.
300. Yuan S, Burrell BD. Endocannabinoid-dependent LTD in a nociceptive synapse requires activation of a presynaptic TRPV-like receptor. J Neurophysiol. 2010;104(5):2766–77.
301. Zhang G, Chen W, Lao L, Marvizon JC. Cannabinoid CB1 receptor facilitation of substance P release in the rat spinal cord, measured as neurokinin 1 receptor internalization. Eur J Neurosci. 2010;31(2):225–37.
302. Zhang HY, Gao M, Liu QR, Bi GH, Li X, Yang HJ, Gardner EL, Wu J, Xi ZX. Cannabinoid CB2 receptors modulate midbrain dopamine neuronal activity and dopamine-related behavior in mice. Proc Natl Acad Sci U S A. 2014;111(46):E5007–15.
303. Zhang J, Chen C. Endocannabinoid 2-arachidonoylglycerol protects neurons by limiting COX-2 elevation. J Biol Chem. 2008;283(33):22601–11.
304. Zhang M, Martin BR, Adler MW, Razdan RK, Ganea D, Tuma RF. Modulation of the balance between cannabinoid CB(1) and CB(2) receptor activation during cerebral ischemic/reperfusion injury. Neuroscience. 2008;152(3):753–60.
305. Zhao P, Abood ME. GPR55 and GPR35 and their relationship to cannabinoid and lysophospholipid receptors. Life Sci. 2013;92(8-9):453–7.
306. Zhou Y, Howell FV, Glebov OO, Albrecht D, Williams G, Doherty P. Regulated endosomal trafficking of Diacylglycerol lipase alpha (DAGLalpha) generates distinct cellular pools; implications for endocannabinoid signaling. Mol Cell Neurosci. 2016;76:76–86.
307. Zhu HJ, Wang JS, Markowitz JS, Donovan JL, Gibson BB, Gefroh HA, Devane CL. Characterization of P-glycoprotein inhibition by major cannabinoids from marijuana. J Pharmacol Exp Ther. 2006;317(2):850–7.
308. Zimmer A, Zimmer AM, Hohmann AG, Herkenham M, Bonner TI. Increased mortality, hypoactivity, and hypoalgesia in cannabinoid CB1 receptor knockout mice. Proc Natl Acad Sci U S A. 1999;96(10):5780–5.
309. Zurier RB, Rossetti RG, Lane JH, Goldberg JM, Hunter SA, Burstein SH. Dimethylheptyl-THC-11 oic acid: a nonpsychoactive antiinflammatory agent with a cannabinoid template structure. Arthritis Rheum. 1998;41(1):163–70.
310. Zygmunt PM, Andersson DA, Hogestatt ED. Delta 9-tetrahydrocannabinol and cannabinol activate capsaicin-sensitive sensory nerves via a CB1 and CB2 cannabinoid receptor-independent mechanism. J Neurosci. 2002;22(11):4720–7.

Chapter 2
Cannabinoid-Based Medicine: Pharmacology and Drug Interactions

Contents

2.1 Introduction 42
2.2 Terminology 43
2.3 Endocannabinoids and Drug Interactions 43
2.4 Endocannabinoids, Cyclooxygenase, and Drug Interactions 44
2.5 Endocannabinoids and Glucocorticoids 45
2.6 Endocannabinoids and Opioids 46
2.7 Clinical and Animal Studies of Cannabinoid Opioid Interactions 46
2.8 Endocannabinoids, Anxiety and Depression 48
2.8.1 Endocannabinoid "Tone": Beyond the Theory 49
2.9 Endocannabinoids and Post-traumatic Stress Disorder 50
2.10 Endocannabinoid System Disruptions and Potential Impact on Treatment with Antipsychotics 51
2.11 The use of Phytoannabinoids as Antipsychotics 53
2.12 Omega-3 Fatty Acids and effects on the Endocannabinoid System 54
2.13 Phytocannabinoid Pharmacokinetics: THC 55
2.14 Phytocannabinoid Pharmacokinetics: CBD 57
2.15 Cannabidiol and Efflux Pumps 59
2.16 Pharmacokinetics of Approved Cannabinoids 60
2.17 Pharmacokinetic Cannabis-Drug Interactions 60
2.18 Pharmacokinetic Cannabis-Drug Interactions: Relevant Examples 62
2.18.1 Corticosteroids 62
2.18.2 Nonsteroidal Anti-inflammatory Drugs 63
2.18.3 Opioids 63
2.18.4 Antidepressants 63
2.18.5 Janus Kinase Inhibitors 63
2.18.6 Antipsychotics 64
2.18.7 Anticonvulsants 64
2.18.8 Benzodiazepines 64
2.18.9 Ethanol 65
2.18.10 Anticoagulants 65
2.18.11 Antiplatelet Medications 65
2.18.12 HIV Medications 65
2.18.13 Theophylline 66
2.18.14 Chemotherapy 66

C. Cyr et al., *Cannabis and Cannabinoid-Based Medicines in Cancer Care*,
https://doi.org/10.1007/978-3-030-89918-9_2

2.19 Conclusion 66
References 66

2.1 Introduction

Phytocannabinoids have generally been considered to be a safe class of compounds with multiple benefits and have not been associated with fatal adverse effects. However, interactions are always a concern with any drug, including cannabinoids. Although cannabis seems to have an enviable safety profile, recent studies have shed new light on the possible negative outcomes associated with concomitant use of checkpoint inhibitors.

Drug-drug interactions depend on the schedule of administration, absorption, method of administration, the capacity of drugs and cannabinoids to inhibit CYP enzymes (inhibitory constant) (IC50), and the ability to upregulate CYP enzymes. Cannabinoid interactions with the immune system are also of particular concern with novel cancer therapeutics, as mentioned previously.

Cannabis can be consumed in many ways and vary according to personal (recreational) use or medical (prescribed) use. Products may be consumed in the form of edibles, inhaled through vaping, or smoked (as heat may change cannabinoid content) or as an oily extract. Labeling accuracy is crucial as the cannabinoid content and quality of the product will influence drug-drug interactions. In unregulated markets, including many US states where physicians "qualify" medical cannabis patients (instead of prescribe it like other medications), it is often extremely difficult to determine the precise content of the products that patients have purchased through dispensaries [28, 176, 178, 179, 227].

Diet is another important factor when oral administration is considered as the fat content influences the absorption of cannabidiol (CBD) [279]. When inhalation is concerned, vaping at temperatures other than 180–200 Celsius will have a measurable effect on cannabinoid blood levels [354].

While both endocannabinoids and phytocannabinoids are metabolized by CYP P450 cytochromes mixed function oxidases found on the endoplasmic reticulum and mitochondria [194, 297, 400], endocannabinoids also have their own specific enzymatic pathways. Subfamilies of P450 cytochrome containing enzymes CYP1A, CYP3A, CYP2B, CYP2C, and CYP2D are the major sites at which drug-drug interactions occur with cannabis [11]. Drug levels may vary 40-fold between individuals with the most important contributing factor being cytochrome levels and function. Levels and function depend on inherited genetic polymorphism within exons and at the promoter site. In addition, epigenetic changes can occur resulting in induction or inhibition of enzyme activity [397]. Inhibition of enzyme activity may be competitive or noncompetitive through allosteric modulation of the enzyme site. Induction involves interactions at the genetic level, at the site where transcription takes place, also known as the *promoter* site. In general, induction usually leads to increased clearance of the "victim" drug that will occur over time such that drug activity diminishes over a week or two [398].

Serum levels of various cannabinoids, principally tetrahydrocannabinol (THC), cannabidiol (CBD), and cannabinol (CBN) may not reflect what is happening within the cell. In addition, basic scientists have described inhibition constants in terms of micromolar (muM), while pharmacokinetic investigators describe serum levels in nanograms per milliliters (ng/ml). What has been considered to be strong inhibition on a strictly biochemical level would require clinically unachievable doses as translated in terms of ng/ml. The discrepancy between cellular and clinical research ends up being confusing when reviewing the literature unless one can translate muM into ng/ml. Hence, one needs to remember that biochemically relevant interactions may not necessarily be clinically significant.

Many medications and the major phytocannabinoids are also subject to glucuronidation via uridine 5′-diphospho-glucuronosyltransferases (UGT), the multiple efflux pumps (MDR1 also known as P-glycoprotein, MDRP1, and the breast cancer resistance protein ABCG2) [18, 158, 159, 181, 236, 273, 283, 405]. The same difficulty arises in squaring cannabinoid achievable doses with inhibitor constants.

2.2 Terminology

The term "endocannabinoidome" is still not widely used by clinicians and researchers, and in order to avoid confusion, its use to describe the *expanded* endocannabinoid system (ECS) will be restricted to the previous chapter. For the present chapter, the more commonly used term "endocannabinoid system (ECS)" will be used to describe most concepts relating to both the more specific canonical receptors and enzymes and the larger system of molecular targets and ligands. The "endocannabinoidome" will only be mentioned in order to point out a clinically relevant difference between these two related concepts.

2.3 Endocannabinoids and Drug Interactions

Endocannabinoid physiology is more complex and promiscuous than originally thought. Ongoing research is providing new clues on the various downstream effects of their metabolites and their possible role in cancer therapy.

The two main endogenous cannabinoids, anandamide (AEA) and 2-arachidonoylglycerol (2-AG), both bind as partial agonists with the CB1 and CB2 receptors, in a somewhat similar but less potent fashion as THC. They are rapidly produced and liberated on the cell surface on demand in one or two enzymatic steps and then quickly catabolized back to their original precursor substrates. This contrasts with classic neurotransmitters which are usually stored in synaptic vesicles.

Anandamide (AEA) is classically metabolized by fatty acid amide hydrolase within the cells, and inhibitors are being studied to increase AEA levels to facilitate symptom management [94, 184]. However, cyclooxygenases, CYP enzymes, and lipoxygenases are also intimately involved in the metabolism of AEA [325]. AEA and 2-arachidonoylglycerol (2-AG) are major sources of arachidonic acid and a major source of prostaglandin [325, 334, 400]. Some of the metabolites derived through CYP enzymes are active ligands for classical cannabinoid receptors CB1 and CB2 [103, 106, 325]. CYP enzymes 2C8, 2C9, 1A2, 3A, and 2B6 convert arachidonic acid to dihydroxyeicosatetraenoic acid (20-HETE) which is a potent vasoconstrictor within cerebral and renal microvascular networks and is increased in ischemic cerebrovascular pathologic processes, cardiac ischemic injury, kidney dysfunction, hypertension, diabetes, and pregnancy [249, 337]. On the other hand, the CYP2C enzyme family metabolize arachidonic acid from AEA into 14,15 epoxyeicosatrienoic acid (ETT) which is a vasodilator and anti-inflammatory metabolite within the vascular endothelium [16]. However, the dark side is that arachidonic acid-derived EETs promote tumor growth and metastasis [68, 205]. Decreases in EETs have been associated with hypertension and endothelial dysfunction [167, 325, 329]. Drug interactions which influence downstream endocannabinoid metabolites will therefore have clinical relevance. Drugs which induce CYP3A4 such as dexamethasone increase AEA clearance 5–15-fold and increase 20-HETE [215]. This may be the mechanism by which dexamethasone causes hypertension [402].

2-AG is metabolized classically through intracellular monoacylglycerol lipase (MAGL) and alpha/beta hydrolase but is also epoxygenated to EET-glycerol by CYP2C19, CYP3A4, and CYP2D6. EET-glycerol has been shown to promote growth of breast cancer [248, 343]. Thus, disrupting this pathway may reduce cancer growth [12, 131]. EET-glycerol has greater affinity for classical cannabinoid receptors than AEA and 2-AG [55, 281]. Blocking fatty acid amide hydrolase and/or monoacylglycerol lipase may have an effect on downstream CYP expression and on drugs that block or induce CYP enzymes [400].

2.4 Endocannabinoids, Cyclooxygenase, and Drug Interactions

As mentioned previously, the primary route of AEA metabolism is through fatty acid amide hydrolase (FAAH) and 2-AG through monoacylglycerol lipase (MAGL). Cyclooxygenase (COX) competes with FAAH for AEA and with MAGL for 2-AG [5, 89, 120]. An inflammatory state favors COX-2 and bypasses FAAH, increasing the production of prostamides (prostaglandin-ethanolamide and prostaglandin-glycerol) [29]. The various prostamides are D2, E2, and Falpha2 [195, 196, 394, 396]. Prostamides essentially have no activity on prostaglandin receptors nor do prostamides activate classical cannabinoid receptors. However, they do activate unique prostamide receptors which have biological importance [193, 296, 385]. Prostamides are more stable than prostaglandins and are often mistaken for prostaglandins if antibody assays are used [117].

Prostamides may be responsible for some of the biologic effects misidentified with AEA. For example, prostamides protect cerebellar neurons from stress-related apoptosis but do not have anti-tumor activity, whereas AEA does not reduce neuron apoptosis from stress but has anti-tumor activity [10]. Prostamides increase miniature inhibitory postsynaptic currents in the hippocampus which may contribute to central analgesic effects [304]. AEA also has a diuretic and natriuretic effect which is in part related to prostamide E2. Prostamide E2 has a renal protective effect which is lost with exposure to nonsteroidal anti-inflammatory (NSAID) drugs [289]. Furthermore, NSAIDs have the potential of altering general endocannabinoid biologic activity through inhibition of prostamide production.

As mentioned before, AEA and 2-AG are major sources of arachidonic acid. When FAAH and MAGL release arachidonic acid from AEA and 2-AG during breakdown, arachidonic acid is then made available to COX1 and COX2 metabolism, resulting in production of various prostaglandins. Multiple effects which branch out from this metabolic pathway have been observed. For example, upregulation of FAAH causes a pro-inflammatory and pro-algesic endocannabinoid effect through downstream prostaglandin production [83, 253, 318]. AEA pulmonary effects and vascular myogenic effects are related to prostaglandin production [75, 366]. Activation of CB1 receptors by AEA, THC, or synthetic cannabinoids upregulates COX2 [56, 100, 247]. Double blockade with FAAH and COX inhibitors synergistically improves edema and pain from carrageenan and formalin injections in animals [129, 130, 170]. Centrally, CB1 agonists cause a depolarization-induced suppression of inhibition which is potentiated by NSAIDs presumably due to prevention of COX2-related prostaglandin production [183, 303]. Certain NSAIDs also inhibit FAAH, including ibuprofen, flurbiprofen, indomethacin, and rofecoxib [65, 160, 306].

AEA may even prevent gastric ulcers caused by NSAIDs. In an animal study, a combination of a FAAH inhibitor and NSAID improves analgesia and reduces the gastrointestinal toxicity caused by NSAIDs relative to an NSAID alone [67]. This synergistic effect increases the therapeutic index (improves analgesia and reduces toxicity). This has not been observed with a combination of THC and an NSAID, however [108, 228]. There is evidence that THC competes with AEA and 2-AG binding with the intracellular carrier protein FABP1. This results in a decrease in AEA and 2-AG metabolism through FAAH and MAGL and an increase in endocannabinoid levels [238].

2.5 Endocannabinoids and Glucocorticoids

Glucocorticoid receptors occur near CB1 and CB2 within the central nervous system and immunocytes. There are interactions between the two receptor systems. In a spinal injury model, dexamethasone increases CB1 receptor expression within the CNS [370]. Glucocorticoids also upregulate CB1 receptors in hematopoietic cells [186]. Dexamethasone acutely inhibits COX 2, shifting arachidonic acid away from prostaglandin production toward endocannabinoid production. Dexamethasone also increases the release of endocannabinoids [87, 88, 369]. The interaction between glucocorticoids and the endocannabinoid system may account for the analgesia observed initially with dexamethasone.

The chronic use of glucocorticoids interacts with the endocannabinoid system quite differently. Chronic glucocorticoids exposure downregulates endocannabinoids and decreases CB1 receptor density within the hippocampus which may contribute to the hyperalgesia seen with corticosteroid withdrawal [41, 146, 147]. Stress increases release of corticosteroids from the hypothalamic-pituitary-adrenal axis. This increases anandamide, upregulates vanilloid receptors (TRPV1), and downregulates CB1 receptors in dorsal root ganglia leading to visceral hyperalgesia [161]. Corticosteroids increase endogenous cannabinoids which chronically causes downregulation of CB1 receptors within the CNS.

The appetite-stimulating effects of corticosteroids may be related to modulation of the endocannabinoid system. Corticosteroids increase endocannabinoids which then suppress the hypothalamic paraventricular nucleus. This is countered by the anorexigenic hormone leptin [229]. This is also the same mechanism by which ghrelin stimulates appetite. Therefore, an intact cannabinoid signaling pathway is necessary for the stimulatory effects of ghrelin [189, 350].

2.6 Endocannabinoids and Opioids

Endocannabinoids modulate opioid responses by several potential mechanisms. Interactions are reported to be synergistic, additive, cross-tolerant, and even antagonistic which reflects the complexity of interactions between the two systems [61, 64, 230, 232, 358, 359].

Opioid receptors and classical cannabinoid receptors form dimers: opioids modulate endocannabinoid release and endocannabinoids modulate downstream opioid signaling [307, 308]. Morphine combined with THC acutely upregulates CB1 receptors more than either ligand alone. In animal models, morphine enhances cannabinoid receptor binding and downstream CB1 receptor signaling [62, 98]. Acutely, opioid receptor antagonists such as naloxone block downstream signaling of THC, also likely through dimer interactions [6].

Chronic use of morphine has been shown to produce several changes in endocannabinoid signaling. It reportedly reduces CB1 receptors within the hippocampus and cerebellum while also diminishing 2-AG levels [360]. Translation of CB1 receptor protein is diminished over time with morphine exposure [119]. Chronic morphine desensitizes both mu and CB1 receptors through dimer interactions [59].

2.7 Clinical and Animal Studies of Cannabinoid Opioid Interactions

The complexity of interactions extends from preclinical to clinical experiences of cannabinoid/opioid combinations, and there are differences between animal models of ligand combinations and human studies which further muddy the waters of understanding. It is worth discussing the complexities if only to illustrate why opioid/cannabinoid combination trials will need to be stringently designed and that safety and efficacy will need to be co-primary outcomes [1].

Synergistic analgesia with combinations of opioid/cannabinoid ligands is clearly observed in animal and clinical studies. In animal studies, either morphine or codeine produces synergistic antinociception when combined with THC [63, 261, 282]. Healthy men subject to thermal pain experience analgesia with a combination of nabilone and morphine but not when either drug is used alone with similar doses [290].

There are also safety concerns with opioid/cannabinoid combinations. Heroin and morphine reinstate cannabinoid drug-seeking behaviors in rats [174, 328]. Conversely, cannabis rewarding effects in rodents are blocked by naloxone [42]. In humans subtherapeutic doses of THC and oxycodone produce analgesia but also increase the drug-liking effects of oxycodone [70]. Hence combinations may "shift left" analgesia curves relative to either opioid or cannabis alone but may also increase "drug-liking" effects.

The conflicting evidence between human and animal studies is yet to be explained but there tends to be species-specific effects with cannabinoid/opioid combinations. In rodents the combination of morphine and THC increases the discriminating effects of THC, whereas in humans hydromorphone does not substitute for THC discrimination. The differences may be related to study design, however [214, 326, 327]. Rodents which have developed tolerance to THC demonstrate cannabis withdrawal behaviors when given an opioid antagonist. This is not observed in monkeys or in individuals who are heavy cannabis users, however [26, 258]. Paradoxically, opioid antagonists enhance cannabis drug-liking effects in heavy cannabis users [71, 137, 138]. Hence, opioid receptor antagonists may potentially become an abusable class of medication in heavy cannabis users.

Cannabinoid-opioid interactions also influence opioid side effects which may be modulated by endocannabinoid levels. In situations where anandamide levels are increased, such as with the FAAH single nucleotide polymorphism rs324420, which reduces FAAH activity, this is associated with increased morphine-related nausea and vomiting and respiratory depression [57, 115, 301, 376]. Paradoxically reductions in MAGL, which increase 2-AG levels, improve opioid analgesia without increasing side effects. Inhibitors to MAGL have shown to exhibit opioid sparing effects [375].

Cannabis is proposed by some as a treatment for opioid withdrawal symptoms. There is some neurophysiological data to support this. Morphine withdrawal causes norepinephrine release from the locus coeruleus which is responsible for many of the symptoms of withdrawal [377]. CB1 receptors on locus coeruleus neurons blunt norepinephrine release [288]. In animals, THC reduces withdrawal behaviors and facilitates enkephalin release [211, 387].

Cannabis may also be useful as a treatment for opioid addiction and abstinence maintenance [66]. In animals, THC enhances opioid self-administration, and CB1 receptor antagonists reduce heroin drug-seeking behavior [93, 258, 327]. Clinically, cannabis doesn't seem to either improve or worsen drug rehabilitation outcomes [50, 257, 307, 308]. However, the frequency of cannabis use may be a factor.

Infrequent or occasional use may improve opioid abstinence during opioid maintenance therapy [97, 220, 284]. Individuals on methadone maintenance who use cannabis have lower plasma levels per dose of methadone suggesting that cannabis increases the clearance of methadone [135].

The topic of cannabinoid/opioid pharmacological interactions is complex and has been covered only in broad strokes here. These interactions are important to pursue in research since this will have important clinical and policy outcomes [34, 105, 225, 269, 324, 365].

2.8 Endocannabinoids, Anxiety and Depression

Data seems to suggest that the endocannabinoid system plays an important role in anxiety and mood disorders. This is a particularly important issue in cancer and palliative care patients.

CB1 receptors have been shown to modulate anxiety. Preclinical evidence suggests that upregulation of CB1 in the CNS reduces anxiety [143, 151, 152, 234, 314, 335]. The anxiolytic effects of THC are mediated through CB1/mu dimers since mu receptor antagonists abolish THC anxiolysis [30]. Benzodiazepines may reduce anxiety, in part, through interactions with the endocannabinoid system. There is a superadditive anxiolytic effect with the combination of a FAAH blocker and a benzodiazepine in animals, and CB1 receptor antagonists reduce the anxiolysis of benzodiazepines [110, 244]. Unfortunately, the combination of a benzodiazepine and THC also impairs verbal recall and increases distractibility and impairs vigilance so the trade-off may not be equatable [76].

Endocannabinoid system dysfunction has also been implicated in the development of depression [323], and preliminary findings have generated more questions than answers.

The endocannabinoid system has shown to be malleable. Overexposure to CB1 receptor agonists such as THC produces a sharp downregulation in receptor expression, which may explain the increased depression risk with prolonged high potency cannabis use. Depressed patients have also been shown to have altered CB1 receptor expression in different areas of the brain. Other intriguing discoveries have led researchers to believe that the role of the endocannabinoid system and depression may be even more promiscuous.

Genetic deletions of CB1 in mice cause depression-associated behaviors [149, 150], while increased expression of prefrontal lobe CB1 receptors has been linked with suicide [164]. Alcoholics who have committed suicide have been found to have reduced levels of AEA in the prefrontal cortex and increased CB1 receptors in the ventral striatum [362]. Depressed women have reduced CNS levels of 2-AG relative to healthy women [154].

Other psychoactive compounds, such as corticosteroids and antidepressants, have also been shown to modulate the endocannabinoid system (ECS). Increase in corticosteroids due to stress and depression reduces CB receptors in the hippocampus and correlates with altered circadian cortisol rhythms in depression [146–150, 155, 200, 286]. Hypothalamus CB1 receptors are down-modulated when the hypothalamic-pituitary-adrenal axis is activated by stress [221]. Indeed, long-term cannabis use is also associated with an increased incidence of depression and suicide which, again, is likely due to down-modulation of CB1 receptors [39, 40, 226].

Further evidence was found when studies looking into the effects of antidepressants on the endocannabinoid system (ECS) began to emerge. It was discovered that regional CB1 receptor expression changes which occur in depression are normalized by antidepressants [146, 147], and antidepressants have been shown to increase CB1 receptors in the prefrontal cortex and decrease receptors in the hippocampus, hypothalamus, and ventral striatum [15, 146, 147, 302, 331].

The brief approval of rimonabant, a CB1 receptor antagonist marketed for weight loss, further illustrates the complex nature of cannabinoid mental health research. Initial preclinical findings on animals had shown that CB1 receptor antagonists reduced stress-induced depression [126, 319]. However, the opposite was true in human post marketing adverse event data. Rimonabant was eventually taken off the market due to depression and anxiety as treatment emerging side effects [58].

Treating depression with cannabis is complex and risky, and data pulled from animal studies may not be reliable. The data suggests that increases in CNS endocannabinoids seem to relieve depression, and there exists an inverse relationship between circulating 2-AG levels and major depression. In animals, FAAH inhibitors increase anandamide levels and promote mood and have antidepressant-like activity [118, 153, 154, 300]. MAGL inhibitors have also been shown to have antidepressant effects by increasing 2-AG [403, 404]. The histopathology observed with depression (reduced signs of neurogenesis and neuroinflammation) is reversed by FAAH or MGL inhibitors as well [262, 403]. Combinations of antidepressants with FAAH blockers are therefore a potentially therapeutic combination which warrant further investigation [146, 147].

2.8.1 *Endocannabinoid "Tone": Beyond the Theory*

The concept of the "endocannabinoid tone" has been proposed to explain many chronic ailments, from fibromyalgia and depression to irritable bowel syndrome, and, according to Raphael Mechoulam, it may be in part responsible for human personality traits [346]. The theory postulates that interindividual differences exist in circulating endocannabinoids, receptor expression, and endocannabinoid enzymatic activity. Considering the complex relationship linking the endocannabinoid system (ECS) with other molecular targets and circulating corticosteroid levels, it's very likely that this theory may indeed provide answers to lingering questions concering interindividual cognitive and emotional regulation and responses to stress. This could certainly help to explain certain other chronic conditions which have no known biological markers such as fibromyalgia. However, this would also add a further layer of necessary exploration. If endocannabinoid tone is in fact associated with certain illnesses, it would require reliable diagnostic criteria for early detection and prevention and specific treatment modalities, not unlike any other dysregulated biological system.

Basal serum concentrations of AEA and 2-AG have indeed been shown to be significantly reduced in women with major depression [153], and rodent studies suggest it may predict antidepressant responses [239, 322]. Anhedonia, a hallmark of depression, is also associated with reduced anandamide in the ventral striatum [146, 147].

Cannabinoid receptor agonists given in low doses (URB597, CP55,940, and AM404) potentiate imipramine and citalopram antidepressant activity in rats [2], and this also occurs with subtherapeutic doses of imipramine. On the other hand, rimonabant, the CB1 receptor antagonist, blocks the antidepressant effects of the combination. CB1 receptor agonists enhance serotonin neuronal activity which may be the reason for synergy with citalopram. The acute antidepressant-like properties of CB1 receptor agonists are mediated by serotonin neuronal activity arising from the ventromedial prefrontal cortex [20], and the antidepressant effects of fluoxetine in animals may be by way of upregulation of CB1 receptors in the prefrontal cortex which in turn increases serotonin neurotransmission through the serotonin receptor 5HT1a [234].

Furthermore, imipramine in animals prevents altered CB1 receptor expression within the CNS associated with depression [146, 147]. The activity associated with desipramine and electroshock therapy also correlates with upregulation of CB1 receptor expression [54, 144, 152]. Desipramine and tranylcypromine have also been shown to upregulate CB1 receptors in the hippocampus [151, 152], while imipramine reverses impaired endocannabinoid binding to CB1 receptors within the amygdala occurring with stress-related depression [146, 147]. Antidepressants increase anandamide levels within the hippocampus and ventral striatum and thereby reduce stress-related depression in animals [180, 280, 321]. Antidepressants increase anandamide with in the ventral striatum.

Endocannabinoid tone may influence the expression of clinical depression and other mental health conditions, and this may help choose a more appropriate treatment. Preclinical evidence seems to suggest that certain antidepressants may be more dependent on a functioning endocannabinoid system than others and may be class dependent. For example, animal studies have shown that antidepressants which block norepinephrine reuptake are more dependent on the endocannabinoid system for antidepressant actions than those which inhibit serotonin reuptake [233, 331].

2.9 Endocannabinoids and Post-traumatic Stress Disorder

The endocannabinoid system (ECS) seems to play an important role in post-traumatic stress disorder (PTSD), which could be relevant in cancer care and aversive memory extinction.

Clinical studies suggest that PTSD (post-traumatic stress disorder) patients may cope better with their symptoms by using cannabis. This may explain the high prevalence of cannabis use among individuals with PTSD. Preliminary studies in humans suggest that treatment with cannabinoids potentially decreases PTSD symptoms including sleep quality, frequency of nightmares, and hyperarousal [250]. Acutely, in patients with a highly traumatic experience, 2AG and AEA are increased in circulation, whereas in chronic PTSD circulating levels of endocannabinoid levels are low [142, 145], which further provides evidence for the theory of individual endocannabinoid tone.

Increasing endocannabinoid tone may therefore help with certain chronic PTSD symptoms. In animals, systemic manipulations of the endocannabinoid system (ECS) alter anxiety-like behavior but not extinction-resistant associative fear memory [361]. Current limited evidence in healthy humans and PTSD patients supports the use of THC to suppress anxiety and aversive memory expression. Combinations with an SSRI or the commercially available medicinal nutraceutical palmitoylethanolamide (PEA) have shown to be helpful as seen in animal models [219]. Standard antidepressants frequently fail to improve PTSD, such that combinations of a low-dose CB1 agonist or FAAH inhibitor with antidepressants may prove to be of interest [104, 260]. Cannabinoids are particularly effective in reducing nightmares and insomnia associated with PTSD [109, 156]. In a randomized trial, nabilone provided significant relief for military personnel with PTSD. To date, no guidelines have been published regarding the most appropriate method for introducing cannabinoids in PTSD. Although adding cannabinoids such as low-dose THC and CBD may become a promising treatment for patients with nightmares and poor response to traditional therapies [169], no specific formulation or dosage guidelines are yet available. As such, very low doses of THC are especially recommended in any clinical setting, particularly in unstable mental health issues.

2.10 Endocannabinoid System Disruptions and Potential Impact on Treatment with Antipsychotics

It has been demonstrated that there is an intrinsic disruption of the endocannabinoid system (ECS) in schizophrenia. Patients with schizophrenia have elevated cerebrospinal fluid (CSF) levels of endocannabinoids which is thought to be a compensatory process to the dysfunction of the endocannabinoid system [207]. CSF levels of AEA are eightfold higher than in healthy individuals, but this is also encountered in patients with dementia and those with a mood disorder. Higher levels of AEA level in the CSF are associated with fewer psychotic symptoms, however, which suggests that endocannabinoid levels can be predictive of disease activity. Patients suffering from schizophrenia also have increased CB1 receptors and/or activity within the anterior and posterior cingulate gyrus and dorsolateral prefrontal cortex [77, 82, 259, 399]. However, not all studies have demonstrated this abnormal distribution of cannabinoid receptors in schizophrenia [90, 91, 188]. Differences may be due to treatment adherence or whether the disease is acute versus chronic. Other factors include comorbidities, pre- or postmortem changes, and cannabinoid agonist therapy (THC, etc.) associated with downregulation and internalization of cannabinoid receptors which may interfere with the type of test used to detect CB1 receptors [209]. Activity may be increased without increasing numbers of receptors secondary to positive allosteric modulation of CB1 receptors as well [363].

Patients who are using antipsychotics which target the dopamine D2 receptor do not exhibit higher AEA levels in the CSF, although they remain elevated in those on atypical antipsychotics which largely target the serotonin 5-HT2A receptor [116]. Other studies have also found elevated plasma AEA levels in schizophrenia which return to normal with remission [80, 187, 207].

Furthermore, complex interactions exist between antipsychotics and the endocannabinoid system (ECS) which is not observed across other drug classes [206, 380]. Antipsychotics do not directly interact with cannabinoid receptors, but there are complex interactions between dopamine D2 receptors and CB1 receptors which lead to alterations in the endocannabinoid system (ECS) [373].

Antipsychotics reduce CB1 receptor expression or activity in the prefrontal cortex [353]. Paradoxically, haloperidol and olanzapine increase CB1 receptor expression within the basal ganglia which has been associated with extrapyramidal side effects [84, 241, 293]. Olanzapine also increases CB1 receptor expression in the secondary somatosensory cortex, auditory and visual cortex, and geniculate nuclei which is suppressed by a high-fat diet [84]. Olanzapine is reported to both increase and decrease CB1 receptors within the hypothalamus, whereas risperidone increases receptors in the hypothalamus [84, 243, 373]. Interestingly the increased expression is a distributional effect of the receptor protein since CB1 receptor mRNA is not increased but is actually reduced [314].

Clozapine exhibits an interesting interaction with the endocannabinoid system (ECS). It is unique among antipsychotics as it reduces CB1 receptor expression in the nucleus accumbens. Clozapine has been recommended by some authors as the antipsychotic of choice for individuals who have cannabis-related psychosis or schizophrenia though this recommendation has not been confirmed in systematic reviews [335, 338, 381]. Cannabis use is associated with deleterious psychotic outcomes which include increased odds of non-remission, prescriptions of unique antipsychotic medications, and cumulative prescriptions with poor treatment trajectories [287]. Withdrawal from haloperidol, olanzapine, and chlorpromazine leads to upregulation of CB1 receptors within the brain which is not observed with clozapine [335]. These observations may have clinical relevance, and there are multiple ongoing trials using combinations of antipsychotics and cannabidiol. However, interactions between antipsychotics and cannabis are complex and should not be lumped together under one category. Each cannabinoid may have unique interactions with individual antipsychotics, and the evidence seems to suggest a very important role for cannabidiol in this condition.

Polymorphisms of the CB1 receptor gene (CNR1) are reported to be associated with a risk of developing cannabis-related schizophrenia [53]. Using the family-based association test, a link was found with the (AAT)n-repeat marker of the CNR1 and judged to be significant [53]. However, the genotype appears to be related to refractoriness to antipsychotic therapy rather than a predisposition to cannabis-related psychosis [136]. Polymorphisms of CNR1 are also associated with weight gain from antipsychotics and tardive dyskinesia [344, 345].

2.11 The use of Phytoannabinoids as Antipsychotics

Two CB1 receptor antagonists have been tested as antipsychotics either alone or as "add-on" therapy [7, 242, 294]. The actions of rimonabant on the brain, particularly C-fos expression, share a similar pattern observed with atypical antipsychotics [7, 272]. However trials of antagonists have been few, and unfortunately the dropout rate with rimonabant was significant [182, 208, 242].

There is reason to believe that CBD may reduce psychotic symptoms. This has been demonstrated in multiple trials, although results are somewhat conflicting. CBD has been used clinically to treat schizophrenia at least in one trial [291], while abnormal functional MRI patterns seen with patients who are at clinical high risk (CHR) for psychosis are partially normalized by CBD [32, 379]. The number of published cannabis trials remains small, however, and it's really too early to adequately summarize these findings in a systematic review or meta-analyses, although this has been attempted [112, 191]. High-dose CBD has been used in these trials, similar to dosing regimens used in anti-seizure studies, although they may not be necessary when looking at inhibitory concentrations (IC50) for the proposed targets. CBD competitively inhibits FAAH which increases AEA CNS levels. Significant inhibition occurs at levels ranging from 10 to 160 umol/l. This is equivalent to plasma levels of 3–50 ng/ml [33, 81, 210, 213, 342, 371]. CBD also inhibits the AEA intracellular FABP transporter which also increases AEA levels. The IC50 for this to occur ranges between 22 and 25 umol/l which is a plasma concentration of 6–8 ng/ml [81, 285]. Other proposed mechanisms include activation of PPAR-alpha which has an IC50 of 5 umol/l or a plasma concentration of 1.6 ng/ml [263, 264]. CBD also increases palmitoylethanolamide (PEA) levels through competitive inhibition of FAAH. Palmitoylethanolamide (PEA) itself is a potent activator of PPAR-alpha [95, 139]. CBD activates the vanilloid receptor TRPV1 which is important in balancing glutaminergic and dopaminergic neurotransmission that is disrupted with schizophrenia [99, 352]. The IC50 binding for this to occur is between 1 and 3.5umol/l which is equivalent to a CBD plasma concentration of 1 ng/ml [81]. CBD also activates the 5-HT1A receptors with an IC50 of 16 umol/l or plasma concentration of 5 ng/ml [299]. Even though CBD is a partial agonist at many of these targets [291], modest doses of CBD are likely to be as effective as high doses. Unfortunately, there are no published dose-response trials available in the literature.

Though the pharmacodynamic profile of CBD resembles that of antipsychotics, not all symptoms of schizophrenia respond in a similar manner to CBD, and some could potentially worsen [294, 295]. In a phencyclidine psychosis animal model which is a surrogate to schizophrenia, social cognitive impairment is related to CB1 receptor inactivation, whereas social withdrawal is associated with CB1 receptor activation [235, 315, 316]. In a small ketamine trial involving healthy individuals, CBD marginally reduces depersonalization but increases psychomotor adverse effects [132]. Therefore CBD responses may benefit certain symptoms and may worsen others or have similar adverse effects. As such, benefits may depend on the cluster of schizophrenic symptoms.

There are published case reports and series starting about 25 years ago which have attempted to utilize CBD as therapy for schizophrenia [291, 305, 311, 406, 407]. A phase II study compared 800 mg of CBD with 800 mg of amisulpride in 39 treatment-naïve schizophrenic patients treated over 4 weeks. CBD responses were equivalent to amisulpride. However, CBD was better tolerated and had fewer extrapyramidal side effects, less weight gain, and sexual dysfunction [210]. Not all trials showed positive results. A three-arm randomized trial consisting of placebo and 300 and 600 mg of CBD in 28 patients with schizophrenia found no benefit with CBD [133]. A study involving 88 patients with partial responses to antipsychotics randomized 88 patients between placebo and 100 mg of CBD. Treatment over 6 weeks demonstrated some benefits to CBD by psychiatric examination but not by standard questionnaires [237]. Another study, however, found no benefit to adding CBD 600 mg daily to stable antipsychotic treatment compared to placebo. Neither cognition nor symptoms improved [35]. There are larger studies in progress, and so it is too early to make any conclusions about CBD in the treatment of schizophrenia [310].

In conclusion, although CBD may be potentially useful in preventing psychosis, there are no clinical studies to validate this hypothesis.

2.12 Omega-3 Fatty Acids and effects on the Endocannabinoid System

Omega-3 fatty acids are popular supplements among patients with cancer. There is some evidence that omega-3 fatty acids reduce sarcopenia related to cancer treatment [24, 51, 86, 217, 357]. Omega-6 fatty acids, particularly linoleic acid, are a source of arachidonic acid needed to produce AEA and 2-AG. Excessive omega-6 fatty acids may lead to overproduction of endocannabinoids which causes subsequent downregulation of CB1 and CB2 receptors over time, however excessive omega-6 fatty acids have also been associated with obesity in mice [8, 240]. On the other hand, the omega-3 fatty acid, eicosapentaenoic acid (EPA), and docosahexaenoic acid (DHA) decrease AEA and 2-AG levels in plasma and tissues [165, 384]. With chronic dosing, omega-3 fatty acids increase CB1 and CB2 receptor expression and upregulate both receptors' mRNA. Endocannabinoid-synthesizing enzymes have also been shown to increase [165]. Deficiencies in omega-3 fatty acids impair endocannabinoid modulation of mood and lead to neuroinflammation and are associated with clinical depression [199, 202]. Omega-3 fatty acids also upregulate production of non-arachidonic acid containing ethanolamides such as palmitoylethanolamide (PEA) which has antidepressant activity [74, 79, 113, 165, 270, 395].

Krill oil may contain a superior omega-3 formulation and produce a greater effect on the endocannabinoid system (ECS). Krill oil has esterified EPA and DHA which have greater bioavailability than fish oil EPA and DHA and as a result a greater effect on AEA and 2-AG. Krill oil reduces circulating AEA in obese individuals to a greater extent than other sources of EPA and DHA [21, 312].

2.13 Phytocannabinoid Pharmacokinetics: THC

THC concentrations in blood are dependent on dose, diet, route of administration, vehicle, and disease state. THC bioavailability in sesame oil is 10–20%, whereas the same dose as the commercial product, dronabinol, has a bioavailability of 6% [265, 267, 268, 367]. Smoked cannabis increases THC levels by bypassing hepatic clearance. The lungs also have limited expression of CYP2C9, the main cytochrome responsible for THC metabolism, resulting in increased bioavailability [162, 204, 298, 374]. THC bioavailability in both vaporized and smoked cannabis is about 25%, but there is a great large variability (2–56%) due to technique and temperature. This marked variation will be influenced by product matrix, ignition temperature, inhalation dynamics, number and depth of inhalations, CYP2C9 genotype, and lung volume [107]. More on this in Chap. 7. Single nucleotide polymorphisms at CYP2C9 influence THC dose to blood concentration, ratios, and half-life. Reduced CYP2C9 activity increases THC exposure 2.3-fold, and poor metabolizers are relatively common among non-Hispanic whites (35%) [45, 203, 368]. This may explain the often unpredictable vulnerability to THC encountered in certain individuals.

The systemic distribution of THC is also time dependent. The volume of distribution ranges between 4 and 14 liters/kilogram which reflects THC lipophilic characteristic and tissue penetration. Plasma protein binding is 97%. Immediately upon absorption, THC rapidly distributes to fatty tissue and highly perfused organs such as the brain, heart, lung, and liver. THC is subsequently slowly released from fat and consequently has a relatively short distribution half-life but a prolonged elimination half-life [38, 163, 222]. After rapid distribution with an initial half-life of 6 minutes, there is a slow redistribution resulting in a terminal half-life of 22 hours [223, 224].

THC is highly extracted by the liver, and the bulk of its clearance is dependent upon hepatic blood flow. This high extraction ratio means that oral cannabis is more likely to have associated drug-drug interactions than other routes of administration of THC which bypasses the liver, such as inhalation [383]. Liver disease and hepatic shunting decrease THC clearance as well [383].

THC bioavailability is also influenced by P-glycoprotein 1 (P-gp 1), also known as multidrug resistance protein 1 (MDR1), is an efflux pump found in the intestinal wall and blood-brain barrier which plays an important role in drug transporter-mediated drug interactions [36]. P-glycoprotein 1, is therefore an important protein of the cell membrane that pumps many foreign substances, including drugs, out of cells. P-gp 1 also plays a significant role in oncology since it is highly expressed in some cancer cells where it is responsible for decreased anti-cancer drug accumulation in multidrug-resistant cancer cells. Compounds being transported (effluxed) out of the cell by P-gp 1 are said to be P-gp *substrates.* Drugs which inhibit P-glycoprotein 1 may increase THC blood and CNS levels. Inhibitors of P-gp 1 such as amiodarone and clarithromycin may increase the serum concentration of P-gp substrates, whereas inducers of P-gp, such as apalutamide and lorlatinib, may decrease serum concentrations of substrates of P-gp. THC is a P-glycoprotein efflux and a P-glycoprotein substrate. Substrates of P-glycoprotein, such as apixaban, cyclosporine, tacrolimus, and THC (but not CBD) are therefore susceptible to changes in pharmacokinetics due to drug interactions with P-gp inhibitors or inducers. Drugs which inhibit P-glycoprotein may increase THC blood and CNS levels. Distribution to the brain is greater in MDR1 knockout mice [330]. Hepatic blood flow is the major factor determining THC clearance rather than P-glycoprotein or CYP2C9 levels. THC is also a substrate for other efflux pumps such as the breast cancer resistance protein (ABCG2) [348]. What role these other various efflux pumps play in THC pharmacokinetics is not established.

The quantity of THC delivered to the brain is less than 1% of inhaled or oral THC. This occurs despite the fact that the brain is highly perfused, and THC is lipophilic. The active metabolite, 11-hydroxy-tetrahydrocannabinol (11-OH-THC), enters the brain more rapidly than THC and achieves higher levels than THC [127, 364, 382]. Thus, 11-OH-THC may contribute more significantly to the psychoactive effects of THC particularly when THC is taken orally. CBD alters THC brain levels as well. In rats, subcutaneous THC and CBD (20 mg each) increase THC brain levels fourfold but reduces CBD brain levels twofold compared to each drug alone. The mechanism behind this is not entirely clear. CBD is not a substrate for P-glycoprotein, whereas THC is a substrate. CBD is an inhibitor of P-glycoprotein but only at very high doses which is unlikely to be clinically relevant [101, 102]. In a study which explored interactions between CBD and p-glycoprotein interactions, 10–25 micromolar concentrations were used. The levels (3140 ng/ml) are about 3 times greater than what can be achieved with high dose CBD (10–20 mg/kg) [73]. CBD at 20 mg/kg produces a maximum serum concentration (C-max) of 1090 ng/ml [277]. CBD also inhibits THC metabolism through CYP2C9 resulting in higher brain levels [157]. Vaporization or smoking cannabis produces rapid peak THC levels followed by rapid decreases. Subcutaneous and oral administration paradoxically produce the highest and longest lasting levels of cannabinoids [60, 157].

THC and its metabolites are eliminated slowly. 11-nor-9-carboxy-THC (THC-COOH) and its glucuronidated conjugate are eliminated in the urine and are often used for drug testing. 11-OH-THC can be detected in plasma for 3 days, while free (unbound) THC and THC-COOH can be detected in plasma for 30 days and 33 days, respectively, following abstinence from chronic daily cannabis use [28]. Fatty acid conjugates of THC and 11-OH-THC are formed which stabilize both cannabinoids [128]. Since THC is quite lipophilic, renal tubular reabsorption is significant leading to low renal excretion of unchanged drug. THC-COOH which is even more hydrophilic such that THC-COOH and THC-COOH glucuronide are the main metabolites found in the urine. Glucuronides of 11-OH-THC and THC-COOH are also excreted in bile and undergo enterohepatic recirculation which contributes to the long half-life of THC-COOH and 11-OH-THC [177, 278].

The distribution of THC metabolites after smoking cannabis is distinctly different from that of oral cannabis. THC and THC metabolites peak in serum at 15 minutes and are largely undetectable after a single exposure 2 hours after administration. The glucuronide metabolite of THC-COOH remains elevated for 3–4 hours then returns to baseline at 22 hours after administration [313]. Smoked THC bioavailability is approximately 25% [107], depending on depth of inhalation and breath hold. More on this in Chap. 7.

Differences in pharmacokinetics between oral and smoked cannabis are largely related to first-pass hepatic clearance and cytochrome distributions which differ between the lung and liver. CYP2C9, CYP2C19, and CYP3A are involved in the hepatic metabolism of THC and CBD, whereas CYP1A1 has negligible influences on clearance. CYP1A1 is the major contributor to THC conversion to 11-OH-THC in the lung [134, 256, 401]. Both cannabis and tobacco smoking induce cytochrome P450 (CYP) 1A2 through activation of the aromatic hydrocarbon receptor, and induction is additive. Smoking cessation rapidly downregulates CYP1A in the lung. On the basis of the estimated half-life of CYP1A2, dose reduction of CYP1A-metabolized drugs may be necessary as early as the first few days after smoking cessation to prevent toxicity [9, 173].

As mentioned, THC is a substrate P-glycoprotein BCRP/ABCG2 efflux pumps [330]. Single nucleotide polymorphisms of the P-glycoprotein gene ABCB1 influence THC serum levels. The polymorphism C3435T (CC > TT) is associated with increased THC serum levels and cannabis dependence [27, 181].

This presentation of THC pharmacokinetics is simpler than what in reality is a complex and dynamic process. There are 80 distinct metabolites of THC, which means that we understand the pharmacokinetic pathways of only a fraction of the many metabolites from this prominent cannabinoid [128, 236].

2.14 Phytocannabinoid Pharmacokinetics: CBD

The pharmacokinetic data on CBD is rather limited. The real gap in understanding involves the lack of pharmacokinetic studies in sick populations such as those who have cancer, AIDS, multiple sclerosis, and epilepsy. What has been published has been in healthy individuals. However, sick populations often have severely altered absorption, distribution, metabolism, and excretion caused either by organ dysfunction, polypharmacy, or cachexia. These conditions influence drug clearance, distribution through altered efflux pumps, and excretion [218]. Known pharmacokinetics are usually studied using single phytocannabinoids, but most individuals are taking a mixture of cannabinoids in cannabis [3]. Studies done with nabiximols, a mixture of THC and CBD, have demonstrated that pharmacokinetics and distribution of THC are altered by the presence of CBD. A dose of 5 mg of CBD increases THC (10 mg) area under the curve (AUC) and C-max by 20% and decreases the formation of the active metabolite 11-OH-THC [254]. This occurs because CBD is a potent inhibitor of multiple cytochromes which alter THC metabolism. At high doses, CBD may also influence P-glycoprotein which further alters THC pharmacokinetics. Thus, CBD-THC interactions have an important impact on THC levels, relative to THC used as a single phytocannabinoid [37].

Data on CBD bioavailability and plasma half-life are also limited. In mice, oral bioavailability has been shown to be approximately 8%, and plasma half-life is between 3 and 5 hours [43]. However, in a systematic review of studies centered on CBD pharmacokinetics, the AUC and C-max are dose dependent, but reach a plateau at high doses (400–800 mg) where saturation to absorption is observed [246]. However, results are conflicting as this has not been observed in very high doses in the most recent study [340]. The half-life of CBD in human studies is between 1.4 and 10.9 h after an oromucosal spray, 2–5 days after chronic oral administration, 24 h after i.v., and 31 h after smoking cannabis with CBD. Bioavailability following smoked CBD is 31%; however, no other studies have attempted to report the absolute bioavailability of CBD following other routes in humans [246]. Oromucosal sprays of 10–20 mg of CBD produce maximum plasma concentrations between 2.5 and 3.3 ng/mL which has been fairly consistent from study to study [246].

Another study demonstrated that oral doses of 10 mg result in a mean C-max of 2.47 ng/mL at 1.27 hours. A CBD dose of 400 mg results in a C-max of 181 ng/mL at 3 hours, and a 800 mg dose produces a C-max of 221 ng/mL at 3 hours [231, 245]. Much higher CBD dosing regimens have also been examined, though are usually encountered in specific clinical settings such as epilepsy. A single 1.5 g, 3 g, 4.5 g, and 6 g dose resulted in a C-max of 292 ng/ml, 533 ng/ml, 722 ng/ml, and 782 ng/ml, respectively [340]. T-max with very high doses occurs later than lower doses, between 4 and 5 hours after the oral dose [340]. Therefore, the T-max concentrations of CBD after oral administration will range between 1.6 and 4.2 hours depending on the dose. Minimal accumulation with chronic dosing occurs over 5–9 days [317]. C-max increases slightly over time with high doses. Patients taking 750 mg of CBD have a C-max of 291 ng/ml on day 1 and 330 ng/ml on day 7, while patients on 1500 mg have a C-max of 362 ng/ml on day 1 and 541 ng/ml on day 7 [340]. It is important to refer to these plasma levels when considering drug-drug interactions which will be discussed later in this chapter.

It is also important to remember that bioavailability of CBD is greater in a fed state [246]. High-fat diets increase CBD C-max 4.85-fold [340].

There is a single study of intravenous CBD pharmacokinetics: 20 mg led to a mean C-max of 686 ng/mL at 3 minutes after injection, while levels at 1 hour were 48 ng/mL [266]. Smoked CBD (19.2 mg) produced plasma levels of 110 ng/mL at 3 minutes and 10.2 ng/mL at 1 hour [266].

Intranasal CBD pharmacokinetics are not available in humans. In rats, CBD bioavailability ranges between 34 and 46% of the intranasal dose. Enhancers do not improve absorption [275]. The highly lipophilic nature of cannabinoids is ideal for developing advanced nanosized delivery systems as a method of drug delivery [47].

Transdermal cannabinoids bypass hepatic clearance and seem to produce sustained cannabinoid levels in circulation, although few human trials have been carried out. THC is more lipophilic than CBD and has greater resistance to diffusion across aqueous tissue layers and thus less suitable to topical administration. THC becomes concentrated in the stratum corneum intercellular lipids. CBD is commonly used as a topical preparation since it readily crosses the skin barrier [332]. Enhancers increase CBD topical bioavailability, and steady-state concentrations increase 3.7-fold with their use [275].

The elimination half-life of CBD is estimated at 2–5 days. As with THC, CBD rapidly distributes into fat and slowly redistributes which is the rate limiting step to elimination [69].

The pharmacokinetics of CBD are unchanged in renal failure [341], but there is very little data about CBD in liver disease, however. Interestingly, in mice subject to fulminant hepatic failure induced by thioacetamide, CBD restores liver function, normalizes serotonin levels, and improves brain pathology [19]. Mice subject to bile duct ligation-induced hepatic failure have improved cognition and locomotion with CBD [19]. The pharmacokinetics and potential benefits of CBD in liver failure should definitely be explored.

CBD metabolites have varying degrees of activity. One of these metabolites, 7-OH-CBD, has demonstrated anti-seizure activity. This active metabolite is then metabolized to 7-COOH-CBD by CYP2C19 [171, 400]. CBD is also metabolized into 6-OH-CBD which is metabolized subsequently into 6-oxo-CBD which may have biologic activity and has been shown to increase pentobarbital sedation [52, 341]. There is also a 4-OH-CBD metabolite that has been identified. The 7-OH-CBD is derived from CYP2C19, and the 6-OH-CBD metabolite is derived from CYP3A4 and CYP2C19, while the 4-OH-CBD is the result of CYP 3A4 [171]. CYP2C19 poor metabolizers will have higher plasma levels of CBD relative to dose [201, 251]. The 7-hydroxylated metabolite exceeds the 6-hydroxylated metabolite in circulation 10–20-fold. The inactive metabolite 7-COOH-CBD is derived from 7-OH-CBD through CYP2C9 and CYP2C19 [171]. The 7-COOH-CBD metabolite exceeds all other metabolites in circulation. There is no evidence in vivo that CBD can be converted to THC [255, 386].

CBD is also glucuronidated by UGT1A9 and UGT2B7 which are minor contributors to CBD metabolism. Drug-drug interactions are much more likely to occur with CYP2C9, CYP2C19, and CYP3A4 than with conjugases [236]. CBD has been assumed to be an efflux pump substrate. Piperine inhibits P-glycoprotein and increases the bioavailability of CBD and also inhibits CYP3A4 which is expressed on intestinal mucosa as well as in the liver [31].

2.15 Cannabidiol and Efflux Pumps

Piperidine, an alkaloid derived from pepper, is known to block P-glycoprotein and increase the bioavailability of CBD 2.5-fold, [168]. Piperidine also inhibits CYP3A4 which is expressed on intestinal mucosa as well as in the liver [31]. ABCB1/MDR1 knockout mice do not express P-glycoprotein, and CBD levels do not differ in the brain or plasma in these knockout mice compared to wild-type mice. The same is true for the efflux pump BCRP (Breast Cancer Resistant Protein)/ABCG2 protein efflux pump [48].

2.16 Pharmacokinetics of Approved Cannabinoids

Dronabinol undergoes first-pass clearance and is metabolized in the liver to an active 11-oic acid metabolite [46, 141]. Nabilone undergoes reduction to a 9-keto moiety and oxidation of the penultimate carbon of the dimethylheptyl side chain. Neither dronabinol nor nabilone are major inhibitors of cytochromes or conjugases [141], and this may influence the choice of cannabinoid in patients with polypharmacy.

2.17 Pharmacokinetic Cannabis-Drug Interactions

The most important cannabinoid drug interactions occur within the cytochrome system and are largely inhibitory (see Table 2.1). In general, CBD is a greater CYP drug-drug interactions (DDI) *perpetrator*, while THC is mostly a DDI *victim*. For example, CBD, but not THC, induces CYP1A2. Most in vitro and in vivo animal studies demonstrate drug enzyme interactions at concentrations of cannabis which are not achievable in humans. There are also interactions which may be allosteric rather than at orthosteric enzyme sites [216].

Cannabis interactions with efflux pumps change with length of exposure. Short-term exposure induces P-glycoprotein, while longer-term exposure inhibits

Table 2.1 Summary of cannabinoid drug interactions

Enzyme	Type of interaction	Cannabinoid
CYP3A4	Inhibition	CBD > THC > CBN
CYP2C8	Inhibition	CBD
CYP2C9	Inhibition	CBN > THC > CBD
CYP2C19	Inhibition	CBD > CBN > THC
CYP2D6	Inhibition	CBD > THC > CBN
CYP1A1	Inhibition/induction	CBD > THC
CYP1A2	Inhibition	CBD, CBN > THC
CYP2B6	Inhibition	CBD > THC > CBN
UGT1A7	Inhibition	CBN
UGT1A8	Inhibition	CBN
UGT1A9	Inhibition	CBD, CBN > THC
UGT2B7	Inhibition	CBD

CBD cannabidiol, *THC* tetrahydrocannabinol, *CBN* cannabinol
[17, 140, 171, 190, 271, 283, 336, 372, 388–393]

P-glycoprotein [13, 14, 101, 102, 330]. P-Glycoprotein interactions normally influence both bioavailability and drug distribution since P-glycoprotein is found along the intestinal wall and the blood-brain barrier [101, 102, 159, 181, 405]. However, CBD concentrations at which P-glycoprotein interactions are reported are not clinically achievable.

Smoked cannabis produces active aryl hydrocarbons, which induce CYP1A2. Secondary non-cannabinoid compounds in cannabis may also contribute to drug interactions, but their role appears to be a minor one. Although terpenoids potently interact with metabolizing enzymes [173, 390, 391], they are a minor component within cannabis and not clinically significant. Flavonoid glycosides inhibit organic anion transporters which influence the clearance of drugs like terfenadine, statins, and beta-antagonists [212].

Once again, it is important to understand that circulating THC and CBD concentrations necessary to produce inhibitory activity involving cytochromes and P-glycoprotein are usually not achievable (Tables 2.2 and 2.3). Thus, anticipating clinically relevant drug-drug interactions will rely less on "potential" drug interactions and depend mostly on achievable drug levels and receptor affinities. For instance, THC may be termed a "potent CYP3A inhibitor" yet based on the IC50 of 1.3 umol/ mL; the serum levels required to produce this inhibition are 400 ng/mL, which are nearly impossible to achieve in practice and are mostly encountered in overdoses. As an example, a dose of 20 mg of THC by mouth will result in a serum level of 4–11 ng/mL [267]. However, this dosage range would be sufficient to inhibit CYP2C9 (Table 2.3). In this case, prodrugs such as clopidogrel, which rely on 2C9 to transform the parent compound to an active metabolite, might need to be changed for another antiplatelet agent such as ticagrelor. Other drugs metabolized by 2C9 and with a narrow therapeutic window such as coumadin may require closer INR monitoring.

Table 2.2 CBD ICD50 [22]

Cytochrome P450	Micromolar/ml	Ng/ml
CYP1A2	0.45	141
CYP2C9	0.17	53
CYP2C19	0.03	9
CYP2D6	0.95	298
CYP3A	0.38	119

Table 2.3 THC IC50 [22]

Cytochrome P450	Micromolar/ml	Ng/ml
CYP1A2	0.06	18.9
CYP2C9	0.012	6.3
CYP2C19	0.57	179.3
CYP2D6	1.28	402.6
CYP3A	1.30	408.9

Combinations of oral CBD and THC (10 mg /10 mg) produce serum levels of 2.5 ng/mL of CBD and 6.4 ng/mL of THC [25, 276]. Nabiximols, at low doses (THC 5.4 mg/CBD 5 mg), produces a THC C-max of 5.1 ng/ml and CBD 1.6 ng/ml. High-dose nabiximols (THC 16.2 mg / CBD 15 mg) produces a THC C-max of 15.3 ng/ml and CBD 6.7 ng/ml [176].

High-dose CBD is sometimes dispensed in American dispensaries and has been a standard for seizures with doses ranging between 5 and 20 mg/kg (GW Pharmaceuticals, Epidiolex ™). A median 5 mg/kg dose produces a C-max of 296 ng/mL, a 10 mg/kg dose will produce a C-max of 598 ng/mL, and a 20 mg/kg dose will produce an average C max of 1180 ng/mL. At 48 hours serum levels will be 10 ng/mL and at 120 hours 5–10 ng/mL by single-dose pharmacokinetics [277]. A second study of a single dose of 750 mg, 1500 mg, and 4500 mg produced a C-max of 336 ng/mL, 524 ng/mL, and 427 ng/mL, respectively.

As seen earlier, saturation to absorption of CBD occurs at higher doses [309]. A fed state will increase CBD absorption. In a fasting state, a dose of 750 mg of CBD produces a C-max of 187 ng/mL, whereas with a high-fat meal, the C-max is 1050 ng/mL with the same dose. Alcohol increases the absorption of CBD as well; a 750 mg dose given with alcohol leading to a C-max is 354 ng/mL [252, 339]. This C-max occurs at 3–5 hours, and blood levels thereafter rapidly decline. A 200 mg dose of the commercially available CBD (Epidiolex ™) produces a C-max between 150 and 200 ng/ml at 3–5 hours which rapidly declines to <10 ng/ml at 12 hours [341]. It is likely that CYP2C enzymes will be inhibited by CBD during this time period. The transient high levels and rapid distribution of CBD suggests that blood levels of CBD for most of the day will be below the IC50 for CYP3A, CYP2D6, and likely CYP1A2. An important point to make, however, is that blood levels of CBD may not reflect tissue levels where cytochrome enzymes are located. Nevertheless CBD has been labeled as a "major inhibitor" of CYP3A4, yet there are no interactions noted clinically between CBD and midazolam, a CYP3A4 substrate [111, 252]. Certainly at usual doses as used with nabiximols, CBD will not have significant drug-drug interactions with CYP1A2, CYP2D6, or CYP3A4.

CBD concentrations reported to inhibit P-glycoprotein range between 3 and 100 umol or approximately 1ug/ml (1000 ng/ml) [69, 166]. A single high CBD dose (800 mg) will produce a C-max in a normal individual of about 221 ng/ml [231]. Thus, CBD is unlikely to block efflux pumps.

2.18 Pharmacokinetic Cannabis-Drug Interactions: Relevant Examples

2.18.1 Corticosteroids

Dexamethasone is metabolized by CYP3A4. As mentioned above, very high doses of CBD may potentially delay clearance of dexamethasone [391]. Interactions will not occur with standard CBD doses, however.

2.18.2 Nonsteroidal Anti-inflammatory Drugs

Naproxen is metabolized by CYP2C9. Both THC and CBD may potentially delay naproxen clearance at standard doses. In vitro studies have confirmed the potential drug-drug interaction with CBD. There are no clinical studies to validate the in vitro studies [391].

2.18.3 Opioids

Tramadol conversion to the active metabolite, desmethyltramadol, is through CYP2D6. Interactions between CBD and tramadol will not occur at standard doses. There are no studies which have evaluated potential drug-drug interactions with high-dose CBD. Fentanyl is metabolized to an inactive metabolite, norfentanyl, through CYP3A4 [378]. The combination of fentanyl 0.5 ug/kg plus CBD (400 and 800 mg) does not produce respiratory depression or cardiovascular complications indirectly implying a lack of drug interaction. CBD pharmacokinetics were obtained in this study, but not for fentanyl. CBD pharmacokinetics were carried out for only 8 hours [231]. Hence there are multiple shortcomings to this study. Further studies will be needed to establish the safety of fentanyl and high-dose CBD. There are no studies which have evaluated CBD and methadone interactions either. Methadone is metabolized through multiple cytochromes which may be blocked by high-dose CBD and thus requires closer monitoring.

2.18.4 Antidepressants

Sertraline is metabolized through CYP3A4; paroxetine through CYP2D6; mirtazapine by CYP1A2, CYP2D6, and CYP3A4; and citalopram by CYP3A4 and CYP2C19. Fluoxetine is metabolized by CYP2D6 and CYP2C9. Except for fluoxetine and citalopram, most commonly used antidepressants will not have drug-drug interactions with standard cannabis doses of either CBD or THC. Amitriptyline is cleared by multiple cytochromes including CYP2D6, CYP2C19, CYP3A4, CYP1A2, and CYP2C9. Metabolism through multiple cytochromes is likely to diminish interactions at CYP2C with standard cannabis doses. However, studies are needed to determine the safety of amitriptyline and high-dose CBD [378].

2.18.5 Janus Kinase Inhibitors

Tofacitinib, used to treat rheumatoid arthritis, is metabolized mainly through CYP3A4 but also by CYP2C19 which may be inhibited by CBD at usual doses [378].

2.18.6 Antipsychotics

Smoked cannabis increases CYP1A2 activity, as previously mentioned. In regular users of cannabis (defined as two cigarettes per week), olanzapine clearance was increased through CYP1A2 [72]. Furthermore, most antipsychotics are P-glycoprotein substrates [36, 92]. THC acutely stimulates P-glycoprotein; risperidone (a P-glycoprotein substrate) and its metabolite 9-hydroxy-risperidone show reduced brain levels with THC [49].

Clozapine is not a P-glycoprotein substrate, and thus it may be preferred in schizophrenic patients who use cannabis [49, 121, 198]. High-dose CBD does inhibit P-glycoprotein and ABCG2 which may potentially increase CNS levels of certain antipsychotics [101, 102].

2.18.7 Anticonvulsants

Epidiolex ™ is approved by the Federal Drug Administration for seizures associated with the Lennox-Gastaut syndrome and the Dravet Syndrome and is available as an extract containing 100 mg/ml of CBD. Benefits were observed in three studies using doses up to 20 milligrams/kilogram per day. Three other antiseizure medications are commonly used in these two syndromes: clobazam, stiripentol, and valproic acid. Clobazam is metabolized to N-desmethylclobazam by CYP3A4, and this metabolite is subsequently metabolized by CYP2C19. Hence, the active metabolite N-desmethylclobazam accumulates with high-dose CBD exposure [85, 122–124, 355]. Stiripentol is an inhibitor of CYP3A4 and CYP2C19 and may contribute to the drug interactions [252, 274, 349]. Valproic acid undergoes glucuronidation and then beta oxidation and thus does not have drug-drug interactions with CBD [114, 252, 355].

CBD increases N-desmethylclobazam exposure (AUC and C-max) by 3.4-fold, and stiripentol increases N-desmethylclobazam exposure 1.7-fold. Clobazam increases the CBD metabolite 7-OH-CBD (C-max 1.7-fold and AUC 1.5-fold). Stiripentol increases clobazam exposure with a C-max and AUC 1.29-fold which is not clinically significant [252].

CBD doses of 5–50 mg/kg increases serum levels of topiramate and rufinamide but not valproic acid, levetiracetam, phenobarbital, clonazepam, phenytoin, carbamazepine, lamotrigine, oxcarbazepine, ethosuximide, vigabatrin, pregabalin, and lacosamide [111]. Brivaracetam is approved in Europe which undergoes CYP2C19 metabolism. Brivaracetam blood levels are increased with CBD 5-20 mg/kg. Dose reductions of brivaracetam are needed if combined with high-dose CBD [185].

2.18.8 Benzodiazepines

Both midazolam and clonazepam are metabolized by CYP3A4. As mentioned, neither midazolam nor clonazepam pharmacokinetics were altered by high-dose CBD [111, 252].

2.18.9 Ethanol

CBD inhibits ethanol glucuronidation by UGT1A9 and UGT2B7 at blood levels of 1.17 ng/ml. Cannabinol (CBN) increases ethanol glucuronidation also and in a concentration-dependent manner [4]. Ethyl glucuronide, the direct metabolite of ethanol, demonstrates lower levels in urine with cannabis use if CBD is the prominent constituent. This may confound urine screening for alcohol. Individuals on CBD should be warned about interactions with alcohol. This may be a particular issue if CBD is used as maintenance therapy for alcoholism where it tends to reduce craving related to alcohol-related cues [351]. Low doses of alcohol have been shown to increase blood THC levels [292]. Ethanol prolongs THC elimination by ethanol-mediated changes in THC distribution [347].

2.18.10 Anticoagulants

Direct oral anticoagulants dabigatran, elexilate, rivaroxaban, edoxaban, and apixaban are P-glycoprotein substrates but not metabolized through the CYP2C family of mixed function oxidases. Drug interactions are unlikely to occur unless patients are on very high doses of CBD. Inhibition of CYP3A4 interferes with rivaroxaban and apixaban [356]. Again, it would require high doses of CBD to inhibit this class of anticoagulants.

Warfarin is metabolized through CYP2C9. Case reports of drug interactions following recreational cannabis have been published. CBD doses of 5 mg/kg increase the INR [44, 78]. Doses of THC in recreational cannabis are likely to interact with warfarin as well, and thus, cannabis use may require more frequent INR monitoring.

2.18.11 Antiplatelet Medications

Clopidogrel is a prodrug which needs to be converted to its active metabolite through CYP2C19. CBD inhibits CYP2C19 and prevents the formation of this active metabolite. Case reports, one in vitro study, and a pharmacokinetic study provide evidence that this interaction is clinically relevant [125]. Patients taking clopidogrel should avoid using cannabis, or switch to another antiplatelet such as ticagrelor, which is not affected by this type of interaction.

2.18.12 HIV Medications

Cannabis users are significantly more likely to have uncontrolled HIV (17%) compared with those who do not use cannabis (4%) [175]. Daily cannabis use does not influence optimal adherence to HIV medications [320].

There are small changes in indinavir and nelfinavir pharmacokinetics with dronabinol (7.5 mg/d) which are not clinically relevant [192].

2.18.13 *Theophylline*

Smoked cannabis upregulates CYP1A2 which increases theophylline clearance. Two "joints" per week increase theophylline clearance by 70% [172, 197, 333].

2.18.14 *Chemotherapy*

A cannabis preparation of 18% THC and 0.8% CBD for 15 days did not interfere with irinotecan pharmacokinetics. Cannabis tea does not influence the clearance of docetaxel, irinotecan, or its metabolites [96].

Cannabis consumption adversely affects checkpoint inhibitor responses. Cannabis consumption correlates with a significant decrease in time to tumor progression and overall survival [23]. As such, cannabis should not be used by patients while undergoing treatment with checkpoint inhibitors.

2.19 Conclusion

Many drug classes have interactions with the endocannabinoid system (ECS) which result in either clinical benefit or toxicity. We know a substantial amount about the pharmacokinetics of CBD and THC but little about the minor phytocannabinoids. THC and CBD drug-drug interactions are largely through the CYP2C family of mixed function oxidases. High-dose CBD has other clinically relevant drug-drug interactions though this is yet to be fully defined clinically. The most clinically significant drug interactions include checkpoint inhibitors, clopidogrel, and warfarin.

References

1. Drug interactions with cannabis. Prescrire Int. 2011;20(115):100.
2. Adamczyk P, Golda A, McCreary AC, Filip M, Przegalinski E. Activation of endocannabinoid transmission induces antidepressant-like effects in rats. J Physiol Pharmacol. 2008;59(2):217–28.
3. Agurell S, Halldin M, Lindgren JE, Ohlsson A, Widman M, Gillespie H, Hollister L. Pharmacokinetics and metabolism of delta 1-tetrahydrocannabinol and other cannabinoids with emphasis on man. Pharmacol Rev. 1986;38(1):21–43.
4. Al Saabi A, Allorge D, Sauvage FL, Tournel G, Gaulier JM, Marquet P, Picard N. Involvement of UDP-glucuronosyltransferases UGT1A9 and UGT2B7 in ethanol glucuronidation, and interactions with common drugs of abuse. Drug Metab Dispos. 2013;41(3):568–74.

5. Alhouayek M, Muccioli GG. COX-2-derived endocannabinoid metabolites as novel inflammatory mediators. Trends Pharmacol Sci. 2014;35(6):284–92.
6. Allen KV, McGregor IS, Hunt GE, Singh ME, Mallet PE. Regional differences in naloxone modulation of Delta(9)-THC induced Fos expression in rat brain. Neuropharmacology. 2003;44(2):264–74.
7. Alonso R, Voutsinos B, Fournier M, Labie C, Steinberg R, Souilhac J, Le Fur G, Soubrie P. Blockade of cannabinoid receptors by SR141716 selectively increases Fos expression in rat mesocorticolimbic areas via reduced dopamine D2 function. Neuroscience. 1999;91(2):607–20.
8. Alvheim AR, Malde MK, Osei-Hyiaman D, Lin YH, Pawlosky RJ, Madsen L, Kristiansen K, Froyland L, Hibbeln JR. Dietary linoleic acid elevates endogenous 2-AG and anandamide and induces obesity. Obesity (Silver Spring). 2012;20(10):1984–94.
9. Anderson GD, Chan LN. Pharmacokinetic drug interactions with tobacco, cannabinoids and smoking cessation products. Clin Pharmacokinet. 2016;55(11):1353–68.
10. Andrianova EL, Genrikhs EE, Bobrov MY, Lizhin AA, Gretskaya NM, Frumkina LE, Khaspekov LG, Bezuglov VV. In vitro effects of anandamide and prostamide e2 on normal and transformed nerve cells. Bull Exp Biol Med. 2011;151(1):30–2.
11. Anzenbacher P, Anzenbacherova E. Cytochromes P450 and metabolism of xenobiotics. Cell Mol Life Sci. 2001;58(5–6):737–47.
12. Apaya MK, Hsiao PW, Yang YC, Shyur LF. Deregulating the CYP2C19/epoxy-Eicosatrienoic acid-associated FABP4/FABP5 Signaling network as a therapeutic approach for metastatic triple-negative breast cancer. Cancers (Basel). 2020;12(1):199.
13. Arnold JC, Boucher AA, Karl T. The yin and yang of cannabis-induced psychosis: the actions of Delta(9)-tetrahydrocannabinol and cannabidiol in rodent models of schizophrenia. Curr Pharm Des. 2012a;18(32):5113–30.
14. Arnold JC, Hone P, Holland ML, Allen JD. CB2 and TRPV1 receptors mediate cannabinoid actions on MDR1 expression in multidrug resistant cells. Pharmacol Rep. 2012b;64(3):751–7.
15. Aso E, Ozaita A, Valdizan EM, Ledent C, Pazos A, Maldonado R, Valverde O. BDNF impairment in the hippocampus is related to enhanced despair behavior in CB1 knockout mice. J Neurochem. 2008;105(2):565–72.
16. Atone J, Wagner K, Hashimoto K, Hammock BD. Cytochrome P450 derived epoxidized fatty acids as a therapeutic tool against neuroinflammatory diseases. Prostaglandins Other Lipid Mediat. 2020;147:106385.
17. Atwal N, Casey SL, Mitchell VA, Vaughan CW. THC and gabapentin interactions in a mouse neuropathic pain model. Neuropharmacology. 2019;144:115–21.
18. Auzmendi J, Palestro P, Blachman A, Gavernet L, Merelli A, Talevi A, Calabrese GC, Ramos AJ, Lazarowski A. Cannabidiol (CBD) inhibited Rhodamine-123 efflux in cultured vascular endothelial cells and astrocytes under hypoxic conditions. Front Behav Neurosci. 2020;14:32.
19. Avraham Y, Grigoriadis N, Poutahidis T, Vorobiev L, Magen I, Ilan Y, Mechoulam R, Berry E. Cannabidiol improves brain and liver function in a fulminant hepatic failure-induced model of hepatic encephalopathy in mice. Br J Pharmacol. 2011;162(7):1650–8.
20. Bambico FR, Katz N, Debonnel G, Gobbi G. Cannabinoids elicit antidepressant-like behavior and activate serotonergic neurons through the medial prefrontal cortex. J Neurosci. 2007;27(43):11700–11.
21. Banni S, Carta G, Murru E, Cordeddu L, Giordano E, Sirigu AR, Berge K, Vik H, Maki KC, Di Marzo V, Griinari M. Krill oil significantly decreases 2-arachidonoylglycerol plasma levels in obese subjects. Nutr Metab (Lond). 2011;8(1):7.
22. Bansal S, Maharao N, Paine MF, Unadkat JD. Predicting the potential for cannabinoids to precipitate pharmacokinetic drug interactions via reversible inhibition or inactivation of major cytochromes P450. Drug Metab Dispos. 2020;48(10):1008–17.
23. Bar-Sela G, Cohen I, Campisi-Pinto S, Lewitus GM, Oz-Ari L, Jehassi A, Peer A, Turgeman I, Vernicova O, Berman P, Wollner M, Moskovitz M, Meiri D. Cannabis consumption used

by cancer patients during immunotherapy correlates with poor clinical outcome. Cancers (Basel). 2020;12(9):2447.
24. Baracos VE, Mazurak VC, Bhullar AS. Cancer cachexia is defined by an ongoing loss of skeletal muscle mass. Ann Palliat Med. 2019;8(1):3–12.
25. Barco S, Fucile C, Manfredini L, De Grandis E, Gherzi M, Martelli A, Tripodi G, Mattioli F, Cangemi G. A UHPLC-MS/MS method for the quantification of Delta9-tetrahydrocannabinol and cannabidiol in decoctions and in plasma samples for therapeutic monitoring of medical cannabis. Bioanalysis. 2018;10(24):2003–14.
26. Beardsley PM, Balster RL, Harris LS. Dependence on tetrahydrocannabinol in rhesus monkeys. J Pharmacol Exp Ther. 1986;239(2):311–9.
27. Benyamina A, Bonhomme-Faivre L, Picard V, Sabbagh A, Richard D, Blecha L, Rahioui H, Karila L, Lukasiewicz M, Farinotti R, Picard V, Marill C, Reynaud M. Association between ABCB1 C3435T polymorphism and increased risk of cannabis dependence. Prog Neuro-Psychopharmacol Biol Psychiatry. 2009;33(7):1270–4.
28. Bergamaschi MM, Karschner EL, Goodwin RS, Scheidweiler KB, Hirvonen J, Queiroz RH, Huestis MA. Impact of prolonged cannabinoid excretion in chronic daily cannabis smokers' blood on per se drugged driving laws. Clin Chem. 2013;59(3):519–26.
29. Berger C, Schmid PC, Schabitz WR, Wolf M, Schwab S, Schmid HH. Massive accumulation of N-acylethanolamines after stroke. Cell signalling in acute cerebral ischemia? J Neurochem. 2004;88(5):1159–67.
30. Berrendero F, Maldonado R. Involvement of the opioid system in the anxiolytic-like effects induced by Delta(9)-tetrahydrocannabinol. Psychopharmacology. 2002;163(1):111–7.
31. Bhardwaj RK, Glaeser H, Becquemont L, Klotz U, Gupta SK, Fromm MF. Piperine, a major constituent of black pepper, inhibits human P-glycoprotein and CYP3A4. J Pharmacol Exp Ther. 2002;302(2):645–50.
32. Bhattacharyya S, Wilson R, Appiah-Kusi E, O'Neill A, Brammer M, Perez J, Murray R, Allen P, Bossong MG, McGuire P. Effect of Cannabidiol on medial temporal, midbrain, and striatal dysfunction in people at clinical high risk of psychosis: a randomized clinical trial. JAMA Psychiat. 2018;75(11):1107–17.
33. Bisogno T, Hanus L, De Petrocellis L, Tchilibon S, Ponde DE, Brandi I, Moriello AS, Davis JB, Mechoulam R, Di Marzo V. Molecular targets for cannabidiol and its synthetic analogues: effect on vanilloid VR1 receptors and on the cellular uptake and enzymatic hydrolysis of anandamide. Br J Pharmacol. 2001;134(4):845–52.
34. Boehnke KF, Scott JR, Litinas E, Sisley S, Williams DA, Clauw DJ. Pills to pot: observational analyses of cannabis substitution among medical cannabis users with chronic pain. J Pain. 2019;20(7):830–41.
35. Boggs DL, Surti T, Gupta A, Gupta S, Niciu M, Pittman B, Schnakenberg Martin AM, Thurnauer H, Davies A, D'Souza DC, Ranganathan M. The effects of cannabidiol (CBD) on cognition and symptoms in outpatients with chronic schizophrenia a randomized placebo controlled trial. Psychopharmacology. 2018;235(7):1923–32.
36. Bonhomme-Faivre L, Benyamina A, Reynaud M, Farinotti R, Abbara C. Disposition of Delta tetrahydrocannabinol in CF1 mice deficient in mdr1a P-glycoprotein. Addict Biol. 2008;13(3–4):295–300.
37. Bornheim LM, Kim KY, Li J, Perotti BY, Benet LZ. Effect of cannabidiol pretreatment on the kinetics of tetrahydrocannabinol metabolites in mouse brain. Drug Metab Dispos. 1995;23(8):825–31.
38. Bouquie R, Deslandes G, Mazare H, Cogne M, Mahe J, Gregoire M, Jolliet P. Cannabis and anticancer drugs: societal usage and expected pharmacological interactions - a review. Fundam Clin Pharmacol. 2018;32(5):462–84.
39. Bovasso G. The long-term treatment outcomes of depression and anxiety comorbid with substance abuse. J Behav Health Serv Res. 2001a;28(1):42–57.
40. Bovasso GB. Cannabis abuse as a risk factor for depressive symptoms. Am J Psychiatry. 2001b;158(12):2033–7.

41. Bowles NP, Hill MN, Bhagat SM, Karatsoreos IN, Hillard CJ, McEwen BS. Chronic, noninvasive glucocorticoid administration suppresses limbic endocannabinoid signaling in mice. Neuroscience. 2012;204:83–9.
42. Braida D, Iosue S, Pegorini S, Sala M. Delta9-tetrahydrocannabinol-induced conditioned place preference and intracerebroventricular self-administration in rats. Eur J Pharmacol. 2004;506(1):63–9.
43. Brenneman DE, Petkanas D, Kinney WA. Pharmacological comparisons between Cannabidiol and KLS-13019. J Mol Neurosci. 2018;66(1):121–34.
44. Brown GW, Bellnier TJ, Janda M, Miskowitz K. Delta-9-tetrahydrocannabinol dose increase leads to warfarin drug interaction and elevated INR. J Am Pharm Assoc (2003). 2020;61(1):e57–60.
45. Brown JD. Potential adverse drug events with tetrahydrocannabinol (THC) due to drug-drug interactions. J Clin Med. 2020;9(4):919.
46. Brown NK, Harvey DJ. In vivo metabolism of the ethyl homologues of delta-8-tetrahydrocannabinol and delta-9-tetrahydrocannabinol in the mouse. Biol Mass Spectrom. 1991;20(5):324–8.
47. Bruni N, Della Pepa C, Oliaro-Bosso S, Pessione E, Gastaldi D, Dosio F. Cannabinoid delivery systems for pain and inflammation treatment. Molecules. 2018;23(10):2478.
48. Brzozowska N, Li KM, Wang XS, Booth J, Stuart J, McGregor IS, Arnold JC. ABC transporters P-gp and Bcrp do not limit the brain uptake of the novel antipsychotic and anticonvulsant drug cannabidiol in mice. PeerJ. 2016;4:e2081.
49. Brzozowska NI, de Tonnerre EJ, Li KM, Wang XS, Boucher AA, Callaghan PD, Kuligowski M, Wong A, Arnold JC. The differential binding of antipsychotic drugs to the ABC transporter P-glycoprotein predicts cannabinoid-antipsychotic drug interactions. Neuropsychopharmacology. 2017;42(11):2222–31.
50. Budney AJ, Bickel WK, Amass L. Marijuana use and treatment outcome among opioid-dependent patients. Addiction. 1998;93(4):493–503.
51. Buoite Stella A, Gortan Cappellari G, Barazzoni R, Zanetti M. Update on the impact of omega 3 fatty acids on inflammation, insulin resistance and sarcopenia: a review. Int J Mol Sci. 2018;19(1):218.
52. Carlini EA, Mechoulam R, Lander N. Anticonvulsant activity of four oxygenated cannabidiol derivatives. Res Commun Chem Pathol Pharmacol. 1975;12(1):1–15.
53. Chavarria-Siles I, Contreras-Rojas J, Hare E, Walss-Bass C, Quezada P, Dassori A, Contreras S, Medina R, Ramirez M, Salazar R, Raventos H, Escamilla MA. Cannabinoid receptor 1 gene (CNR1) and susceptibility to a quantitative phenotype for hebephrenic schizophrenia. Am J Med Genet B Neuropsychiatr Genet. 2008;147(3):279–84.
54. Chen C, Bazan NG. Lipid signaling: sleep, synaptic plasticity, and neuroprotection. Prostaglandins Other Lipid Mediat. 2005;77(1–4):65–76.
55. Chen J, Chen JK, Falck JR, Guthi JS, Anjaiah S, Capdevila JH, Harris RC. Mitogenic activity and signaling mechanism of 2-(14,15- epoxyeicosatrienoyl)glycerol, a novel cytochrome p450 arachidonate metabolite. Mol Cell Biol. 2007;27(8):3023–34.
56. Chen P, Hu S, Yao J, Moore SA, Spector AA, Fang X. Induction of cyclooxygenase-2 by anandamide in cerebral microvascular endothelium. Microvasc Res. 2005;69(1–2):28–35.
57. Chidambaran V, Pilipenko V, Spruance K, Venkatasubramanian R, Niu J, Fukuda T, Mizuno T, Zhang K, Kaufman K, Vinks AA, Martin LJ, Sadhasivam S. Fatty acid amide hydrolase-morphine interaction influences ventilatory response to hypercapnia and postoperative opioid outcomes in children. Pharmacogenomics. 2017;18(2):143–56.
58. Christensen R, Kristensen PK, Bartels EM, Bliddal H, Astrup A. Efficacy and safety of the weight-loss drug rimonabant: a meta-analysis of randomised trials. Lancet. 2007;370(9600):1706–13.
59. Chu J, Zheng H, Zhang Y, Loh HH, Law PY. Agonist-dependent mu-opioid receptor signaling can lead to heterologous desensitization. Cell Signal. 2010;22(4):684–96.

60. Church SH, Rothenberg JL, Sullivan MA, Bornstein G, Nunes EV. Concurrent substance use and outcome in combined behavioral and naltrexone therapy for opiate dependence. Am J Drug Alcohol Abuse. 2001;27(3):441–52.
61. Cichewicz DL. Synergistic interactions between cannabinoid and opioid analgesics. Life Sci. 2004;74(11):1317–24.
62. Cichewicz DL, Haller VL, Welch SP. Changes in opioid and cannabinoid receptor protein following short-term combination treatment with delta(9)-tetrahydrocannabinol and morphine. J Pharmacol Exp Ther. 2001;297(1):121–7.
63. Cichewicz DL, Martin ZL, Smith FL, Welch SP. Enhancement mu opioid antinociception by oral delta9-tetrahydrocannabinol: dose-response analysis and receptor identification. J Pharmacol Exp Ther. 1999;289(2):859–67.
64. Cichewicz DL, Welch SP. Modulation of oral morphine antinociceptive tolerance and naloxone-precipitated withdrawal signs by oral Delta 9-tetrahydrocannabinol. J Pharmacol Exp Ther. 2003;305(3):812–7.
65. Cipriano M, Bjorklund E, Wilson AA, Congiu C, Onnis V, Fowler CJ. Inhibition of fatty acid amide hydrolase and cyclooxygenase by the N-(3-methylpyridin-2-yl)amide derivatives of flurbiprofen and naproxen. Eur J Pharmacol. 2013;720(1–3):383–90.
66. Clem SN, Bigand TL, Wilson M. Cannabis use motivations among adults prescribed opioids for pain versus opioid addiction. Pain Manag Nurs. 2020;21(1):43–7.
67. Cocco MT, Congiu C, Onnis V, Morelli M, Cauli O. Synthesis of ibuprofen heterocyclic amides and investigation of their analgesic and toxicological properties. Eur J Med Chem. 2003;38(5):513–8.
68. Colombero C, Cardenas S, Venara M, Martin A, Pennisi P, Barontini M, Nowicki S. Cytochrome 450 metabolites of arachidonic acid (20-HETE, 11,12-EET and 14,15-EET) promote pheochromocytoma cell growth and tumor associated angiogenesis. Biochimie. 2020;171–172:147–57.
69. Consroe P, Kennedy K, Schram K. Assay of plasma cannabidiol by capillary gas chromatography/ion trap mass spectroscopy following high-dose repeated daily oral administration in humans. Pharmacol Biochem Behav. 1991;40(3):517–22.
70. Cooper ZD, Bedi G, Ramesh D, Balter R, Comer SD, Haney M. Impact of co-administration of oxycodone and smoked cannabis on analgesia and abuse liability. Neuropsychopharmacology. 2018;43(10):2046–55.
71. Cooper ZD, Haney M. Opioid antagonism enhances marijuana's effects in heavy marijuana smokers. Psychopharmacology. 2010;211(2):141–8.
72. Cox EJ, Maharao N, Patilea-Vrana G, Unadkat JD, Rettie AE, McCune JS, Paine MF. A marijuana-drug interaction primer: precipitants, pharmacology, and pharmacokinetics. Pharmacol Ther. 2019;201:25–38.
73. Crockett J, Critchley D, Tayo B, Berwaerts J, Morrison G. A phase 1, randomized, pharmacokinetic trial of the effect of different meal compositions, whole milk, and alcohol on cannabidiol exposure and safety in healthy subjects. Epilepsia. 2020;61(2):267–77.
74. Crupi R, Paterniti I, Ahmad A, Campolo M, Esposito E, Cuzzocrea S. Effects of palmitoylethanolamide and luteolin in an animal model of anxiety/depression. CNS Neurol Disord Drug Targets. 2013;12(7):989–1001.
75. Czikora A, Lizanecz E, Boczan J, Darago A, Papp Z, Edes I, Toth A. Vascular metabolism of anandamide to arachidonic acid affects myogenic constriction in response to intraluminal pressure elevation. Life Sci. 2012;90(11–12):407–15.
76. D'Souza DC, Pittman B, Perry E, Simen A. Preliminary evidence of cannabinoid effects on brain-derived neurotrophic factor (BDNF) levels in humans. Psychopharmacology. 2009;202(4):569–78.
77. Dalton VS, Long LE, Weickert CS, Zavitsanou K. Paranoid schizophrenia is characterized by increased CB1 receptor binding in the dorsolateral prefrontal cortex. Neuropsychopharmacology. 2011;36(8):1620–30.

78. Damkier P, Lassen D, Christensen MMH, Madsen KG, Hellfritzsch M, Pottegard A. Interaction between warfarin and cannabis. Basic Clin Pharmacol Toxicol. 2019;124(1):28–31.
79. De Gregorio D, Manchia M, Carpiniello B, Valtorta F, Nobile M, Gobbi G, Comai S. Role of palmitoylethanolamide (PEA) in depression: Translational evidence: Special Section on "Translational and Neuroscience Studies in Affective Disorders". Section Editor, Maria Nobile MD, PhD. This Section of JAD focuses on the relevance of translational and neuroscience studies in providing a better understanding of the neural basis of affective disorders. The main aim is to briefly summaries relevant research findings in clinical neuroscience with particular regards to specific innovative topics in mood and anxiety disorders. J Affect Disord. 2019;255:195–200.
80. De Marchi N, De Petrocellis L, Orlando P, Daniele F, Fezza F, Di Marzo V. Endocannabinoid signalling in the blood of patients with schizophrenia. Lipids Health Dis. 2003;2:5.
81. De Petrocellis L, Ligresti A, Moriello AS, Allara M, Bisogno T, Petrosino S, Stott CG, Di Marzo V. Effects of cannabinoids and cannabinoid-enriched cannabis extracts on TRP channels and endocannabinoid metabolic enzymes. Br J Pharmacol. 2011;163(7):1479–94.
82. Dean B, Sundram S, Bradbury R, Scarr E, Copolov D. Studies on [3H]CP-55940 binding in the human central nervous system: regional specific changes in density of cannabinoid-1 receptors associated with schizophrenia and cannabis use. Neuroscience. 2001;103(1):9–15.
83. Dean C, Hillard CJ, Seagard JL, Hopp FA, Hogan QH. Upregulation of fatty acid amide hydrolase in the dorsal periaqueductal gray is associated with neuropathic pain and reduced heart rate in rats. Am J Physiol Regul Integr Comp Physiol. 2017;312(4):R585–96.
84. Delis F, Rosko L, Shroff A, Leonard KE, Thanos PK. Oral haloperidol or olanzapine intake produces distinct and region-specific increase in cannabinoid receptor levels that is prevented by high fat diet. Prog Neuropsychopharmacol Biol Psychiatry. 2017;79(Pt B):268–80.
85. Devinsky O, Patel AD, Thiele EA, Wong MH, Appleton R, Harden CL, Greenwood S, Morrison G, Sommerville K, G. P. A. S. Group. Randomized, dose-ranging safety trial of cannabidiol in Dravet syndrome. Neurology. 2018;90(14):e1204–11.
86. Di Girolamo FG, Situlin R, Mazzucco S, Valentini R, Toigo G, Biolo G. Omega-3 fatty acids and protein metabolism: enhancement of anabolic interventions for sarcopenia. Curr Opin Clin Nutr Metab Care. 2014;17(2):145–50.
87. Di S, Malcher-Lopes R, Halmos KC, Tasker JG. Nongenomic glucocorticoid inhibition via endocannabinoid release in the hypothalamus: a fast feedback mechanism. J Neurosci. 2003;23(12):4850–7.
88. Di S, Malcher-Lopes R, Marcheselli VL, Bazan NG, Tasker JG. Rapid glucocorticoid-mediated endocannabinoid release and opposing regulation of glutamate and gamma-aminobutyric acid inputs to hypothalamic magnocellular neurons. Endocrinology. 2005;146(10):4292–301.
89. Dinh TP, Carpenter D, Leslie FM, Freund TF, Katona I, Sensi SL, Kathuria S, Piomelli D. Brain monoglyceride lipase participating in endocannabinoid inactivation. Proc Natl Acad Sci U S A. 2002;99(16):10819–24.
90. Eggan SM, Hashimoto T, Lewis DA. Reduced cortical cannabinoid 1 receptor messenger RNA and protein expression in schizophrenia. Arch Gen Psychiatry. 2008;65(7):772–84.
91. Eggan SM, Stoyak SR, Verrico CD, Lewis DA. Cannabinoid CB1 receptor immunoreactivity in the prefrontal cortex: comparison of schizophrenia and major depressive disorder. Neuropsychopharmacology. 2010;35(10):2060–71.
92. Elkhayat HA, Aly RH, Elagouza IA, El-Kabarity RH, Galal YI. Role of P-glycoprotein inhibitors in children with drug-resistant epilepsy. Acta Neurol Scand. 2017;136(6):639–44.
93. Ellgren M, Spano SM, Hurd YL. Adolescent cannabis exposure alters opiate intake and opioid limbic neuronal populations in adult rats. Neuropsychopharmacology. 2007;32(3):607–15.
94. Endo T, Takeuchi T, Maehara S. Pharmacological characterization of a novel, potent, selective, and orally active fatty acid amide hydrolase inhibitor, PKM-833 [(R)-N-(pyridazin-3-yl)-4-(7-(trifluoromethyl)chroman-4-yl)piperazine-1-carboxami de] in rats: potential for the treatment of inflammatory pain. Pharmacol Res Perspect. 2020;8(2):e00569.

95. Endocannabinoid Research, G, De Filippis D, D'Amico A, Cipriano M, Petrosino S, Orlando P, Di Marzo V, Iuvone T. Levels of endocannabinoids and palmitoylethanolamide and their pharmacological manipulation in chronic granulomatous inflammation in rats. Pharmacol Res. 2010;61(4):321–8.
96. Engels FK, de Jong FA, Sparreboom A, Mathot RA, Loos WJ, Kitzen JJ, de Bruijn P, Verweij J, Mathijssen RH. Medicinal cannabis does not influence the clinical pharmacokinetics of irinotecan and docetaxel. Oncologist. 2007;12(3):291–300.
97. Epstein DH, Preston KL. Does cannabis use predict poor outcome for heroin-dependent patients on maintenance treatment? Past findings and more evidence against. Addiction. 2003;98(3):269–79.
98. Fattore L, Vigano D, Fadda P, Rubino T, Fratta W, Parolaro D. Bidirectional regulation of mu-opioid and CB1-cannabinoid receptor in rats self-administering heroin or WIN 55,212-2. Eur J Neurosci. 2007;25(7):2191–200.
99. Fawley JA, Hofmann ME, Andresen MC. Cannabinoid 1 and transient receptor potential vanilloid 1 receptors discretely modulate evoked glutamate separately from spontaneous glutamate transmission. J Neurosci. 2014;34(24):8324–32.
100. Fechtner S, Singh AK, Ahmed S. Role of cannabinoid receptor 2 in mediating interleukin-1beta-induced inflammation in rheumatoid arthritis synovial fibroblasts. Clin Exp Rheumatol. 2019;37(6):1026–35.
101. Feinshtein V, Erez O, Ben-Zvi Z, Erez N, Eshkoli T, Sheizaf B, Sheiner E, Huleihel M, Holcberg G. Cannabidiol changes P-gp and BCRP expression in trophoblast cell lines. PeerJ. 2013b;1:e153.
102. Feinshtein V, Erez O, Ben-Zvi Z, Eshkoli T, Sheizaf B, Sheiner E, Holcberg G. Cannabidiol enhances xenobiotic permeability through the human placental barrier by direct inhibition of breast cancer resistance protein: an ex vivo study. Am J Obstet Gynecol. 2013a;209(6):573.e571–15.
103. Fezza F, Bari M, Florio R, Talamonti E, Feole M, Maccarrone M. Endocannabinoids, related compounds and their metabolic routes. Molecules. 2014;19(11):17078–106.
104. Fidelman S, Mizrachi Zer-Aviv T, Lange R, Hillard CJ, Akirav I. Chronic treatment with URB597 ameliorates post-stress symptoms in a rat model of PTSD. Eur Neuropsychopharmacol. 2018;28(5):630–42.
105. Finn K. Why marijuana won't fix the opioid epidemic. Mo Med. 2019;116(5):363.
106. Fonseca BM, Costa MA, Almada M, Correia-da-Silva G, Teixeira NA. Endogenous cannabinoids revisited: a biochemistry perspective. Prostaglandins Other Lipid Mediat. 2013;102–103:13–30.
107. Foster BC, Abramovici H, Harris CS. Cannabis and cannabinoids: kinetics and interactions. Am J Med. 2019;132(11):1266–70.
108. Fowler CJ, Naidu PS, Lichtman A, Onnis V. The case for the development of novel analgesic agents targeting both fatty acid amide hydrolase and either cyclooxygenase or TRPV1. Br J Pharmacol. 2009;156(3):412–9.
109. Fraser GA. The use of a synthetic cannabinoid in the management of treatment-resistant nightmares in posttraumatic stress disorder (PTSD). CNS Neurosci Ther. 2009;15(1):84–8.
110. Garcia-Gutierrez MS, Manzanares J. The cannabinoid CB1 receptor is involved in the anxiolytic, sedative and amnesic actions of benzodiazepines. J Psychopharmacol. 2010;24(5):757–65.
111. Gaston TE, Bebin EM, Cutter GR, Liu Y, Szaflarski JP, Program UC. Interactions between cannabidiol and commonly used antiepileptic drugs. Epilepsia. 2017;58(9):1586–92.
112. Ghabrash MF, Coronado-Montoya S, Aoun J, Gagne AA, Mansour F, Ouellet-Plamondon C, Trepanier A, Jutras-Aswad D. Cannabidiol for the treatment of psychosis among patients with schizophrenia and other primary psychotic disorders: a systematic review with a risk of bias assessment. Psychiatry Res. 2020;286:112890.
113. Ghazizadeh-Hashemi M, Ghajar A, Shalbafan MR, Ghazizadeh-Hashemi F, Afarideh M, Malekpour F, Ghaleiha A, Ardebili ME, Akhondzadeh S. Palmitoylethanolamide as

adjunctive therapy in major depressive disorder: a double-blind, randomized and placebo-controlled trial. J Affect Disord. 2018;232:127–33.
114. Ghodke-Puranik Y, Thorn CF, Lamba JK, Leeder JS, Song W, Birnbaum AK, Altman RB, Klein TE. Valproic acid pathway: pharmacokinetics and pharmacodynamics. Pharmacogenet Genomics. 2013;23(4):236–41.
115. Giang DK, Cravatt BF. Molecular characterization of human and mouse fatty acid amide hydrolases. Proc Natl Acad Sci U S A. 1997;94(6):2238–42.
116. Giuffrida A, Leweke FM, Gerth CW, Schreiber D, Koethe D, Faulhaber J, Klosterkotter J, Piomelli D. Cerebrospinal anandamide levels are elevated in acute schizophrenia and are inversely correlated with psychotic symptoms. Neuropsychopharmacology. 2004;29(11):2108–14.
117. Glass M, Hong J, Sato TA, Mitchell MD. Misidentification of prostamides as prostaglandins. J Lipid Res. 2005;46(7):1364–8.
118. Gobbi G, Bambico FR, Mangieri R, Bortolato M, Campolongo P, Solinas M, Cassano T, Morgese MG, Debonnel G, Duranti A, Tontini A, Tarzia G, Mor M, Trezza V, Goldberg SR, Cuomo V, Piomelli D. Antidepressant-like activity and modulation of brain monoaminergic transmission by blockade of anandamide hydrolysis. Proc Natl Acad Sci U S A. 2005;102(51):18620–5.
119. Gonzalez S, Fernandez-Ruiz J, Sparpaglione V, Parolaro D, Ramos JA. Chronic exposure to morphine, cocaine or ethanol in rats produced different effects in brain cannabinoid CB(1) receptor binding and mRNA levels. Drug Alcohol Depend. 2002;66(1):77–84.
120. Goparaju SK, Ueda N, Yamaguchi H, Yamamoto S. Anandamide amidohydrolase reacting with 2-arachidonoylglycerol, another cannabinoid receptor ligand. FEBS Lett. 1998;422(1):69–73.
121. Green AI, Burgess ES, Dawson R, Zimmet SV, Strous RD. Alcohol and cannabis use in schizophrenia: effects of clozapine vs. risperidone. Schizophr Res. 2003;60(1):81–5.
122. Greenblatt DJ, Divoll M, Abernethy DR, Ochs HR, Shader RI. Clinical pharmacokinetics of the newer benzodiazepines. Clin Pharmacokinet. 1983a;8(3):233–52.
123. Greenblatt DJ, Divoll M, Puri SK, Ho I, Zinny MA, Shader RI. Clobazam kinetics in the elderly. Br J Clin Pharmacol. 1981;12(5):631–6.
124. Greenblatt DJ, Divoll M, Puri SK, Ho I, Zinny MA, Shader RI. Reduced single-dose clearance of clobazam in elderly men predicts increased multiple-dose accumulation. Clin Pharmacokinet. 1983b;8(1):83–94.
125. Greger J, Bates V, Mechtler L, Gengo F. A review of cannabis and interactions with anticoagulant and antiplatelet agents. J Clin Pharmacol. 2020;60(4):432–8.
126. Griebel G, Stemmelin J, Scatton B. Effects of the cannabinoid CB1 receptor antagonist rimonabant in models of emotional reactivity in rodents. Biol Psychiatry. 2005;57(3):261–7.
127. Gronewold A, Skopp G. A preliminary investigation on the distribution of cannabinoids in man. Forensic Sci Int. 2011;210(1–3):e7–e11.
128. Grotenhermen F. Pharmacokinetics and pharmacodynamics of cannabinoids. Clin Pharmacokinet. 2003;42(4):327–60.
129. Guindon J, De Lean A, Beaulieu P. Local interactions between anandamide, an endocannabinoid, and ibuprofen, a nonsteroidal anti-inflammatory drug, in acute and inflammatory pain. Pain. 2006a;121(1–2):85–93.
130. Guindon J, LoVerme J, De Lean A, Piomelli D, Beaulieu P. Synergistic antinociceptive effects of anandamide, an endocannabinoid, and nonsteroidal anti-inflammatory drugs in peripheral tissue: a role for endogenous fatty-acid ethanolamides? Eur J Pharmacol. 2006b;550(1–3):68–77.
131. Guo Z, Johnson V, Barrera J, Porras M, Hinojosa D, Hernandez I, McGarrah P, Potter DA. Targeting cytochrome P450-dependent cancer cell mitochondria: cancer associated CYPs and where to find them. Cancer Metastasis Rev. 2018;37(2–3):409–23.
132. Hallak JE, Dursun SM, Bosi DC, de Macedo LR, Machado-de-Sousa JP, Abrao J, Crippa JA, McGuire P, Krystal JH, Baker GB, Zuardi AW. The interplay of cannabinoid and NMDA

glutamate receptor systems in humans: preliminary evidence of interactive effects of cannabidiol and ketamine in healthy human subjects. Prog Neuro-Psychopharmacol Biol Psychiatry. 2011;35(1):198–202.
133. Hallak JE, Machado-de-Sousa JP, Crippa JA, Sanches RF, Trzesniak C, Chaves C, Bernardo SA, Regalo SC, Zuardi AW. Performance of schizophrenic patients in the Stroop Color Word Test and electrodermal responsiveness after acute administration of cannabidiol (CBD). Braz J Psychiatry. 2010;32(1):56–61.
134. Halldin MM, Isaac H, Widman M, Nilsson E, Ryrfeldt A. A comparison between the metabolism of delta 1-tetrahydrocannabinol by perfused lung and liver of rat and Guinea-pig. Xenobiotica. 1984;14(3):277–82.
135. Hallinan R, Crettol S, Agho K, Attia J, Besson J, Croquette-Krokar M, Hammig R, Deglon JJ, Byrne A, Ray J, Somogyi AA, Eap CB. Cannabis and benzodiazepines as determinants of methadone trough plasma concentration variability in maintenance treatment: a transnational study. Eur J Clin Pharmacol. 2009;65(11):1113–20.
136. Hamdani N, Tabeze JP, Ramoz N, Ades J, Hamon M, Sarfati Y, Boni C, Gorwood P. The CNR1 gene as a pharmacogenetic factor for antipsychotics rather than a susceptibility gene for schizophrenia. Eur Neuropsychopharmacol. 2008;18(1):34–40.
137. Haney M. Opioid antagonism of cannabinoid effects: differences between marijuana smokers and nonmarijuana smokers. Neuropsychopharmacology. 2007;32(6):1391–403.
138. Haney M, Bisaga A, Foltin RW. Interaction between naltrexone and oral THC in heavy marijuana smokers. Psychopharmacology. 2003;166(1):77–85.
139. Hansen HS. Palmitoylethanolamide and other anandamide congeners. Proposed role in the diseased brain. Exp Neurol. 2010;224(1):48–55.
140. Hartman RL, Brown TL, Milavetz G, Spurgin A, Gorelick DA, Gaffney G, Huestis MA. Controlled cannabis vaporizer administration: blood and plasma cannabinoids with and without alcohol. Clin Chem. 2015;61(6):850–69.
141. Harvey DJ, Brown NK. In vitro metabolism of the equatorial C11-methyl isomer of hexahydrocannabinol in several mammalian species. Drug Metab Dispos. 1991;19(3):714–6.
142. Hauer D, Schelling G, Gola H, Campolongo P, Morath J, Roozendaal B, Hamuni G, Karabatsiakis A, Atsak P, Vogeser M, Kolassa IT. Plasma concentrations of endocannabinoids and related primary fatty acid amides in patients with post-traumatic stress disorder. PLoS One. 2013;8(5):e62741.
143. Hesketh SA, Brennan AK, Jessop DS, Finn DP. Effects of chronic treatment with citalopram on cannabinoid and opioid receptor-mediated G-protein coupling in discrete rat brain regions. Psychopharmacology. 2008;198(1):29–36.
144. Hill MN, Barr AM, Ho WS, Carrier EJ, Gorzalka BB, Hillard CJ. Electroconvulsive shock treatment differentially modulates cortical and subcortical endocannabinoid activity. J Neurochem. 2007;103(1):47–56.
145. Hill MN, Bierer LM, Makotkine I, Golier JA, Galea S, McEwen BS, Hillard CJ, Yehuda R. Reductions in circulating endocannabinoid levels in individuals with post-traumatic stress disorder following exposure to the World Trade Center attacks. Psychoneuroendocrinology. 2013;38(12):2952–61.
146. Hill MN, Carrier EJ, Ho WS, Shi L, Patel S, Gorzalka BB, Hillard CJ. Prolonged glucocorticoid treatment decreases cannabinoid CB1 receptor density in the hippocampus. Hippocampus. 2008c;18(2):221–6.
147. Hill MN, Carrier EJ, McLaughlin RJ, Morrish AC, Meier SE, Hillard CJ, Gorzalka BB. Regional alterations in the endocannabinoid system in an animal model of depression: effects of concurrent antidepressant treatment. J Neurochem. 2008a;106(6):2322–36.
148. Hill MN, Gorzalka BB. Enhancement of anxiety-like responsiveness to the cannabinoid CB(1) receptor agonist HU-210 following chronic stress. Eur J Pharmacol. 2004;499(3):291–5.
149. Hill MN, Gorzalka BB. Is there a role for the endocannabinoid system in the etiology and treatment of melancholic depression? Behav Pharmacol. 2005a;16(5–6):333–52.

150. Hill MN, Gorzalka BB. Pharmacological enhancement of cannabinoid CB1 receptor activity elicits an antidepressant-like response in the rat forced swim test. Eur Neuropsychopharmacol. 2005b;15(6):593–9.
151. Hill MN, Ho WS, Hillard CJ, Gorzalka BB. Differential effects of the antidepressants tranylcypromine and fluoxetine on limbic cannabinoid receptor binding and endocannabinoid contents. J Neural Transm (Vienna). 2008b;115(12):1673–9.
152. Hill MN, Ho WS, Sinopoli KJ, Viau V, Hillard CJ, Gorzalka BB. Involvement of the endocannabinoid system in the ability of long-term tricyclic antidepressant treatment to suppress stress-induced activation of the hypothalamic-pituitary-adrenal axis. Neuropsychopharmacology. 2006;31(12):2591–9.
153. Hill MN, Miller GE, Carrier EJ, Gorzalka BB, Hillard CJ. Circulating endocannabinoids and N-acyl ethanolamines are differentially regulated in major depression and following exposure to social stress. Psychoneuroendocrinology. 2009;34(8):1257–62.
154. Hill MN, Miller GE, Ho WS, Gorzalka BB, Hillard CJ. Serum endocannabinoid content is altered in females with depressive disorders: a preliminary report. Pharmacopsychiatry. 2008d;41(2):48–53.
155. Hill MN, Patel S, Carrier EJ, Rademacher DJ, Ormerod BK, Hillard CJ, Gorzalka BB. Downregulation of endocannabinoid signaling in the hippocampus following chronic unpredictable stress. Neuropsychopharmacology. 2005;30(3):508–15.
156. Hindocha C, Cousijn J, Rall M, Bloomfield MAP. The effectiveness of cannabinoids in the treatment of Posttraumatic Stress Disorder (PTSD): a systematic review. J Dual Diagn. 2020;16(1):120–39.
157. Hlozek T, Uttl L, Kaderabek L, Balikova M, Lhotkova E, Horsley RR, Novakova P, Sichova K, Stefkova K, Tyls F, Kuchar M, Palenicek T. Pharmacokinetic and behavioural profile of THC, CBD, and THC+CBD combination after pulmonary, oral, and subcutaneous administration in rats and confirmation of conversion in vivo of CBD to THC. Eur Neuropsychopharmacol. 2017;27(12):1223–37.
158. Holland ML, Lau DT, Allen JD, Arnold JC. The multidrug transporter ABCG2 (BCRP) is inhibited by plant-derived cannabinoids. Br J Pharmacol. 2007;152(5):815–24.
159. Holland ML, Panetta JA, Hoskins JM, Bebawy M, Roufogalis BD, Allen JD, Arnold JC. The effects of cannabinoids on P-glycoprotein transport and expression in multidrug resistant cells. Biochem Pharmacol. 2006;71(8):1146–54.
160. Holt S, Paylor B, Boldrup L, Alajakku K, Vandevoorde S, Sundstrom A, Cocco MT, Onnis V, Fowler CJ. Inhibition of fatty acid amide hydrolase, a key endocannabinoid metabolizing enzyme, by analogues of ibuprofen and indomethacin. Eur J Pharmacol. 2007;565(1–3):26–36.
161. Hong S, Fan J, Kemmerer ES, Evans S, Li Y, Wiley JW. Reciprocal changes in vanilloid (TRPV1) and endocannabinoid (CB1) receptors contribute to visceral hyperalgesia in the water avoidance stressed rat. Gut. 2009;58(2):202–10.
162. Huestis MA, Cone EJ. Relationship of Delta 9-tetrahydrocannabinol concentrations in oral fluid and plasma after controlled administration of smoked cannabis. J Anal Toxicol. 2004;28(6):394–9.
163. Huestis MA, Scheidweiler KB, Saito T, Fortner N, Abraham T, Gustafson RA, Smith ML. Excretion of Delta9-tetrahydrocannabinol in sweat. Forensic Sci Int. 2008;174(2–3):173–7.
164. Hungund BL, Vinod KY, Kassir SA, Basavarajappa BS, Yalamanchili R, Cooper TB, Mann JJ, Arango V. Upregulation of CB1 receptors and agonist-stimulated [35S]GTPgammaS binding in the prefrontal cortex of depressed suicide victims. Mol Psychiatry. 2004;9(2):184–90.
165. Hutchins-Wiese HL, Li Y, Hannon K, Watkins BA. Hind limb suspension and long-chain omega-3 PUFA increase mRNA endocannabinoid system levels in skeletal muscle. J Nutr Biochem. 2012;23(8):986–93.
166. Ibeas Bih C, Chen T, Nunn AV, Bazelot M, Dallas M, Whalley BJ. Molecular targets of Cannabidiol in neurological disorders. Neurotherapeutics. 2015;12(4):699–730.

167. Imig JD. Epoxide hydrolase and epoxygenase metabolites as therapeutic targets for renal diseases. Am J Physiol Renal Physiol. 2005;289(3):F496–503.
168. Izgelov D, Domb AJ, Hoffman A. The effect of piperine on oral absorption of cannabidiol following acute vs. chronic administration. Eur J Pharm Sci. 2020;148:105313.
169. Jetly R, Heber A, Fraser G, Boisvert D. The efficacy of nabilone, a synthetic cannabinoid, in the treatment of PTSD-associated nightmares: a preliminary randomized, double-blind, placebo-controlled cross-over design study. Psychoneuroendocrinology. 2015;51:585–8.
170. Jhaveri MD, Richardson D, Robinson I, Garle MJ, Patel A, Sun Y, Sagar DR, Bennett AJ, Alexander SP, Kendall DA, Barrett DA, Chapman V. Inhibition of fatty acid amide hydrolase and cyclooxygenase-2 increases levels of endocannabinoid related molecules and produces analgesia via peroxisome proliferator-activated receptor-alpha in a model of inflammatory pain. Neuropharmacology. 2008;55(1):85–93.
171. Jiang R, Yamaori S, Takeda S, Yamamoto I, Watanabe K. Identification of cytochrome P450 enzymes responsible for metabolism of cannabidiol by human liver microsomes. Life Sci. 2011;89(5–6):165–70.
172. Jusko WJ, Gardner MJ, Mangione A, Schentag JJ, Koup JR, Vance JW. Factors affecting theophylline clearances: age, tobacco, marijuana, cirrhosis, congestive heart failure, obesity, oral contraceptives, benzodiazepines, barbiturates, and ethanol. J Pharm Sci. 1979;68(11):1358–66.
173. Jusko WJ, Schentag JJ, Clark JH, Gardner M, Yurchak AM. Enhanced biotransformation of theophylline in marihuana and tobacco smokers. Clin Pharmacol Ther. 1978;24(4):405–10.
174. Justinova Z, Munzar P, Panlilio LV, Yasar S, Redhi GH, Tanda G, Goldberg SR. Blockade of THC-seeking behavior and relapse in monkeys by the cannabinoid CB(1)-receptor antagonist rimonabant. Neuropsychopharmacology. 2008;33(12):2870–7.
175. Kalichman SC, Washington C, Kegler C, Grebler T, Kalichman MO, Cherry C, Eaton L. Continued substance use among people living with HIV-hepatitis-C co-infection and receiving antiretroviral therapy. Subst Use Misuse. 2015;50(12):1536–43.
176. Karschner EL, Darwin WD, Goodwin RS, Wright S, Huestis MA. Plasma cannabinoid pharmacokinetics following controlled oral delta9-tetrahydrocannabinol and oromucosal cannabis extract administration. Clin Chem. 2011;57(1):66–75.
177. Karschner EL, Schwilke EW, Lowe RH, Darwin WD, Pope HG, Herning R, Cadet JL, Huestis MA. Do Delta9-tetrahydrocannabinol concentrations indicate recent use in chronic cannabis users? Addiction. 2009;104(12):2041–8.
178. Karschner EL, Schwope DM, Schwilke EW, Goodwin RS, Kelly DL, Gorelick DA, Huestis MA. Predictive model accuracy in estimating last Delta9-tetrahydrocannabinol (THC) intake from plasma and whole blood cannabinoid concentrations in chronic, daily cannabis smokers administered subchronic oral THC. Drug Alcohol Depend. 2012;125(3):313–9.
179. Karschner EL, Swortwood MJ, Hirvonen J, Goodwin RS, Bosker WM, Ramaekers JG, Huestis MA. Extended plasma cannabinoid excretion in chronic frequent cannabis smokers during sustained abstinence and correlation with psychomotor performance. Drug Test Anal. 2016;8(7):682–9.
180. Kathuria S, Gaetani S, Fegley D, Valino F, Duranti A, Tontini A, Mor M, Tarzia G, La Rana G, Calignano A, Giustino A, Tattoli M, Palmery M, Cuomo V, Piomelli D. Modulation of anxiety through blockade of anandamide hydrolysis. Nat Med. 2003;9(1):76–81.
181. Kebir O, Lafaye G, Blecha L, Chaumette B, Mouaffak F, Laqueille X, Benyamina A. ABCB1 C3435T polymorphism is associated with tetrahydrocannabinol blood levels in heavy cannabis users. Psychiatry Res. 2018;262:357–8.
182. Kelly DL, Gorelick DA, Conley RR, Boggs DL, Linthicum J, Liu F, Feldman S, Ball MP, Wehring HJ, McMahon RP, Huestis MA, Heishman SJ, Warren KR, Buchanan RW. Effects of the cannabinoid-1 receptor antagonist rimonabant on psychiatric symptoms in overweight people with schizophrenia: a randomized, double-blind, pilot study. J Clin Psychopharmacol. 2011;31(1):86–91.

183. Kim J, Alger BE. Inhibition of cyclooxygenase-2 potentiates retrograde endocannabinoid effects in hippocampus. Nat Neurosci. 2004;7(7):697–8.
184. Kiso T, Watabiki T, Sekizawa T. ASP8477, a fatty acid amide hydrolase inhibitor, exerts analgesic effects in rat models of neuropathic and dysfunctional pain. Eur J Pharmacol. 2020;881:173194.
185. Klotz KA, Hirsch M, Heers M, Schulze-Bonhage A, Jacobs J. Effects of cannabidiol on brivaracetam plasma levels. Epilepsia. 2019;60(7):e74–7.
186. Ko JY, Wu RW, Kuo SJ, Chen MW, Yeh DW, Ke HC, Wu SL, Wang FS. Cannabinoid receptor 1 mediates glucocorticoid-induced bone loss in rats by perturbing bone mineral acquisition and marrow adipogenesis. Arthritis Rheum. 2012;64(4):1204–14.
187. Koethe D, Giuffrida A, Schreiber D, Hellmich M, Schultze-Lutter F, Ruhrmann S, Klosterkotter J, Piomelli D, Leweke FM. Anandamide elevation in cerebrospinal fluid in initial prodromal states of psychosis. Br J Psychiatry. 2009;194(4):371–2.
188. Koethe D, Llenos IC, Dulay JR, Hoyer C, Torrey EF, Leweke FM, Weis S. Expression of CB1 cannabinoid receptor in the anterior cingulate cortex in schizophrenia, bipolar disorder, and major depression. J Neural Transm (Vienna). 2007;114(8):1055–63.
189. Kola B, Farkas I, Christ-Crain M, Wittmann G, Lolli F, Amin F, Harvey-White J, Liposits Z, Kunos G, Grossman AB, Fekete C, Korbonits M. The orexigenic effect of ghrelin is mediated through central activation of the endogenous cannabinoid system. PLoS One. 2008;3(3):e1797.
190. Kong TY, Kim JH, Kim DK, Lee HS. Synthetic cannabinoids are substrates and inhibitors of multiple drug-metabolizing enzymes. Arch Pharm Res. 2018;41(7):691–710.
191. Kopelli E, Samara M, Siargkas A, Goulas A, Papazisis G, Chourdakis M. The role of cannabidiol oil in schizophrenia treatment. A systematic review and meta-analysis. Psychiatry Res. 2020;291:113246.
192. Kosel BW, Aweeka FT, Benowitz NL, Shade SB, Hilton JF, Lizak PS, Abrams DI. The effects of cannabinoids on the pharmacokinetics of indinavir and nelfinavir. AIDS. 2002;16(4):543–50.
193. Kozak KR, Crews BC, Ray JL, Tai HH, Morrow JD, Marnett LJ. Metabolism of prostaglandin glycerol esters and prostaglandin ethanolamides in vitro and in vivo. J Biol Chem. 2001;276(40):36993–8.
194. Kozak KR, Marnett LJ. Oxidative metabolism of endocannabinoids. Prostaglandins Leukot Essent Fatty Acids. 2002;66(2–3):211–20.
195. Kozak KR, Prusakiewicz JJ, Rowlinson SW, Prudhomme DR, Marnett LJ. Amino acid determinants in cyclooxygenase-2 oxygenation of the endocannabinoid anandamide. Biochemistry. 2003;42(30):9041–9.
196. Kozak KR, Rowlinson SW, Marnett LJ. Oxygenation of the endocannabinoid, 2-arachidonylglycerol, to glyceryl prostaglandins by cyclooxygenase-2. J Biol Chem. 2000;275(43):33744–9.
197. Kozak PP Jr. Factors that influence theophylline metabolism. West J Med. 1979;131(4):319–20.
198. Kreyenbuhl J, Nossel IR, Dixon LB. Disengagement from mental health treatment among individuals with schizophrenia and strategies for facilitating connections to care: a review of the literature. Schizophr Bull. 2009;35(4):696–703.
199. Lafourcade M, Larrieu T, Mato S, Duffaud A, Sepers M, Matias I, De Smedt-Peyrusse V, Labrousse VF, Bretillon L, Matute C, Rodriguez-Puertas R, Laye S, Manzoni OJ. Nutritional omega-3 deficiency abolishes endocannabinoid-mediated neuronal functions. Nat Neurosci. 2011;14(3):345–50.
200. Lai JCL, Lee DYH, Leung MOY, Lam YW. Daily hassles, loneliness, and diurnal salivary cortisol in emerging adults. Horm Behav. 2019;115:104558.
201. Landmark CJ, Brandl U. Pharmacology and drug interactions of cannabinoids. Epileptic Disord. 2020;22(S1):16–22.
202. Larrieu T, Madore C, Joffre C, Laye S. Nutritional n-3 polyunsaturated fatty acids deficiency alters cannabinoid receptor signaling pathway in the brain and associated anxiety-like behavior in mice. J Physiol Biochem. 2012;68(4):671–81.

203. Lee CR, Goldstein JA, Pieper JA. Cytochrome P450 2C9 polymorphisms: a comprehensive review of the in-vitro and human data. Pharmacogenetics. 2002;12(3):251–63.
204. Lee D, Bergamaschi MM, Milman G, Barnes AJ, Queiroz RH, Vandrey R, Huestis MA. Plasma cannabinoid pharmacokinetics after controlled smoking and ad libitum cannabis smoking in chronic frequent users. J Anal Toxicol. 2015;39(8):580–7.
205. Leineweber CG, Pietzner A, Zhang IW, Blessin UB, Rothe M, Schott E, Schebb NH, Weylandt KH. Assessment of the effect of Sorafenib on Omega-6 and Omega-3 Epoxyeicosanoid formation in patients with hepatocellular carcinoma. Int J Mol Sci. 2020;21(5):1875.
206. Leweke FM, Giuffrida A, Koethe D, Schreiber D, Nolden BM, Kranaster L, Neatby MA, Schneider M, Gerth CW, Hellmich M, Klosterkotter J, Piomelli D. Anandamide levels in cerebrospinal fluid of first-episode schizophrenic patients: impact of cannabis use. Schizophr Res. 2007;94(1–3):29–36.
207. Leweke FM, Giuffrida A, Wurster U, Emrich HM, Piomelli D. Elevated endogenous cannabinoids in schizophrenia. Neuroreport. 1999;10(8):1665–9.
208. Leweke FM, Mueller JK, Lange B, Fritze S, Topor CE, Koethe D, Rohleder C. Role of the endocannabinoid system in the pathophysiology of schizophrenia: implications for pharmacological intervention. CNS Drugs. 2018;32(7):605–19.
209. Leweke FM, Mueller JK, Lange B, Rohleder C. Therapeutic potential of cannabinoids in psychosis. Biol Psychiatry. 2016;79(7):604–12.
210. Leweke FM, Piomelli D, Pahlisch F, Muhl D, Gerth CW, Hoyer C, Klosterkotter J, Hellmich M, Koethe D. Cannabidiol enhances anandamide signaling and alleviates psychotic symptoms of schizophrenia. Transl Psychiatry. 2012;2:e94.
211. Lichtman AH, Sheikh SM, Loh HH, Martin BR. Opioid and cannabinoid modulation of precipitated withdrawal in delta(9)-tetrahydrocannabinol and morphine-dependent mice. J Pharmacol Exp Ther. 2001;298(3):1007–14.
212. Lies B, Martens S, Schmidt S, Boll M, Wenzel U. Flavone potently stimulates an apical transporter for flavonoids in human intestinal Caco-2 cells. Mol Nutr Food Res. 2012;56(11):1627–35.
213. Ligresti A, Moriello AS, Starowicz K, Matias I, Pisanti S, De Petrocellis L, Laezza C, Portella G, Bifulco M, Di Marzo V. Antitumor activity of plant cannabinoids with emphasis on the effect of cannabidiol on human breast carcinoma. J Pharmacol Exp Ther. 2006;318(3):1375–87.
214. Lile JA, Kelly TH, Pinsky DJ, Hays LR. Substitution profile of Delta9-tetrahydrocannabinol, triazolam, hydromorphone, and methylphenidate in humans discriminating Delta9-tetrahydrocannabinol. Psychopharmacology. 2009;203(2):241–50.
215. Lin F, Abraham NG, Schwartzman ML. Cytochrome P450 arachidonic acid omega-hydroxylation in the proximal tubule of the rat kidney. Ann N Y Acad Sci. 1994;744:11–24.
216. Liu J, Tawa GJ, Wallqvist A. Identifying cytochrome p450 functional networks and their allosteric regulatory elements. PLoS One. 2013;8(12):e81980.
217. Liu S, Baracos VE, Quinney HA, Clandinin MT. Dietary omega-3 and polyunsaturated fatty acids modify fatty acyl composition and insulin binding in skeletal-muscle sarcolemma. Biochem J. 1994;299(Pt 3):831–7.
218. Liu Z, Martin JH. Gaps in predicting clinical doses for cannabinoids therapy: overview of issues for pharmacokinetics and pharmacodynamics modelling. Br J Clin Pharmacol. 2018;84(11):2483–7.
219. Locci A, Geoffroy P, Miesch M, Mensah-Nyagan AG, Pinna G. Social isolation in early versus late adolescent mice is associated with persistent Behavioral deficits that can be improved by Neurosteroid-based treatment. Front Cell Neurosci. 2017;11:208.
220. Lopez-Moreno JA, Lopez-Jimenez A, Gorriti MA, de Fonseca FR. Functional interactions between endogenous cannabinoid and opioid systems: focus on alcohol, genetics and drug-addicted behaviors. Curr Drug Targets. 2010;11(4):406–28.
221. Lopez JF, Chalmers DT, Little KY, Watson SJ. A.E. Bennett Research Award. Regulation of serotonin1A, glucocorticoid, and mineralocorticoid receptor in rat and human hippocampus: implications for the neurobiology of depression. Biol Psychiatry. 1998;43(8):547–73.

222. Lowe RH, Karschner EL, Schwilke EW, Barnes AJ, Huestis MA. Simultaneous quantification of Delta9-tetrahydrocannabinol, 11-hydroxy-Delta9-tetrahydrocannabinol, and 11-nor-Delta9-tetrahydrocannabinol-9-carboxylic acid in human plasma using two-dimensional gas chromatography, cryofocusing, and electron impact-mass spectrometry. J Chromatogr A. 2007;1163(1–2):318–27.
223. Lucas CJ, Galettis P, Schneider J. The pharmacokinetics and the pharmacodynamics of cannabinoids. Br J Clin Pharmacol. 2018b;84(11):2477–82.
224. Lucas CJ, Galettis P, Song S, Solowij N, Reuter SE, Schneider J, Martin JH. Cannabinoid disposition after human intraperitoneal use: AnInsight into intraperitoneal pharmacokinetic properties in metastatic cancer. Clin Ther. 2018a;40(9):1442–7.
225. Lucas P, Baron EP, Jikomes N. Medical cannabis patterns of use and substitution for opioids & other pharmaceutical drugs, alcohol, tobacco, and illicit substances; results from a cross-sectional survey of authorized patients. Harm Reduct J. 2019;16(1):9.
226. Lynskey MT, Glowinski AL, Todorov AA, Bucholz KK, Madden PA, Nelson EC, Statham DJ, Martin NG, Heath AC. Major depressive disorder, suicidal ideation, and suicide attempt in twins discordant for cannabis dependence and early-onset cannabis use. Arch Gen Psychiatry. 2004;61(10):1026–32.
227. Madras BK. Are THC levels in oral fluids and blood plasma comparable after oral ingestion of edibles containing cannabis or THC? Clin Chem. 2017;63(3):629–31.
228. Maia J, Fonseca BM, Cunha SC, Braga J, Goncalves D, Teixeira N, Correia-da-Silva G. Impact of tetrahydrocannabinol on the endocannabinoid 2-arachidonoylglycerol metabolism: ABHD6 and ABHD12 as novel players in human placenta. Biochim Biophys Acta Mol Cell Biol Lipids. 2020;1865:158807.
229. Malcher-Lopes R, Di S, Marcheselli VS, Weng FJ, Stuart CT, Bazan NG, Tasker JG. Opposing crosstalk between leptin and glucocorticoids rapidly modulates synaptic excitation via endocannabinoid release. J Neurosci. 2006;26(24):6643–50.
230. Maldonado R, Valverde O. Participation of the opioid system in cannabinoid-induced antinociception and emotional-like responses. Eur Neuropsychopharmacol. 2003;13(6):401–10.
231. Manini AF, Yiannoulos G, Bergamaschi MM, Hernandez S, Olmedo R, Barnes AJ, Winkel G, Sinha R, Jutras-Aswad D, Huestis MA, Hurd YL. Safety and pharmacokinetics of oral cannabidiol when administered concomitantly with intravenous fentanyl in humans. J Addict Med. 2015;9(3):204–10.
232. Manzanares J, Corchero J, Romero J, Fernandez-Ruiz JJ, Ramos JA, Fuentes JA. Pharmacological and biochemical interactions between opioids and cannabinoids. Trends Pharmacol Sci. 1999;20(7):287–94.
233. Mato S, Aso E, Castro E, Martin M, Valverde O, Maldonado R, Pazos A. CB1 knockout mice display impaired functionality of 5-HT1A and 5-HT2A/C receptors. J Neurochem. 2007;103(5):2111–20.
234. Mato S, Vidal R, Castro E, Diaz A, Pazos A, Valdizan EM. Long-term fluoxetine treatment modulates cannabinoid type 1 receptor-mediated inhibition of adenylyl cyclase in the rat prefrontal cortex through 5-hydroxytryptamine 1A receptor-dependent mechanisms. Mol Pharmacol. 2010;77(3):424–34.
235. Matricon J, Seillier A, Giuffrida A. Distinct neuronal activation patterns are associated with PCP-induced social withdrawal and its reversal by the endocannabinoid-enhancing drug URB597. Neurosci Res. 2016;110:49–58.
236. Mazur A, Lichti CF, Prather PL, Zielinska AK, Bratton SM, Gallus-Zawada A, Finel M, Miller GP, Radominska-Pandya A, Moran JH. Characterization of human hepatic and extrahepatic UDP-glucuronosyltransferase enzymes involved in the metabolism of classic cannabinoids. Drug Metab Dispos. 2009;37(7):1496–504.
237. McGuire P, Robson P, Cubala WJ, Vasile D, Morrison PD, Barron R, Taylor A, Wright S. Cannabidiol (CBD) as an adjunctive therapy in schizophrenia: a multicenter randomized controlled trial. Am J Psychiatry. 2018;175(3):225–31.
238. McIntosh AL, Martin GG, Huang H, Landrock D, Kier AB, Schroeder F. Delta(9)-tetrahydrocannabinol induces endocannabinoid accumulation in mouse hepatocytes: antagonism by Fabp1 gene ablation. J Lipid Res. 2018;59(4):646–57.

239. McLaughlin RJ, Hill MN, Morrish AC, Gorzalka BB. Local enhancement of cannabinoid CB1 receptor signalling in the dorsal hippocampus elicits an antidepressant-like effect. Behav Pharmacol. 2007;18(5–6):431–8.
240. McPartland JM, Guy GW, Di Marzo V. Care and feeding of the endocannabinoid system: a systematic review of potential clinical interventions that upregulate the endocannabinoid system. PLoS One. 2014;9(3):e89566.
241. Medeiros P, de Freitas RL, Silva MO, Coimbra NC, Melo-Thomas L. CB1 cannabinoid receptor-mediated anandamide signaling mechanisms of the inferior colliculus modulate the haloperidol-induced catalepsy. Neuroscience. 2016;337:17–26.
242. Meltzer HY, Arvanitis L, Bauer D, Rein W, G. Meta-Trial Study. Placebo-controlled evaluation of four novel compounds for the treatment of schizophrenia and schizoaffective disorder. Am J Psychiatry. 2004;161(6):975–84.
243. Menzies JR, Ludwig M, Leng G. Direct and indirect effects of cannabinoids on in vitro GABA release in the rat arcuate nucleus. J Neuroendocrinol. 2010;22(6):585–92.
244. Micale V, Cristino L, Tamburella A, Petrosino S, Leggio GM, Drago F, Di Marzo V. Anxiolytic effects in mice of a dual blocker of fatty acid amide hydrolase and transient receptor potential vanilloid type-1 channels. Neuropsychopharmacology. 2009;34(3):593–606.
245. Millar SA, Stone NL, Bellman ZD, Yates AS, England TJ, O'Sullivan SE. A systematic review of cannabidiol dosing in clinical populations. Br J Clin Pharmacol. 2019;85(9):1888–900.
246. Millar SA, Stone NL, Yates AS, O'Sullivan SE. A systematic review on the pharmacokinetics of Cannabidiol in humans. Front Pharmacol. 2018;9:1365.
247. Mitchell MD, Sato TA, Wang A, Keelan JA, Ponnampalam AP, Glass M. Cannabinoids stimulate prostaglandin production by human gestational tissues through a tissue- and CB1-receptor-specific mechanism. Am J Physiol Endocrinol Metab. 2008;294(2):E352–6.
248. Mitra R, Guo Z, Milani M, Mesaros C, Rodriguez M, Nguyen J, Luo X, Clarke D, Lamba J, Schuetz E, Donner DB, Puli N, Falck JR, Capdevila J, Gupta K, Blair IA, Potter DA. CYP3A4 mediates growth of estrogen receptor-positive breast cancer cells in part by inducing nuclear translocation of phospho-Stat3 through biosynthesis of (+/−)-14,15-epoxyeicosatrienoic acid (EET). J Biol Chem. 2011;286(20):17543–59.
249. Miyata N, Seki T, Tanaka Y, Omura T, Taniguchi K, Doi M, Bandou K, Kametani S, Sato M, Okuyama S, Cambj-Sapunar L, Harder DR, Roman RJ. Beneficial effects of a new 20-hydroxyeicosatetraenoic acid synthesis inhibitor, TS-011 [N-(3-chloro-4-morpholin-4-yl) phenyl-N'-hydroxyimido formamide], on hemorrhagic and ischemic stroke. J Pharmacol Exp Ther. 2005;314(1):77–85.
250. Mizrachi Zer-Aviv T, Segev A, Akirav I. Cannabinoids and post-traumatic stress disorder: clinical and preclinical evidence for treatment and prevention. Behav Pharmacol. 2016;27(7):561–9.
251. Morano A, Fanella M, Albini M, Cifelli P, Palma E, Giallonardo AT, Di Bonaventura C. Cannabinoids in the treatment of epilepsy: current status and future prospects. Neuropsychiatr Dis Treat. 2020;16:381–96.
252. Morrison G, Crockett J, Blakey G, Sommerville K. A phase 1, open-label, pharmacokinetic trial to investigate possible drug-drug interactions between Clobazam, Stiripentol, or valproate and Cannabidiol in healthy subjects. Clin Pharmacol Drug Dev. 2019;8(8):1009–31.
253. Murphy N, Cowley TR, Blau CW, Dempsey CN, Noonan J, Gowran A, Tanveer R, Olango WM, Finn DP, Campbell VA, Lynch MA. The fatty acid amide hydrolase inhibitor URB597 exerts anti-inflammatory effects in hippocampus of aged rats and restores an age-related deficit in long-term potentiation. J Neuroinflammation. 2012;9:79.
254. Nadulski T, Pragst F, Weinberg G, Roser P, Schnelle M, Fronk EM, Stadelmann AM. Randomized, double-blind, placebo-controlled study about the effects of cannabidiol (CBD) on the pharmacokinetics of Delta9-tetrahydrocannabinol (THC) after oral application of THC verses standardized cannabis extract. Ther Drug Monit. 2005;27(6):799–810.
255. Nahler G, Grotenhermen F, Zuardi AW, Crippa JAS. A conversion of oral Cannabidiol to Delta9-tetrahydrocannabinol seems not to occur in humans. Cannabis Cannabinoid Res. 2017;2(1):81–6.

256. Nakazawa K, Costa E. Metabolism of delta 9 -tetrahydrocannabinol by lung and liver homogenates of rats treated with methylcholanthrene. Nature. 1971;234(5323):48–9.
257. Nava F, Manzato E, Lucchini A. Chronic cannabis use does not affect the normalization of hypothalamic-pituitary-adrenal (HPA) axis induced by methadone in heroin addicts. Prog Neuro-Psychopharmacol Biol Psychiatry. 2007;31(5):1089–94.
258. Navarro M, Carrera MR, Fratta W, Valverde O, Cossu G, Fattore L, Chowen JA, Gomez R, del Arco I, Villanua MA, Maldonado R, Koob GF, Rodriguez de Fonseca F. Functional interaction between opioid and cannabinoid receptors in drug self-administration. J Neurosci. 2001;21(14):5344–50.
259. Newell KA, Deng C, Huang XF. Increased cannabinoid receptor density in the posterior cingulate cortex in schizophrenia. Exp Brain Res. 2006;172(4):556–60.
260. Ney LJ, Matthews A, Bruno R, Felmingham KL. Cannabinoid interventions for PTSD: where to next? Prog Neuro-Psychopharmacol Biol Psychiatry. 2019;93:124–40.
261. Nielsen S, Sabioni P, Trigo JM, Ware MA, Betz-Stablein BD, Murnion B, Lintzeris N, Khor KE, Farrell M, Smith A, Le Foll B. Opioid-sparing effect of cannabinoids: a systematic review and meta-analysis. Neuropsychopharmacology. 2017;42(9):1752–65.
262. Nomura DK, Morrison BE, Blankman JL, Long JZ, Kinsey SG, Marcondes MC, Ward AM, Hahn YK, Lichtman AH, Conti B, Cravatt BF. Endocannabinoid hydrolysis generates brain prostaglandins that promote neuroinflammation. Science. 2011;334(6057):809–13.
263. O'Sullivan SE, Kendall DA. Cannabinoid activation of peroxisome proliferator-activated receptors: potential for modulation of inflammatory disease. Immunobiology. 2010;215(8):611–6.
264. O'Sullivan SE, Sun Y, Bennett AJ, Randall MD, Kendall DA. Time-dependent vascular actions of cannabidiol in the rat aorta. Eur J Pharmacol. 2009;612(1–3):61–8.
265. Oh DA, Parikh N, Khurana V, Cognata Smith C, Vetticaden S. Effect of food on the pharmacokinetics of dronabinol oral solution versus dronabinol capsules in healthy volunteers. Clin Pharmacol. 2017;9:9–17.
266. Ohlsson A, Lindgren JE, Andersson S, Agurell S, Gillespie H, Hollister LE. Single-dose kinetics of deuterium-labelled cannabidiol in man after smoking and intravenous administration. Biomed Environ Mass Spectrom. 1986;13(2):77–83.
267. Ohlsson A, Lindgren JE, Wahlen A, Agurell S, Hollister LE, Gillespie HK. Plasma delta-9 tetrahydrocannabinol concentrations and clinical effects after oral and intravenous administration and smoking. Clin Pharmacol Ther. 1980a;28(3):409–16.
268. Ohlsson A, Widman M, Carlsson S, Ryman T, Strid C. Plasma and brain levels of delta 6-THC and seven monooxygenated metabolites correlated to the cataleptic effect in the mouse. Acta Pharmacol Toxicol (Copenh). 1980b;47(4):308–17.
269. Okusanya BO, Asaolu IO, Ehiri JE, Kimaru LJ, Okechukwu A, Rosales C. Medical cannabis for the reduction of opioid dosage in the treatment of non-cancer chronic pain: a systematic review. Syst Rev. 2020;9(1):167.
270. Olatinsu AO, Sihag J, Jones PJH. Relationship between circulating fatty acids and fatty acid Ethanolamide levels after a single 2-h dietary fat feeding in male Sprague-Dawley rats : elevated levels of oleoylethanolamide, palmitoylethanolamide, linoleoylethanolamide, arachidonoylethanolamide and docosahexanoylethanolamide after a single 2 h dietary fat feeding in male Sprague Dawley rats. Lipids. 2017;52(11):901–6.
271. Olfson M, Wall MM, Liu SM, Blanco C. Cannabis use and risk of prescription opioid use disorder in the United States. Am J Psychiatry. 2018;175(1):47–53.
272. Patel S, Gerrits R, Muthian S, Greene AS, Hillard CJ. The CB1 receptor antagonist SR141716 enhances stimulus-induced activation of the primary somatosensory cortex of the rat. Neurosci Lett. 2002;335(2):95–8.
273. Patilea Vrana GI, Anoshchenko O, Unadkat JD. Hepatic enzymes relevant to the disposition of (−)-(9)-tetrahydrocannabinol (THC) and its psychoactive metabolite, 11-OH-THC. Drug Metab Dispos. 2019;47(3):249–56.
274. Patsalos PN, Szaflarski JP, Gidal B, VanLandingham K, Critchley D, Morrison G. Clinical implications of trials investigating drug-drug interactions between cannabidiol and enzyme inducers or inhibitors or common antiseizure drugs. Epilepsia. 2020;61:1854–68.

275. Paudel KS, Hammell DC, Agu RU, Valiveti S, Stinchcomb AL. Cannabidiol bioavailability after nasal and transdermal application: effect of permeation enhancers. Drug Dev Ind Pharm. 2010;36(9):1088–97.
276. Perez J. Combined cannabinoid therapy via an oromucosal spray. Drugs Today (Barc). 2006;42(8):495–503.
277. Perkins D, Butler J, Ong K, Nguyen TH, Cox S, Francis B, McIntosh M, Lilley B. A phase 1, randomised, placebo-controlled, dose escalation study to investigate the safety, tolerability and pharmacokinetics of Cannabidiol in fed healthy volunteers. Eur J Drug Metab Pharmacokinet. 2020a;45(5):575–86.
278. Pertwee RG. Cannabinoid pharmacology: the first 66 years. Br J Pharmacol. 2006;147(Suppl 1):S163–71.
279. Perucca E, Bialer M. Critical aspects affecting Cannabidiol oral bioavailability and metabolic elimination, and related clinical implications. CNS Drugs. 2020;34(8):795–800.
280. Piomelli D, Tarzia G, Duranti A, Tontini A, Mor M, Compton TR, Dasse O, Monaghan EP, Parrott JA, Putman D. Pharmacological profile of the selective FAAH inhibitor KDS-4103 (URB597). CNS Drug Rev. 2006;12(1):21–38.
281. Pratt-Hyatt M, Zhang H, Snider NT, Hollenberg PF. Effects of a commonly occurring genetic polymorphism of human CYP3A4 (I118V) on the metabolism of anandamide. Drug Metab Dispos. 2010;38(11):2075–82.
282. Pugh G Jr, Smith PB, Dombrowski DS, Welch SP. The role of endogenous opioids in enhancing the antinociception produced by the combination of delta 9-tetrahydrocannabinol and morphine in the spinal cord. J Pharmacol Exp Ther. 1996;279(2):608–16.
283. Qian Y, Gurley BJ, Markowitz JS. The potential for pharmacokinetic interactions between cannabis products and conventional medications. J Clin Psychopharmacol. 2019;39(5): 462–71.
284. Raby WN, Carpenter KM, Rothenberg J, Brooks AC, Jiang H, Sullivan M, Bisaga A, Comer S, Nunes EV. Intermittent marijuana use is associated with improved retention in naltrexone treatment for opiate-dependence. Am J Addict. 2009;18(4):301–8.
285. Rakhshan F, Day TA, Blakely RD, Barker EL. Carrier-mediated uptake of the endogenous cannabinoid anandamide in RBL-2H3 cells. J Pharmacol Exp Ther. 2000;292(3):960–7.
286. Rector JL, Tay L, Wiese CW, Friedman EM. Relative sensitivity of cortisol indices to psychosocial and physical health factors. PLoS One. 2019;14(4):e0213513.
287. Reid S, Bhattacharyya S. Antipsychotic treatment failure in patients with psychosis and comorbid cannabis use: a systematic review. Psychiatry Res. 2019;280:112523.
288. Rios C, Gomes I, Devi LA. mu opioid and CB1 cannabinoid receptor interactions: reciprocal inhibition of receptor signaling and neuritogenesis. Br J Pharmacol. 2006;148(4):387–95.
289. Ritter JK, Li C, Xia M, Poklis JL, Lichtman AH, Abdullah RA, Dewey WL, Li PL. Production and actions of the anandamide metabolite prostamide E2 in the renal medulla. J Pharmacol Exp Ther. 2012;342(3):770–9.
290. Roberts JD, Gennings C, Shih M. Synergistic affective analgesic interaction between delta-9-tetrahydrocannabinol and morphine. Eur J Pharmacol. 2006;530(1–2):54–8.
291. Rohleder C, Muller JK, Lange B, Leweke FM. Cannabidiol as a potential new type of an antipsychotic. A critical review of the evidence. Front Pharmacol. 2016;7:422.
292. Ronen A, Chassidim HS, Gershon P, Parmet Y, Rabinovich A, Bar-Hamburger R, Cassuto Y, Shinar D. The effect of alcohol, THC and their combination on perceived effects, willingness to drive and performance of driving and non-driving tasks. Accid Anal Prev. 2010;42(6):1855–65.
293. Ropke J, Busanello A, Leal CQ, de Moraes Reis E, de Freitas CM, Villarinho JG, Figueira FH, Mello CF, Ferreira J, Fachinetto R. Anandamide attenuates haloperidol-induced vacuous chewing movements in rats. Prog Neuro-Psychopharmacol Biol Psychiatry. 2014;54: 195–9.
294. Roser P, Haussleiter IS. Antipsychotic-like effects of cannabidiol and rimonabant: systematic review of animal and human studies. Curr Pharm Des. 2012;18(32):5141–55.

295. Roser P, Vollenweider FX, Kawohl W. Potential antipsychotic properties of central cannabinoid (CB1) receptor antagonists. World J Biol Psychiatry. 2010;11(2 Pt 2):208–19.
296. Ross RA, Craib SJ, Stevenson LA, Pertwee RG, Henderson A, Toole J, Ellington HC. Pharmacological characterization of the anandamide cyclooxygenase metabolite: prostaglandin E2 ethanolamide. J Pharmacol Exp Ther. 2002;301(3):900–7.
297. Rouzer CA, Marnett LJ. Endocannabinoid oxygenation by cyclooxygenases, lipoxygenases, and cytochromes P450: cross-talk between the eicosanoid and endocannabinoid signaling pathways. Chem Rev. 2011;111(10):5899–921.
298. Rubin K, Ewing P, Backstrom E, Abrahamsson A, Bonn B, Kamata S, Grime K. Pulmonary metabolism of substrates for key drug-metabolizing enzymes by human alveolar type II cells, human and rat lung Microsomes, and the isolated perfused rat lung model. Pharmaceutics. 2020;12(2):117.
299. Russo EB, Burnett A, Hall B, Parker KK. Agonistic properties of cannabidiol at 5-HT1a receptors. Neurochem Res. 2005;30(8):1037–43.
300. Rutkowska M, Jachimczuk O. Antidepressant--like properties of ACEA (arachidonyl-2-chloroethylamide), the selective agonist of CB1 receptors. Acta Pol Pharm. 2004;61(2):165–7.
301. Sadhasivam S, Zhang X, Chidambaran V, Mavi J, Pilipenko V, Mersha TB, Meller J, Kaufman KM, Martin LJ, McAuliffe J. Novel associations between FAAH genetic variants and postoperative central opioid-related adverse effects. Pharmacogenomics J. 2015;15(5):436–42.
302. Sanchis-Segura C, Cline BH, Marsicano G, Lutz B, Spanagel R. Reduced sensitivity to reward in CB1 knockout mice. Psychopharmacology. 2004;176(2):223–32.
303. Sang N, Chen C. Lipid signaling and synaptic plasticity. Neuroscientist. 2006;12(5):425–34.
304. Sang N, Zhang J, Chen C. PGE2 glycerol ester, a COX-2 oxidative metabolite of 2-arachidonoyl glycerol, modulates inhibitory synaptic transmission in mouse hippocampal neurons. J Physiol. 2006;572(Pt 3):735–45.
305. Sarris J, Sinclair J, Karamacoska D, Davidson M, Firth J. Medicinal cannabis for psychiatric disorders: a clinically-focused systematic review. BMC Psychiatry. 2020;20(1):24.
306. Scarpelli R, Sasso O, Piomelli D. A double whammy: targeting both fatty acid amide hydrolase (FAAH) and cyclooxygenase (COX) to treat pain and inflammation. ChemMedChem. 2016;11(12):1242–51.
307. Scavone JL, Sterling RC, Van Bockstaele EJ. Cannabinoid and opioid interactions: implications for opiate dependence and withdrawal. Neuroscience. 2013b;248:637–54.
308. Scavone JL, Sterling RC, Weinstein SP, Van Bockstaele EJ. Impact of cannabis use during stabilization on methadone maintenance treatment. Am J Addict. 2013a;22(4):344–51.
309. Schoedel KA, Szeto I, Setnik B, Sellers EM, Levy-Cooperman N, Mills C, Etges T, Sommerville K. Abuse potential assessment of cannabidiol (CBD) in recreational polydrug users: a randomized, double-blind, controlled trial. Epilepsy Behav. 2018;88:162–71.
310. Schoevers J, Leweke JE, Leweke FM. Cannabidiol as a treatment option for schizophrenia: recent evidence and current studies. Curr Opin Psychiatry. 2020;33(3):185–91.
311. Schubart CD, Sommer IE, Fusar-Poli P, de Witte L, Kahn RS, Boks MP. Cannabidiol as a potential treatment for psychosis. Eur Neuropsychopharmacol. 2014;24(1):51–64.
312. Schuchardt JP, Schneider I, Meyer H, Neubronner J, von Schacky C, Hahn A. Incorporation of EPA and DHA into plasma phospholipids in response to different omega-3 fatty acid formulations–a comparative bioavailability study of fish oil vs. krill oil. Lipids Health Dis. 2011;10:145.
313. Schwope DM, Karschner EL, Gorelick DA, Huestis MA. Identification of recent cannabis use: whole-blood and plasma free and glucuronidated cannabinoid pharmacokinetics following controlled smoked cannabis administration. Clin Chem. 2011;57(10):1406–14.
314. Secher A, Husum H, Holst B, Egerod KL, Mellerup E. Risperidone treatment increases CB1 receptor binding in rat brain. Neuroendocrinology. 2010;91(2):155–68.
315. Seillier A, Giuffrida A. Disruption of social cognition in the sub-chronic PCP rat model of schizophrenia: possible involvement of the endocannabinoid system. Eur Neuropsychopharmacol. 2016;26(2):298–309.

316. Seillier A, Martinez AA, Giuffrida A. Phencyclidine-induced social withdrawal results from deficient stimulation of cannabinoid CB(1) receptors: implications for schizophrenia. Neuropsychopharmacology. 2013;38(9):1816–24.
317. Sellers EM, Schoedel K, Bartlett C, Romach M, Russo EB, Stott CG, Wright S, White L, Duncombe P, Chen CF. A multiple-dose, randomized, double-blind, placebo-controlled, parallel-group QT/QTc study to evaluate the Electrophysiologic effects of THC/CBD spray. Clin Pharmacol Drug Dev. 2013;2(3):285–94.
318. Shang VC, O'Sullivan SE, Kendall DA, Roberts RE. The endogenous cannabinoid anandamide increases human airway epithelial cell permeability through an arachidonic acid metabolite. Pharmacol Res. 2016;105:152–63.
319. Shearman LP, Rosko KM, Fleischer R, Wang J, Xu S, Tong XS, Rocha BA. Antidepressant-like and anorectic effects of the cannabinoid CB1 receptor inverse agonist AM251 in mice. Behav Pharmacol. 2003;14(8):573–82.
320. Slawson G, Milloy MJ, Balneaves L, Simo A, Guillemi S, Hogg R, Montaner J, Wood E, Kerr T. High-intensity cannabis use and adherence to antiretroviral therapy among people who use illicit drugs in a Canadian setting. AIDS Behav. 2015;19(1):120–7.
321. Smaga I, Bystrowska B, Gawlinski D, Pomierny B, Stankowicz P, Filip M. Antidepressants and changes in concentration of endocannabinoids and N-acylethanolamines in rat brain structures. Neurotox Res. 2014;26(2):190–206.
322. Smaga I, Gawlinski D, Brodowicz J, Filip M. Brain region-dependent changes in the expression of endocannabinoid-metabolizing enzymes in rats following antidepressant drugs. J Physiol Pharmacol. 2019;70(5) https://doi.org/10.26402/jpp.2019.5.06.
323. Smaga I, Jastrzebska J, Zaniewska M, Bystrowska B, Gawlinski D, Faron-Gorecka A, Broniowska Z, Miszkiel J, Filip M. Changes in the brain endocannabinoid system in rat models of depression. Neurotox Res. 2017;31(3):421–35.
324. Smart R, Pacula RL. Early evidence of the impact of cannabis legalization on cannabis use, cannabis use disorder, and the use of other substances: findings from state policy evaluations. Am J Drug Alcohol Abuse. 2019;45(6):644–63.
325. Snider NT, Walker VJ, Hollenberg PF. Oxidation of the endogenous cannabinoid arachidonoyl ethanolamide by the cytochrome P450 monooxygenases: physiological and pharmacological implications. Pharmacol Rev. 2010;62(1):136–54.
326. Solinas M, Goldberg SR. Motivational effects of cannabinoids and opioids on food reinforcement depend on simultaneous activation of cannabinoid and opioid systems. Neuropsychopharmacology. 2005;30(11):2035–45.
327. Solinas M, Panlilio LV, Goldberg SR. Exposure to delta-9-tetrahydrocannabinol (THC) increases subsequent heroin taking but not heroin's reinforcing efficacy: a self-administration study in rats. Neuropsychopharmacology. 2004;29(7):1301–11.
328. Spano MS, Fattore L, Cossu G, Deiana S, Fadda P, Fratta W. CB1 receptor agonist and heroin, but not cocaine, reinstate cannabinoid-seeking behaviour in the rat. Br J Pharmacol. 2004;143(3):343–50.
329. Spector AA. Arachidonic acid cytochrome P450 epoxygenase pathway. J Lipid Res. 2009;50(Suppl):S52–6.
330. Spiro AS, Wong A, Boucher AA, Arnold JC. Enhanced brain disposition and effects of Delta9-tetrahydrocannabinol in P-glycoprotein and breast cancer resistance protein knockout mice. PLoS One. 2012;7(4):e35937.
331. Steiner MA, Marsicano G, Nestler EJ, Holsboer F, Lutz B, Wotjak CT. Antidepressant-like behavioral effects of impaired cannabinoid receptor type 1 signaling coincide with exaggerated corticosterone secretion in mice. Psychoneuroendocrinology. 2008;33(1):54–67.
332. Stinchcomb AL, Valiveti S, Hammell DC, Ramsey DR. Human skin permeation of Delta8-tetrahydrocannabinol, cannabidiol and cannabinol. J Pharm Pharmacol. 2004;56(3):291–7.
333. Stout SM, Cimino NM. Exogenous cannabinoids as substrates, inhibitors, and inducers of human drug metabolizing enzymes: a systematic review. Drug Metab Rev. 2014;46(1): 86–95.

334. Sugiura T, Kobayashi Y, Oka S, Waku K. Biosynthesis and degradation of anandamide and 2-arachidonoylglycerol and their possible physiological significance. Prostaglandins Leukot Essent Fatty Acids. 2002;66(2–3):173–92.
335. Sundram S, Copolov D, Dean B. Clozapine decreases [3H] CP 55940 binding to the cannabinoid 1 receptor in the rat nucleus accumbens. Naunyn Schmiedeberg's Arch Pharmacol. 2005;371(5):428–33.
336. Tai S, Fantegrossi WE. Pharmacological and toxicological effects of synthetic cannabinoids and their metabolites. Curr Top Behav Neurosci. 2017;32:249–62.
337. Takeuchi K, Renic M, Bohman QC, Harder DR, Miyata N, Roman RJ. Reversal of delayed vasospasm by an inhibitor of the synthesis of 20-HETE. Am J Physiol Heart Circ Physiol. 2005;289(5):H2203–11.
338. Tang SM, Ansarian A, Courtney DB. Clozapine treatment and cannabis use in adolescents with psychotic disorders – a retrospective cohort chart review. J Can Acad Child Adolesc Psychiatry. 2017;26(1):51–8.
339. Taylor L, Crockett J, Tayo B, Morrison G. A phase 1, open-label, parallel-group, single-dose trial of the pharmacokinetics and safety of Cannabidiol (CBD) in subjects with mild to severe hepatic impairment. J Clin Pharmacol. 2019;59(8):1110–9.
340. Taylor L, Gidal B, Blakey G, Tayo B, Morrison G. A phase I, randomized, double-blind, placebo-controlled, single ascending dose, multiple dose, and food effect trial of the safety, tolerability and pharmacokinetics of highly purified Cannabidiol in healthy subjects. CNS Drugs. 2018;32(11):1053–67.
341. Tayo B, Taylor L, Sahebkar F, Morrison G. A phase I, open-label, parallel-group, single-dose trial of the pharmacokinetics, safety, and tolerability of Cannabidiol in subjects with mild to severe renal impairment. Clin Pharmacokinet. 2020;59(6):747–55.
342. Thomas A, Baillie GL, Phillips AM, Razdan RK, Ross RA, Pertwee RG. Cannabidiol displays unexpectedly high potency as an antagonist of CB1 and CB2 receptor agonists in vitro. Br J Pharmacol. 2007;150(5):613–23.
343. Thuy Phuong NT, Kim JW, Kim JA, Jeon JS, Lee JY, Xu WJ, Yang JW, Kim SK, Kang KW. Role of the CYP3A4-mediated 11,12-epoxyeicosatrienoic acid pathway in the development of tamoxifen-resistant breast cancer. Oncotarget. 2017;8(41):71054–69.
344. Tiwari AK, Zai CC, Likhodi O, Lisker A, Singh D, Souza RP, Batra P, Zaidi SH, Chen S, Liu F, Puls I, Meltzer HY, Lieberman JA, Kennedy JL, Muller DJ. A common polymorphism in the cannabinoid receptor 1 (CNR1) gene is associated with antipsychotic-induced weight gain in schizophrenia. Neuropsychopharmacology. 2010;35(6):1315–24.
345. Tiwari AK, Zai CC, Likhodi O, Voineskos AN, Meltzer HY, Lieberman JA, Potkin SG, Remington G, Muller DJ, Kennedy JL. Association study of cannabinoid receptor 1 (CNR1) gene in tardive dyskinesia. Pharmacogenomics J. 2012;12(3):260–6.
346. Toczek M, Malinowska B. Enhanced endocannabinoid tone as a potential target of pharmacotherapy. Life Sci. 2018;204:20–45.
347. Toennes SW, Schneider K, Kauert GF, Wunder C, Moeller MR, Theunissen EL, Ramaekers JG. Influence of ethanol on cannabinoid pharmacokinetic parameters in chronic users. Anal Bioanal Chem. 2011;400(1):145–52.
348. Tournier N, Chevillard L, Megarbane B, Pirnay S, Scherrmann JM, Decleves X. Interaction of drugs of abuse and maintenance treatments with human P-glycoprotein (ABCB1) and breast cancer resistance protein (ABCG2). Int J Neuropsychopharmacol. 2010;13(7):905–15.
349. Tran A, Rey E, Pons G, Rousseau M, d'Athis P, Olive G, Mather GG, Bishop FE, Wurden CJ, Labroo R, Trager WF, Kunze KL, Thummel KE, Vincent JC, Gillardin JM, Lepage F, Levy RH. Influence of stiripentol on cytochrome P450-mediated metabolic pathways in humans: in vitro and in vivo comparison and calculation of in vivo inhibition constants. Clin Pharmacol Ther. 1997;62(5):490–504.
350. Tucci SA, Rogers EK, Korbonits M, Kirkham TC. The cannabinoid CB1 receptor antagonist SR141716 blocks the orexigenic effects of intrahypothalamic ghrelin. Br J Pharmacol. 2004;143(5):520–3.

351. Turna J, Syan SK, Frey BN, Rush B, Costello MJ, Weiss M, MacKillop J. Cannabidiol as a novel candidate alcohol use disorder pharmacotherapy: a systematic review. Alcohol Clin Exp Res. 2019;43(4):550–63.
352. Tzavara ET, Li DL, Moutsimilli L, Bisogno T, Di Marzo V, Phebus LA, Nomikos GG, Giros B. Endocannabinoids activate transient receptor potential vanilloid 1 receptors to reduce hyperdopaminergia-related hyperactivity: therapeutic implications. Biol Psychiatry. 2006;59(6):508–15.
353. Uriguen L, Garcia-Fuster MJ, Callado LF, Morentin B, La Harpe R, Casado V, Lluis C, Franco R, Garcia-Sevilla JA, Meana JJ. Immunodensity and mRNA expression of A2A adenosine, D2 dopamine, and CB1 cannabinoid receptors in postmortem frontal cortex of subjects with schizophrenia: effect of antipsychotic treatment. Psychopharmacology. 2009;206(2):313–24.
354. Vandrey R, Herrmann ES, Mitchell JM, Bigelow GE, Flegel R, LoDico C, Cone EJ. Pharmacokinetic profile of oral cannabis in humans: blood and oral fluid disposition and relation to Pharmacodynamic outcomes. J Anal Toxicol. 2017;41(2):83–99.
355. VanLandingham KE, Crockett J, Taylor L, Morrison G. A phase 2, double-blind, placebo-controlled trial to investigate potential drug-drug interactions between Cannabidiol and Clobazam. J Clin Pharmacol. 2020;60(10):1304–13.
356. Vazquez SR. Drug-drug interactions in an era of multiple anticoagulants: a focus on clinically relevant drug interactions. Hematology Am Soc Hematol Educ Program. 2018;2018(1):339–47.
357. Vega OM, Abkenari S, Tong Z, Tedman A, Huerta-Yepez S. Omega-3 polyunsaturated fatty acids and lung cancer: nutrition or pharmacology? Nutr Cancer. 2020;73(4):541–61.
358. Vigano D, Rubino T, Parolaro D. Molecular and cellular basis of cannabinoid and opioid interactions. Pharmacol Biochem Behav. 2005b;81(2):360–8.
359. Vigano D, Rubino T, Vaccani A, Bianchessi S, Marmorato P, Castiglioni C, Parolaro D. Molecular mechanisms involved in the asymmetric interaction between cannabinoid and opioid systems. Psychopharmacology. 2005a;182(4):527–36.
360. Vigano D, Valenti M, Cascio MG, Di Marzo V, Parolaro D, Rubino T. Changes in endocannabinoid levels in a rat model of behavioural sensitization to morphine. Eur J Neurosci. 2004;20(7):1849–57.
361. Vimalanathan A, Gidyk DC, Diwan M, Gouveia FV, Lipsman N, Giacobbe P, Nobrega JN, Hamani C. Endocannabinoid modulating drugs improve anxiety but not the expression of conditioned fear in a rodent model of post-traumatic stress disorder. Neuropharmacology. 2020;166:107965.
362. Vinod KY, Arango V, Xie S, Kassir SA, Mann JJ, Cooper TB, Hungund BL. Elevated levels of endocannabinoids and CB1 receptor-mediated G-protein signaling in the prefrontal cortex of alcoholic suicide victims. Biol Psychiatry. 2005;57(5):480–6.
363. Volk DW, Eggan SM, Horti AG, Wong DF, Lewis DA. Reciprocal alterations in cortical cannabinoid receptor 1 binding relative to protein immunoreactivity and transcript levels in schizophrenia. Schizophr Res. 2014;159(1):124–9.
364. Vozella V, Zibardi C, Ahmed F, Piomelli D. Fast and sensitive quantification of Delta(9)-tetrahydrocannabinol and its Main oxidative metabolites by liquid chromatography/tandem mass spectrometry. Cannabis Cannabinoid Res. 2019;4(2):110–23.
365. Vyas MB, LeBaron VT, Gilson AM. The use of cannabis in response to the opioid crisis: a review of the literature. Nurs Outlook. 2018;66(1):56–65.
366. Wahn H, Wolf J, Kram F, Frantz S, Wagner JA. The endocannabinoid arachidonyl ethanolamide (anandamide) increases pulmonary arterial pressure via cyclooxygenase-2 products in isolated rabbit lungs. Am J Physiol Heart Circ Physiol. 2005;289(6):H2491–6.
367. Wall ME, Sadler BM, Brine D, Taylor H, Perez-Reyes M. Metabolism, disposition, and kinetics of delta-9-tetrahydrocannabinol in men and women. Clin Pharmacol Ther. 1983;34(3):352–63.
368. Wang B, Wang J, Huang SQ, Su HH, Zhou SF. Genetic polymorphism of the human cytochrome P450 2C9 gene and its clinical significance. Curr Drug Metab. 2009;10(7):781–834.

369. Wang J, Shen RY, Haj-Dahmane S. Endocannabinoids mediate the glucocorticoid-induced inhibition of excitatory synaptic transmission to dorsal raphe serotonin neurons. J Physiol. 2012;590(22):5795–808.
370. Wang S, Lim G, Mao J, Sung B, Yang L, Mao J. Central glucocorticoid receptors regulate the upregulation of spinal cannabinoid-1 receptors after peripheral nerve injury in rats. Pain. 2007;131(1–2):96–105.
371. Watanabe K, Kayano Y, Matsunaga T, Yamamoto I, Yoshimura H. Inhibition of anandamide amidase activity in mouse brain microsomes by cannabinoids. Biol Pharm Bull. 1996;19(8):1109–11.
372. Watanabe K, Yamaori S, Funahashi T, Kimura T, Yamamoto I. Cytochrome P450 enzymes involved in the metabolism of tetrahydrocannabinols and cannabinol by human hepatic microsomes. Life Sci. 2007;80(15):1415–9.
373. Weston-Green K, Huang XF, Deng C. Alterations to melanocortinergic, GABAergic and cannabinoid neurotransmission associated with olanzapine-induced weight gain. PLoS One. 2012;7(3):e33548.
374. Wheeler CW, Wrighton SA, Guenthner TM. Detection of human lung cytochromes P450 that are immunochemically related to cytochrome P450IIE1 and cytochrome P450IIIA. Biochem Pharmacol. 1992;44(1):183–7.
375. Wilkerson JL, Ghosh S, Mustafa M, Abdullah RA, Niphakis MJ, Cabrera R, Maldonado RL, Cravatt BF, Lichtman AH. The endocannabinoid hydrolysis inhibitor SA-57: intrinsic antinociceptive effects, augmented morphine-induced antinociception, and attenuated heroin seeking behavior in mice. Neuropharmacology. 2017;114:156–67.
376. Willoughby KA, Moore SF, Martin BR, Ellis EF. The biodisposition and metabolism of anandamide in mice. J Pharmacol Exp Ther. 1997;282(1):243–7.
377. Wills KL, Parker LA. Effect of pharmacological modulation of the Endocannabinoid system on opiate withdrawal: a review of the preclinical animal literature. Front Pharmacol. 2016;7:187.
378. Wilson-Morkeh H, Al-Abdulla A, Sien L, Mohamed H, Youngstein T. Important drug interactions exist between cannabidiol oil and commonly prescribed drugs in rheumatology practice. Rheumatology (Oxford). 2020;59(1):249–51.
379. Wilson R, Bossong MG, Appiah-Kusi E, Petros N, Brammer M, Perez J, Allen P, McGuire P, Bhattacharyya S. Cannabidiol attenuates insular dysfunction during motivational salience processing in subjects at clinical high risk for psychosis. Transl Psychiatry. 2019;9(1):203.
380. Wilson RI, Nicoll RA. Endocannabinoid signaling in the brain. Science. 2002;296(5568):678–82.
381. Wilson RP, Bhattacharyya S. Antipsychotic efficacy in psychosis with co-morbid cannabis misuse: a systematic review. J Psychopharmacol. 2016;30(2):99–111.
382. Withey SL, Bergman J, Huestis MA, George SR, Madras BK. THC and CBD blood and brain concentrations following daily administration to adolescent primates. Drug Alcohol Depend. 2020;213:108129.
383. Wolowich WR, Greif R, Kleine-Brueggeney M, Bernhard W, Theiler L. Minimal physiologically based pharmacokinetic model of intravenously and orally Administered Delta-9-tetrahydrocannabinol in healthy volunteers. Eur J Drug Metab Pharmacokinet. 2019;44(5):691–711.
384. Wood JT, Williams JS, Pandarinathan L, Janero DR, Lammi-Keefe CJ, Makriyannis A. Dietary docosahexaenoic acid supplementation alters select physiological endocannabinoid-system metabolites in brain and plasma. J Lipid Res. 2010;51(6):1416–23.
385. Woodward DF, Liang Y, Krauss AH. Prostamides (prostaglandin-ethanolamides) and their pharmacology. Br J Pharmacol. 2008;153(3):410–9.
386. Wray L, Stott C, Jones N, Wright S. Cannabidiol Does Not Convert to Delta(9)-Tetrahydrocannabinol in an In Vivo Animal Model. Cannabis Cannabinoid Res. 2017;2(1):282–7.

387. Yamaguchi T, Hagiwara Y, Tanaka H, Sugiura T, Waku K, Shoyama Y, Watanabe S, Yamamoto T. Endogenous cannabinoid, 2-arachidonoylglycerol, attenuates naloxone-precipitated withdrawal signs in morphine-dependent mice. Brain Res. 2001;909(1–2):121–6.
388. Yamaori S, Ebisawa J, Okushima Y, Yamamoto I, Watanabe K. Potent inhibition of human cytochrome P450 3A isoforms by cannabidiol: role of phenolic hydroxyl groups in the resorcinol moiety. Life Sci. 2011a;88(15–16):730–6.
389. Yamaori S, Ishii H, Chiba K, Yamamoto I, Watanabe K. Delta-tetrahydrocannabinol induces cytotoxicity in macrophage J774-1 cells: involvement of cannabinoid receptor 2 and p38 MAPK. Toxicology. 2013;314(2–3):254–61.
390. Yamaori S, Kinugasa Y, Jiang R, Takeda S, Yamamoto I, Watanabe K. Cannabidiol induces expression of human cytochrome P450 1A1 that is possibly mediated through aryl hydrocarbon receptor signaling in HepG2 cells. Life Sci. 2015;136:87–93.
391. Yamaori S, Koeda K, Kushihara M, Hada Y, Yamamoto I, Watanabe K. Comparison in the in vitro inhibitory effects of major phytocannabinoids and polycyclic aromatic hydrocarbons contained in marijuana smoke on cytochrome P450 2C9 activity. Drug Metab Pharmacokinet. 2012;27(3):294–300.
392. Yamaori S, Kushihara M, Yamamoto I, Watanabe K. Characterization of major phytocannabinoids, cannabidiol and cannabinol, as isoform-selective and potent inhibitors of human CYP1 enzymes. Biochem Pharmacol. 2010;79(11):1691–8.
393. Yamaori S, Okamoto Y, Yamamoto I, Watanabe K. Cannabidiol, a major phytocannabinoid, as a potent atypical inhibitor for CYP2D6. Drug Metab Dispos. 2011b;39(11):2049–56.
394. Yang W, Ni J, Woodward DF, Tang-Liu DD, Ling KH. Enzymatic formation of prostamide F2alpha from anandamide involves a newly identified intermediate metabolite, prostamide H2. J Lipid Res. 2005;46(12):2745–51.
395. Yu HL, Deng XQ, Li YJ, Li YC, Quan ZS, Sun XY. N-palmitoylethanolamide, an endocannabinoid, exhibits antidepressant effects in the forced swim test and the tail suspension test in mice. Pharmacol Rep. 2011;63(3):834–9.
396. Yu M, Ives D, Ramesha CS. Synthesis of prostaglandin E2 ethanolamide from anandamide by cyclooxygenase-2. J Biol Chem. 1997;272(34):21181–6.
397. Zanger UM, Klein K, Thomas M, Rieger JK, Tremmel R, Kandel BA, Klein M, Magdy T. Genetics, epigenetics, and regulation of drug-metabolizing cytochrome p450 enzymes. Clin Pharmacol Ther. 2014;95(3):258–61.
398. Zanger UM, Schwab M. Cytochrome P450 enzymes in drug metabolism: regulation of gene expression, enzyme activities, and impact of genetic variation. Pharmacol Ther. 2013;138(1):103–41.
399. Zavitsanou K, Garrick T, Huang XF. Selective antagonist [3H]SR141716A binding to cannabinoid CB1 receptors is increased in the anterior cingulate cortex in schizophrenia. Prog Neuro-Psychopharmacol Biol Psychiatry. 2004;28(2):355–60.
400. Zendulka O, Dovrtelova G, Noskova K, Turjap M, Sulcova A, Hanus L, Jurica J. Cannabinoids and cytochrome P450 interactions. Curr Drug Metab. 2016;17(3):206–26.
401. Zhang JY, Wang Y, Prakash C. Xenobiotic-metabolizing enzymes in human lung. Curr Drug Metab. 2006;7(8):939–48.
402. Zhang Y, Hu L, Mori TA, Barden A, Croft KD, Whitworth JA. Arachidonic acid metabolism in glucocorticoid-induced hypertension. Clin Exp Pharmacol Physiol. 2008;35(5–6): 557–62.
403. Zhang Z, Wang W, Zhong P, Liu SJ, Long JZ, Zhao L, Gao HQ, Cravatt BF, Liu QS. Blockade of 2-arachidonoylglycerol hydrolysis produces antidepressant-like effects and enhances adult hippocampal neurogenesis and synaptic plasticity. Hippocampus. 2015;25(1):16–26.
404. Zhong P, Wang W, Pan B, Liu X, Zhang Z, Long JZ, Zhang HT, Cravatt BF, Liu QS. Monoacylglycerol lipase inhibition blocks chronic stress-induced depressive-like behaviors via activation of mTOR signaling. Neuropsychopharmacology. 2014;39(7):1763–76.

405. Zhu HJ, Wang JS, Markowitz JS, Donovan JL, Gibson BB, Gefroh HA, Devane CL. Characterization of P-glycoprotein inhibition by major cannabinoids from marijuana. J Pharmacol Exp Ther. 2006;317(2):850–7.
406. Zuardi AW, Hallak JE, Dursun SM, Morais SL, Sanches RF, Musty RE, Crippa JA. Cannabidiol monotherapy for treatment-resistant schizophrenia. J Psychopharmacol. 2006;20(5): 683–6.
407. Zuardi AW, Morais SL, Guimaraes FS, Mechoulam R. Antipsychotic effect of cannabidiol. J Clin Psychiatry. 1995;56(10):485–6.

Chapter 3
Future Therapeutic Potential of Synthetic Cannabinoids and Endocannabinoid System Modulators

Contents

3.1 Introduction 91
3.2 Terminology 93
3.3 Part 1: Synthetic Cannabinoids 93
3.3.1 Synthetic Cannabinoid Use in the Community 93
3.3.2 Pharmacology 94
3.3.3 Conclusion 100
3.4 Part 2: Palmitoylethanolamide (PEA) and the Role of Future Endocannabinoid Modulators in Cancer Care 100
3.4.1 Pharmacodynamics 101
3.4.2 Pharmacokinetics 101
3.4.3 Safety 103
3.5 Conclusion 105
References (Synthetic Cannabinoids) 106

3.1 Introduction

Synthetic cannabinoids (SC) were originally manufactured for research purposes. The first compound was synthesized in 1965, soon after the discovery of THC. Today, they number in the hundreds, and though many are being studied in preclinical trials, some have been manufactured in clandestine laboratories and have made it to the street where they have been given names such as "spice", "black mamba," or "K2." The first evidence of synthetics in the community appeared in Europe in the early 2000s and around 2008 in the USA [26]. Surveys have estimated that between 6% and 17% of college students in the USA have used synthetic cannabinoids [24]. Another survey demonstrated a prevalence of SC use over a 6-month period ranging from 29% to 35% of healthy cannabis smokers [26].

C. Cyr et al., *Cannabis and Cannabinoid-Based Medicines in Cancer Care*,
https://doi.org/10.1007/978-3-030-89918-9_3

Synthetics narrowly target classical cannabinoid receptors and do not interact with serotonin, norepinephrine, dopamine, GABA, sigma, or opioid receptors and thus differ from endocannabinoids. Based on animal studies, SCs are 2–100 times more potent than phytocannabinoids when comparing outcomes such as antinociception, anti-seizure activity, weight loss, anti-inflammatory responses, and anticancer activity. The affinity (Ki) of SCs is in sub-nanomolar concentrations whereas THC affinity (Ki) ranges between 4.9 and 41 nanomolar. Because most synthetics are metabolized through cytochrome P450 enzymes, drug-drug interactions are also likely to occur. Unlike phytocannabinoids, however, synthetic cannabinoids have been clearly associated with fatalities. Other adverse effects include severe malignant hypertension with intracranial hemorrhage, tachycardia and fatal arrhythmias, visual and/or auditory hallucinations, psychosis, and seizures. Withdrawal symptoms have also been shown to be severe with daily users. These compounds, like phytocannabinoids, have also been shown to exhibit in vitro anticancer activity, but evidence for safety and efficacy are lacking.

There are two available synthetic cannabinoids (SCs) on the market, nabilone and dronabinol. The first part of this chapter will briefly cover novel synthetic cannabinoids (SC) with therapeutic potential as well as the risks involved in their recreational use.

Synthetic cannabinoids were originally manufactured in 1965 [1, 2, 85]. On the street they have been given names such as "spice," "black mamba" or "K2," "Yucatan Fire," "Tropical Synergy," and other names. Synthetics are sold in packets as incense, herb blends, and potpourri with disclaimers that they are not made for human consumption. The chemical constituents vary significantly between and within individual packets [119]. Synthetics are readily available in retail or "head" shops and on Internet websites despite being Schedule 1 designated. Synthetics are often mixed with plant material such as "Wild Dagga" and "Indian Warrior" [44, 120, 141]. The compounds are often dissolved in acetone or alcohol which saturates the plant material and then dried. The final product is sold for about 30–40 United States dollars [44, 56]. Standard toxicology immunoassays do not detect synthetic cannabinoids. Gas or chromatography liquid with mass spectrometry is needed, though there is a lack of standardization to testing [109].

Black market manufacturers are constantly changing the chemical structure of synthetic cannabinoids (SC) in order to stay ahead of the legislature which avoids Schedule 1 status and legal entanglement. In addition, and because these compounds are not detected in standard urine toxicology, it is difficult for healthcare professionals to treat or recognize synthetic cannabinoid toxicities. Synthetics are highly potent-specific CB1 agonists as a rule. They possess highly potent efficacy, toxicity, and duration of action. They are often found mixed with street cannabis and heroin or consumed with alcohol [26, 68]. The rewarding effects and significant withdrawal adverse effects lead to significant dependence and chronic use more than seen with phytocannabinoids [26].

Endocannabinoid system modulators act upon the endocannabinoidome via an indirect route, bypassing the canonical CB1 and CB2 receptors (considered as major components of the original endocannabinoid system and now part of the larger endocannabinoidome). They include many potential drugs which are under development, including endocannabinoid catabolic enzyme inhibitors and cannabinoid-like receptor ligands. Of these, palmitoylethanolamide (PEA) is a prominent figure, since it is an available and relatively inexpensive nutraceutical and will be the focus of the second part of this chapter. PEA is a member of the n-acylethanolamine (NAE) family of bioactive fatty acids that are found in all animal tissues. PEA down-modulates mast cell responses to tissue injury and activates peroxisome proliferator activated receptor-alpha (PPAR-alpha) resulting in an anti-inflammatory and analgesic response. It does not interact directly with cannabinoid receptors CB1 and CB2, but it does have an impact on the endocannabinoid system. Though there are few pharmacokinetic studies with PEA, bioavailability has been shown to be around 20–30% in normal individuals. In animal tissues, concentrations are generally higher than in plasma with circulating levels varying markedly during the day. Tissue and plasma concentrations can also increase with injury, particularly with inflammation and in disease processes associated with neurodegeneration. PEA is quite safe by standard in vitro tests, in animal studies, and clinically. There are two meta-analyses published recently which have confirmed PEA analgesia in various pain phenotypes. Although the role of PEA has not yet been determined in cancer care, the low cost and ease of access to this nutraceutical may make this an interesting adjuvant treatment for patients experiencing any type of chronic pain. For this reason, it is important to consider when evaluating patients on the use of natural products.

3.2 Terminology

The term "endocannabinoidome" is still not widely used by clinicians and researchers, and in order to avoid confusion, its use to describe the *expanded* endocannabinoid system (ECS) will be restricted to the first chapter of his book. For this chapter, the more commonly used term "endocannabinoid system (ECS)" will be used to describe most concepts relating to both the more specific canonical receptors and enzymes and the larger system of molecular targets and ligands. The "endocannabinoidome" will only be mentioned in order to point out a clinically relevant difference between these two related concepts.

3.3 Part 1: Synthetic Cannabinoids

3.3.1 Synthetic Cannabinoid Use in the Community

Many of the early synthetic cannabinoids manufactured for research are identified by the initials of the names of the researchers who discovered them or the company or institution where they originated: HU (Hebrew University), JWH (John

W. Hoffman), CP (Charles Pfizer), and AM (Alexandros Makriyannis). The first evidence of synthetics in the community appeared around 2009, and a spike in use occurred in 2010. The majority of samples acquired by law enforcement were identified as the compound JWH-018. Soon after, other compounds such as JWH-073 and CP-47-497 and others began to emerge. These were already known and scheduled. However, the compounds UR-144, XLR-11, and AKB-48, which had unique structures, did not fall under Schedule 1 designation and thus avoided prohibition at the time of discovery [47]. By 2015, synthetic cannabinoid use had become widespread (290 of 1432 tested cannabis street products). Most recently, the highly potent synthetic, AB-CHMINACA, has appeared laced with either heroin or fentanyl [19, 31, 47]. Adolescent deaths of unknown causes may be related to synthetic cannabinoids, which require specialized testing. Compounds detected are PB-22 (1.1 ng/mL), JWH-210 (12 ng/mL), XLR-11 (1.3 ng/mL), JWH-122, AB-CHMINACA (8.2 ng/mL), UR-144 (12.3 ng/mL), and JWH-022 (3 ng/mL). With synthetic drug use on the rise, forensic experts must have a high index of suspicion for the possibility of SC intoxication in adolescent fatalities [105].

Synthetic cannabinoids are tried at least once by most cannabis users and in approximately 1/3 of cannabis users; synthetics are used on a semi-regular basis [26]. Users are usually younger, and there are no gender or ethnic differences between phytocannabinoid and synthetic cannabinoid use [26]. Between 2012 and 2015, there was a stable prevalence of synthetic users among cannabis consumers which ranged between 29% and 35%. About 32.5% of these are occasional users, 6.6% frequent users defined as 10–50 times a year, and 3.7% regular SC users defined as greater than 50 times per year. Most try synthetics and dislike the experience (56.4%), while 12.3% find synthetics a neutral experience [26, 114]. SC users have a higher prevalence of neuroticism and lower agreeableness and extraversion than phytocannabis users and non-users. The prevalence of schizophrenic symptoms is also greater in SC users [23]. There are several reasons that SC users provide for their preference: avoiding detection of cannabis use, lower costs of synthetics, greater availability, as a means of quitting natural cannabis, and because it is considered "legal" [26].

3.3.2 Pharmacology

3.3.2.1 Pharmacodynamics of Synthetic Cannabinoids

The high potency of synthetic cannabinoids (SC) leads to greater reinforcing effects but also greater drug withdrawal reactions relative to phytocannabinoids. Synergistic effects of combined reinforcement and withdrawal occur when synthetics are combined with THC [41, 43, 82, 93, 139]. Based on animal studies, SC are 2–100 times more potent than phytocannabinoids when comparing outcomes such as antinociception, anti-seizure activity, weight loss, anti-inflammatory responses, and anticancer activity [18]. There is also a synergistic effect when certain synthetics are combined. For example, the combination of JWH-018 and JWH-073 has synergistic or additive antinociception in animals based on the ratio of the two synthetics [13].

Not only are synthetics more potent, but in general they have a greater affinity for CB1 and CB2 receptors. The affinity (Ki) is in sub-nanomolar concentrations, whereas THC affinity (Ki) ranges between 4.9 and 41 nanomolar [17, 33, 61, 121, 127, 133]. THC is a partial CB1 agonist, whereas most synthetics are full agonists for G-protein activation and downstream signaling [27, 33, 84]. Secondary metabolites derived from SC can also be active at classical cannabinoid receptors and are often *more* active than the parent compound or may have similar or even greater affinity for the receptor [12, 25, 48, 118]. The major hydroxylase-derived metabolite of JWH-018 and AM-2201 are full agonists at CB1 and CB2 at nanomolar concentrations [125], while the compounds AB-PINACA and 4OH-AB-PINACA are active in vivo, producing CB1 receptor-mediated hypothermia in mice. The pharmacodynamic properties of AB-PINACA at the CB1 receptor relative to THC (e.g., higher potency/efficacy and greater production of desensitization), coupled with production of metabolically stable and active phase I metabolites, contribute to the pronounced adverse effects observed with abuse of this SC compared to marijuana [67].

Affinity and potency of SC has been explored using discriminating effects in non-human primates. The compounds JWH-122, JWN-250, AM-2201, and CP-47,497 were studied because along with JWH-018, JWH-073, and HU-210 are the most commonly found synthetics found in "spice." The synthetics AM2201, JWH-122, CP-47,497, and JWH-250 produce a 10- to 15-fold right shift in rimonabant's ability to block THC discrimination [65]. CP-55.940 has higher affinity for cloned CB1 than CB2 receptors at 2.6 and 3.7 nM, respectively, and CP 55,940 is equally efficacious at CB1 and CB2. WIN 55212–2 and cannabinol have a higher affinity for CB2 than for CB1, while HU 210 has a higher affinity for CB1 than for the CB2 receptor [45].

In a mouse brain, efficacy, as measured by activation of G-proteins in rank order is, CP 55,940 > HU-210 > AEA > THC. The last two ligands are partial agonists [14]. The rank order of potencies as measured by forskolin-stimulated cAMP accumulation is HU-210 > CP-55,940 > THC > WIN-55212–2 > anandamide [10]. As an antiemetic in rats, HU-210 is more potent than THC [46]. In regard to receptor internalization, WIN 55,212–2, CP 55,940, and HU 210 cause rapid internalization, methanandamide less so, whereas high concentrations of THC are needed to cause internalization (3 uM) [66]. 2-AG is as potent at activating the receptor as HU-210 and CP55,940 as measured by calcium flux. 2-AG activity occurred at 0.3 nm, which is similar to the two synthetic ligands. The important point in interpreting these studies is that potency and efficacy are dependent on the type of assay which may lead to confusion or conflicting statements in the literature.

Though several mono-hydroxylated metabolites of JWH-018, JWH-073, and AM-2201 are active agonists, certain oxidative metabolites of JWH-018 are CB1 receptor antagonists, while certain glucuronidated metabolites also prevent CB1 activation [125]. This further complicates the predictability of many of these compounds.

Synthetics narrowly target classical cannabinoid receptors and do not interact with serotonin, norepinephrine, dopamine, GABA, sigma, or opioid receptors [132]. The CB1 receptor antagonist, rimonabant, has been shown to reverse synthetic cannabinoid toxicity in animals [99, 130]. There is cross-tolerance between THC and synthetics which reduce some of the toxicity related to synthetic cannabinoids in chronic THC users. The combination of THC and SC selectively downregulates CB1 receptors. Cross-tolerance develops to certain side effects with phytocannabinoid SC combinations which encourages greater utilization, increased doses, and frequency. Tolerance, however, is not uniform and differ for cardiac, renal, and neurologic side effects [7, 40, 47, 57, 81, 126]. SC tolerance to the rewarding effects is greater than to cardiac, renal, or respiratory adverse effects with a dose-dependent increase in risk of fatality [57, 126].

Prolonged CB2 activation by SC results in upregulation of 5HT2A receptors in the prefrontal lobe. These 5HT2A receptors are primary targets for hallucinatory drugs, and dysregulation causes anxiety and panic attacks [42, 54, 89]. The atypical antipsychotic compound pimavanserin, which is a 5HT2A receptor inverse agonist and antagonist, may therefore be a reasonable option in treating psychosis related to synthetic cannabinoids. This antipsychotic is licensed for Parkinson's disease-related hallucinations and psychosis [29, 34, 92].

The cardiac toxicity of synthetic cannabinoids is in part related to delayed cardiac repolarization. AM 2201, JWH-018, JWH-073, JWH-167, and JWH-391 have low affinity but high efficacy for cardiac hERG potassium-related channels and prolong the QTc interval leading to an arrhythmia [58, 59, 132].

Synthetic cannabinoid levels of 100–600 nM concentrations are reported to activate the serotonin receptor 5HT2B and strychnine-sensitive alpha-1 glycine receptors. However, these levels are not thought to be achievable in humans without severe or fatal toxicity (35 ng/ml) [35].

Synthetic cannabinoid classes with examples and associated metabolizing enzymes are listed in Table 3.1.

Because most synthetics are metabolized through cytochrome P450 enzymes, drug-drug interactions are likely to occur. JWH-018 metabolism is influenced by CYP2C9 polymorphisms [104]. There are no published studies which have demonstrated, at least clinically, the delayed clearance of synthetic cannabinoids by cytochrome or conjugase inhibiting drugs. UGT1A1, UGT1A3, UGT1A9, UGT1A10, and UGT2B7 have been shown to have a relatively high affinity with a K(m) ranging from 12 to 18 uM for some hydroxylated synthetic cannabinoid metabolites. These conjugases exhibit a high metabolic capacity for some of these compounds, and glucuronidated metabolites can be the main metabolites eliminated from the body [20].

There is little data about SC oral bioavailability, half-life, and volume of distribution. Two and 3 mg of smoked JWH-018 in six subjects produces a maximum concentration of JWH-018 of 2.2 to 36 (median 25.7) ng/mL after inhalation which decreases dramatically over the next hour to 0.08–8.42 (median 0.89) ng/mL. The median half-life is 1.69 hours. The elimination phase is a median of 8 hours after

Table 3.1 Synthetic cannabinoid class and metabolizing enzymes

Class	Synthetic cannabinoid examples	Metabolizing cytochrome/ enzyme
Naphthoylindoles	JWH-018	CYP2C9, CYP1A2
Halogenated Naphthoylindoles	AM-2201, MAM-2201, EAM-2201	CYP2C9, CYP1A2, CYP2B6
Indazine carboxamides	AKB-48, AB-CHMINACA	CYP3A4
Tetramethyl cyclopropyl ketone indoles	VR-144, XLR-11	CYP2C19, CYP1A2, CYP3A4, CYP2D6
Quinolinyl ester indoles	QUPIC	Carboxy esterases
Cyclohexylphenol	CP-47,497, CP-55,940	Mixed function oxidases
Phenylacetylindole	JWH-250	Mixed function oxidases and UGT
Tetrahydrocannabinol-dimethylheptyl	HU-210	NA
Aminoalkylindole	WIN 55,212–2	Mixed function oxidases
Carboxamide	STS-135	? CYP3A4, CYP3A5

Refs. [21, 38, 69, 77, 78, 138]

inhalation with the limits of detection at 0.024 ng/mL. Oral fluid/serum ratios vary considerably between individuals with a range of 0.05–555 (median 1.38) [129]. The (S)-isomer of the JWH-018-hydroxylated metabolite is predominantly excreted (>87%) in urine as the glucuronide conjugate, whereas the relative amount of the glucuronidated AM2201 metabolite is low (<5%) and does not demonstrate enantiospecificity [103]. In rhesus monkeys, using drug discrimination duration for AM-2201, JWH-122, and JWH-250, the biologic effect is 1–2 hours, whereas the effect of THC and CP-47,497 is 4–6 hours [65]. On the other hand, HU-210 has a long half-life (1–2 days) and very slow dissociation or pseudo-irreversible binding effect on cannabinoid receptors [64].

Synthetics are noted to inhibit cytochrome enzymes, but the concentration at which this occurs in vitro in animal studies is not thought to be achievable clinically. AM-2201 is reported to inhibit cytochrome P450 and uridine 5′-diphosphoglucuronosyltransferases at 3.9–10 uM. Clinical equivalents would be 1400 ng/ml (using the molecular weight of 359 and IC50 of 3.9uM). This would require a dose which is not tolerated and likely fatal [74]. Certain synthetics like AM-2201 inhibit enzymes that catabolize CBD and THC and may prolong the half-life of both phytocannabinoids [77]. Again, it would depend on whether doses of synthetic cannabinoid necessary to produce these levels are achievable. The in vitro Ki for synthetic EAM-2201 to inhibit CYP2C8, CYP2C9, CYP2C19, CYP3A4, and UGT1A3 is in the 3–4 uM range and thus unlikely to be achievable clinically without serious adverse events [78]. Another synthetic APINACA inhibits CYP3A enzymes and UGT1A9 in a time-dependent manner but does not interact with P-glycoprotein. The Ki for CYP3A is 4.5 uM and UGT1A9 5.9uM and thus doses to achieve this level are also too high [75].

3.3.2.2 Potential Uses of Synthetic Cannabinoids: Anticancer Activity

A multitude of cancers express cannabinoid receptors. In vitro studies suggest that cannabinoids have anticancer activity and can even overcome chemotherapy resistance [32, 102]. Cannabinoid receptors are highly expressed in general in more aggressive cancers which correlates with poor clinical outcomes [16, 22, 70, 72, 76, 83, 86, 101, 112, 136, 140].

There are multiple mechanisms by which phytocannabinoids and synthetic cannabinoids produce anticancer responses. WIN 55,212–2 by activating CB1 receptors also downregulates phosphor-AKT expression and inhibits VEGF-A and metalloprotease expression [135]. Hexahydrocannabinol analogues inhibit VEGF, NF- kappa-B, transcription, and angiogenesis in breast cancer cell lines [128]. This activity is observed whether P53 is mutated or not and independent of CB1 and CB2 receptor expression [128]. Other mechanisms include alterations in p38 mitogen-activated protein kinases, C-JUN, N-terminal kinases, protein kinase B pathways, and cell cycle regulators p27, Cdk4, and pRb [15, 36, 95, 113, 123, 131].

In vitro physiological responses to cannabinoids on cancer cells vary depending on concentration. THC at concentrations of 100–300 nanomoles in vitro actually stimulates lung cancer and glioblastoma cell lines while at concentrations of 1–20 uM causes cancer cells to undergo apoptosis [60, 116]. The concentrations of THC which stimulate cancer cell lines are nearly impossible to obtain clinically. The increased potency and efficacy of SC alone or in combination with THC may therefore improve cannabinoid anticancer activity and provide more feasible administration regimens [9, 30, 50, 62, 111].

However, not all synthetic cannabinoids have been shown to exhibit anticancer activity. For example, WIN 55,212–2 produces anticancer activity in vitro in renal cell cancer cell lines, but not JWH-133, which largely targets CB2 receptors [73]. Both WIN 55,212–2 and JWH-133 reduce tumor implants and the number of lung metastases in mice injected with the breast cancer cell lines which express CB1 and CB2 receptors: MDA-MB231, MDA-MB231-luc, and MDA-MB468 [110].

Conversely, some cancers may respond better to endocannabinoids than to certain synthetics. A gastric cancer cell line has been shown to respond with apoptosis to AEA and CP 55,940 but less so with methanandamide [98]. Therefore, greater efficacy at classical cannabinoid receptors does not always predict anticancer activity.

The clinical feasibility of using synthetics as anticancer agents or adjuvants depends foremost on determining the therapeutic window and achieving a safe dose. This may not be achievable in some cases. For example, WIN 55,212–2 reduces breast cancer viability at an IC50 concentration of 11–18-uM which is not clinically achievable without severe toxicity [37]. This same compound reduces prostate cancer viability when used as a single agent in vitro at an IC50 of 5–6 uM, but again these doses are unlikely to be tolerated [117]. Athymic mice treated with WIN 55,212–2 (5 mg/kg), delivered by intraperitoneal injection three times per week for 3 weeks reduced prostate cancer cell proliferation, migration, invasion, induced apoptosis, and arrested cells in Go/G1 phase in a dose-dependent manner [113].

However, synthetic cannabinoids which selectively target CB2 may improve anticancer therapy with less toxicity [88]. A quinone/cannabinoid pharmacophore, chromenopyrazolediones, is highly selective for the CB2 cannabinoid receptor, inducing death of human triple-negative breast cancer cell lines [88]. The anandamide analogue, methanandamide and JWH-015, both CB2 receptor agonists, exert antiproliferative effects on PC-3 cell lines [97].

Another way of reducing synthetic cannabinoid toxicity may be through unique nanotechnology delivery systems. Nano-micelles containing WIN 55,212–2 dramatically reduce breast cancer growth in mice also receiving doxorubicin and produced relatively tolerable toxicity to animals [55]. Styrene maleic acid conjugated WIN 55,212–2 delivered in nano-micelles have been developed in light of dramatic responses observed against triple-negative breast cancer (MDA-MB-231), hormone receptor-positive breast cancer (MCF-7), and castration-resistant prostate cancer (PC3) cell lines [134]. This also may be an effective therapy for lung gastric and testicular cancer [91, 96]. Clinical studies have not been done to date, however.

3.3.2.3 Synthetic Cannabinoid Toxicity

Unlike phytocannabinoids, synthetic cannabinoids have clearly been linked with human fatalities. Patients present to emergency departments with severe toxic reactions, which include severe malignant hypertension with intracranial hemorrhage, tachycardia and fatal arrhythmias, visual and/or auditory hallucinations, psychosis, and seizures [6, 79, 90, 100]. Toxic psychosis induced by SC is also more profound and prevalent than seen with THC [39, 63, 122, 137]. In addition, hallucinations, paranoia, and suicide ideation last much longer than with THC, and major depression is more profound.

In a cohort of 353 patients presenting for acute medical care following SC intoxication, the median age was 25 (IQR: 18, 36), and the majority were males (84%). The most common symptoms were agitation, delirium, and toxic psychosis, $n = 146$ (41%). Forty-four (12.5%) had tachycardia defined as 140 beats per minute. Bradycardia was the second most commonly reported severe cardiac abnormality with 20 (5.7%) having heart rates of less than 50 beats per minute. Fifteen (4.2%) patients had hypotension and 59 (17%) had seizures. The most common treatments used were benzodiazepines ($n = 131$, 37%) followed by antipsychotics ($n = 36$, 10%). Forty-two (15%) were admitted to the hospital floor, and 67 (24%) were admitted to the ICU [87]. In another study, deaths occurred in 0.2%, strokes in 0.1%, and myocardial infarctions in 0.09% of subjects [28]. The synthetic cannabinoid known as ACHMINACA is particularly dangerous. Seizures occur with this synthetic in 27%, and sudden collapse is reported in 25% [31]. Another particularly dangerous synthetic is AM2201, which causes seizures through release of glutamate within the hippocampus. Other effects such as memory deficits, lightheadedness, perioral and facial numbness, dry mouth, difficulty focusing, giggling, sluggishness, tachycardia, and hypertension have been known to accompany seizures [11, 53].

Synthetic cannabinoid toxicity also includes acute kidney injury. The pathology consists of either acute tubular necrosis or interstitial nephritis. Patients who present in acute renal failure are usually male, ages 15–33 years, and have symptoms of nausea, vomiting, abdominal pain, and/or flank pain plus diarrhea [71]. Renal failure may occur secondarily from rhabdomyolysis and dehydration from hyperemesis [5]. Patients with rhabdomyolysis often present with hyperthermia and renal failure [124].

Furthermore, some synthetic cannabinoids have been tainted with the rodenticide, brodifacoum, which causes severe bleeding [4, 49, 52, 115].

3.3.2.4 Withdrawal

Withdrawal symptoms are severe with daily users of synthetic cannabinoids. The most common withdrawal symptoms are anxiety, mood swings, irritability, agitation, as well as loss of appetite. Nausea and vomiting occur in 40–50%. Withdrawal can begin within 1–2 hours after the last dose and repeated doses throughout the day are required to avoid symptoms from appearing. The symptoms peak on day 2 of abstinence and persist at least for the first 5 days. In one study, most patients who entered medical treatment were prescribed benzodiazepines and quetiapine. Doses of quetiapine ranged from 25 to 475 mg daily though most require less than 200 mg. Nabilone may also reduce craving [26, 80].

3.3.3 Conclusion

Synthetic cannabinoid use in the community is increasing though detection is difficult due to the need for specialized testing. Oncologists should be aware of the signs and symptoms of synthetic cannabinoid toxicities which may overlap with chemotherapy-related toxicities. Synthetics have anticancer activity, but the therapeutic index is likely to be quite narrow. Unique delivery systems are needed to explore the anticancer activity. Synthetics are likely to have significant drug-drug interactions with palliative medications which may compound the risk for toxicities. Clinical studies are needed to understand the pharmacokinetics and dose tolerance to this class of compounds.

3.4 Part 2: Palmitoylethanolamide (PEA) and the Role of Future Endocannabinoid Modulators in Cancer Care

N-(2-Acylethanolamine)-hexadecanamide, also commonly called palmitoylethanolamide or PEA, is a prominent member of the n-acylethanolamine (NAE) family. It is an autacoid local injury antagonist amide (ALIAmide) which are endogenous bioactive ethanolamides with anti-inflammatory properties [144, 165]. These compounds are produced as a reaction to injury and are generated and metabolized in the same cells and tissue. The Nobel Prize winner Rita Levi Montalcini first described the accumulation of NAE under pathologic and degenerative conditions resulting in down-modulation of cellular inflammation and mast cell activation [143, 147, 169]. Down-modulation of inflammation, neuroinflammation, and mast cell activity is associated with antinociception in animals and analgesia in clinical studies [161, 173].

3.4.1 Pharmacodynamics

The pharmacodynamics of PEA related to analgesia are protean [146, 148, 149, 152, 157, 162–164, 167]:

1. Down-modulation of mast cell responses to tissue injury.
2. Activation of peroxisome proliferator activated receptor-alpha (PPAR-alpha).
3. Activation and desensitization of the vanilloid receptor, TRPV1.
4. An entourage effect with anandamide through competition with fatty acid amide hydrolase (FAAH) resulting in indirect activation of the cannabinoid receptors CB1 and CB2.
5. Microglia Inhibition.

3.4.2 Pharmacokinetics

The advantages of ALIAmides over traditional analgesics are that ALIAmides modulate neurotransmitter and inflammatory pathways within tissues rather than targeting single receptors. ALIAmides have no toxic metabolites nor interact with mixed function oxidases and thus do not have drug-drug interactions. Traditional analgesics often alter physiologic processes and cause "collateral" damage through toxic metabolites or off-target effects (constipation, respiratory depression) as seen with opioid analgesics [153, 154].

PEA is a highly lipophilic compound with limited absorption, which is why micronization to less than 10 microns has been shown to increase bioavailability and efficacy [156, 158, 159]. Almost all trials published have used micronized PEA.

Barriers to achieving accurate estimates of PEA pharmacokinetics are fluctuating blood levels and tissue that normally occur and which change with diseases. Circulating levels may vary independent of oral pharmacokinetics. Levels are expressions of second- and third-order pathways or local and circulating levels that are influenced by endocannabinoids competing for intracellular binding and fatty acid amide hydrolase. The local expression of enzymes responsible for PEA production will also influence circulating levels [108, 155, 162, 170]. There are few human pharmacokinetic studies, but fortunately, there are a sizable number of animal studies using radiolabeled micronized PEA in oral and parenteral form which provides useful information about PEA bioavailability and distribution [159].

Concentrations in tissues are generally higher than in plasma with circulating levels varying markedly during the day [159]. Concentrations in tissues and plasma usually increase with injury, particularly with inflammation and in disease processes associated with neurodegeneration [3, 8, 51, 94, 106, 107]. In the pig brain, PEA levels far exceed those of anandamide (205 ng/gram versus 6 ng/gram brain tissue) [166].

Caco-2 is an immortalized cell line of human colorectal adenocarcinoma cells which is widely used in vitro to estimate drug bioavailability. By this method, micronized PEA absorption begins at 30 minutes, and approximately 20–30% of PEA is projected to be bioavailable. Maximum absorption is observed at 3 hours [3, 8, 51, 94, 106, 107]. In a small study of 10 healthy individuals, 300 mg of micronized PEA produced peak concentrations at 2 hours, with a twofold increase in circulating PEA levels over baseline. A second peak occurring later is assumed to be due to enterohepatic recirculation [108].

In rats, oral micronized PEA in corn oil (100 mg/kg) produces plasma levels that are 20-fold higher in concentration within 15 minutes relative to baseline. Plasma levels return to baseline in approximately 2 hours [171]. Beagle dogs given 30 mg/kg of micronized PEA have a sixfold increase in circulating PEA levels [163]. Animals experiencing inflammatory pain have greater absorption of oral micronized PEA than healthy animals. In one study, plasma levels are 4.3-fold higher at 15 minutes in animals with inflammation than in healthy animals, and circulating levels are 4.9-fold higher than healthy controls [162]. Spinal cord concentrations are 26–110-fold higher as measured by $[^{13}C]_4$-labeled micronized PEA. Inflammation reduces the spinal cord barrier to distribution allowing greater amounts of PEA to enter the central nervous system [174].

A 4-arm randomized trial involving Sprague Dawley rats illustrates this point. Standardized and micronized radiolabeled PEA 30 mg/kg used in healthy animals and animals subject to carrageenan paw injections significantly increased radiolabeled PEA levels in injured animals relative to healthy controls, and oral bioavailability was greater than standardized PEA at the same dose [162]. Tissue levels were significantly higher in the carrageenan-treated animals relative to controls measured at 15, 30, 60, and 360 minutes after PEA administration. Significant injured tissue (paw) levels were seen at 15, 30, and 60 minutes. Tissue levels in those receiving micronized PEA subjected to carrageenan were sixfold higher than healthy controls. Rats subjected to carrageenan had radiolabeled PEA levels in the spinal cord that were 110-fold higher than normal controls (11.1 pmol/gm tissue versus 0.10 pmol/gm tissue). Brain levels increased over baseline at 5 minutes through 60 minutes after administration. Levels though were not higher than those seen in healthy controls. Biopsies of the carrageenan injected paws given oral micronized PEA at a dose of 10 mg/kg demonstrated reduced mast cell degradation and reduced TNF-alpha levels, IL-6 levels, and IL-1 beta levels. Expression of NF-kappa-B p65 and cyclooxygenase-2 levels were reduced compared to controls.

These findings correlated with reduced edema and hyperalgesia [162]. Injections of PEA 10 mg/kg produces significant tissue levels in the bowel and prevents radiation enteritis in mast cell-deficient but not wild-type rats suggesting that significant tissue levels are achieved by systemic administration. Paradoxically mast cells are needed to reduce radiation injury. PEA benefits were independent of mast cell modulation [172].

Intraperitoneal emulsified micronized PEA (10 mg/kg) injected in DBA/2 mice produces significant brain, blood, heart, and retina levels which persist at 24 and 48 hours [151]. Brain levels in rodents after oral administration of 30 mg/kg micronized PEA produce levels ranging between 21 and 16 pmol/gm of brain tissue within 15 minutes of administration [162, 168]. Oral administration of radiolabeled micronized PEA at a dose of 100 mg/kg produced significant levels within the pituitary, hypothalamus, and adrenal gland within 20 minutes [150].

In summary, though human studies are few and limited, oral micronized PEA appears to exhibit appreciable bioavailability, which is estimated to be 20–30% by standard in vitro studies. In multiple animal models, micronized PEA is rapidly absorbed, and bioavailability is improved in disease states. PEA penetrates tissues and produces measurable levels in the peripheral tissues and central nervous system.

PEA is catabolized by two enzymes in tissues, fatty acid amide hydrolase (FAAH) and N-acylethanolamine acid amidase. Pharmacokinetics have not been done in end-organ failure, but PEA is likely to be safe in hepatic, renal, and heart failure due to the lack of drug-drug interactions and absence of active metabolite.

3.4.3 *Safety*

PEA is quite safe by standard in vitro tests, in animal studies and clinically. In vitro, PEA is not mutagenic, since it does not induce a two-fold increase in revertant colonies at 30, 90, 300, and 3000 mcg per plate cultures in the Ames test [160]. PEA does not induce biologically significant increases in the percentage incidence of micronuclei in binucleated cells at any dose [160]. PEA does not cause cytotoxicity as measured by the cytokinesis-block proliferation index [160].

The NOEL effect is the highest dose or exposure of a drug that produces no noticeable or observable toxic effect. Animal studies with PEA have shown no NOEL effect at doses greater than 1000 mg per kg twice daily. PEA is not lethal in Sprague Dawley rats at doses as high as 2000 mg/kg for 15 days [160]. There is no toxicity noted using doses of 1000 mg per kg for 90 days [160], and animal survival is 100% at 90 days. There is also no significant loss or gain in weight and there are no differences in blood counts when compared to controls. Furthermore, there were no biologically significant changes in other blood chemistries [160]. Finally, there are no gross anatomical or histopathological changes noted in treated animals [160]. It certainly looks like PEA is safe.

There are a large number of micronized PEA human trials that have been carried out, mostly centered on pain. Daily doses ranged from 300 to 1200 mg per day.

Table 3.2 Clinical toxicity noted in PEA trials

Study	Days on treatment	Number of participants	Toxicity
Canteri (2010)	21	112	0
Guida (2010)	21	626	0
Schifilliti (2014)	60	30	0
Bacci (2011)	15	26	1 -unrelated to PEA
Pescosolido (2011)	15	15	0
Truini (2011)	60	20	0
Costagliola (2014)	180	32	0
Marini (2012)	14	12	0
Barbieri (2010)	4	90	0
Calabro (2010)	14	1	0
Conigliaro (2011)	30	26	0
Affini (2010)	60	50	0
Desio (2010)	45	30	0

Thirteen studies listed below reported no adverse events (Table 3.2), though one study noted a single adverse event, but was unrelated to PEA [160].

Three publications are particularly illustrative of the safety and efficacy of PEA in treating pain. A post hoc analysis of a multi-center double-blind, placebo-controlled, 3-armed trial involving patients with lumbosacral pain with two treatment arms: micronized PEA, 300 and 600 mg daily, and a third placebo arm [145]. Treatment duration was 21 days. The primary outcomes were changes in the visual analogue scale (VAS) (0 no pain 10 severe pain) and the Roland-Morris Disability Questionnaire (RMDQ). The number needed to treat to benefit a single individual (NNT) was calculated using the response criteria of a 50% improvement in pain relief and a 50% improvement in the RMDQ. Attrition due to side effects and the number needed to harm due to discontinuation for reasons of adverse effects were safety outcomes. This study registered 626 patients of which 619 were evaluable. Both treatment arms were superior to placebo ($P < 0.001$). Efficacy was particularly superior in the subgroup with neuropathic pain. For the 300 mg arm, the NNT was 9 (95% confidence intervals 5–29) and the RMDQ NNT 6.4 (95% confidence interval 4–14) ($P < 0.02$). For the 600 mg treatment arm, the NNT was 1.7 (95% confidence intervals 1.4–2), and the RMDQ NNT was 1.5 (1.4–1.7) ($P < 0.001$). The NNH was not different between treatment arms and placebo. Dropouts were 19 from placebo, 2 from the 300 mg treatment arm, and 1 from the 600 mg treatment arm [145].

There are also two meta-analyses that have been published recently. The first pulled raw data available from clinical trials of micronized PEA published between 2010 and 2014 [161]. Patients had either chronic or neuropathic pain. Pain reduction over time was the main measured outcome. Timeframes were divided into baseline (T0), days 7–10 (T1), days 11–14 (T2), days 15 through 21 (T3), days 22–45 (T4), and days 46–60 (T5). Analysis used generalized linear mixed modeling and linear regression. Cox modeling assessed the influence of gender, age, pain etiology, and study design on pain outcomes. Of 26 clinical trials retrieved, 12 met the inclusion criteria. A total of 1484 participants were included using doses ranging from 100 to 1200 mg daily. Pain reduction was seen in both the active and control groups. The pain reduction was superior with PEA with differences that were evident at T1 ($P < 0.05$) which increased over time ($P < 0.001$). The average pain reduction using a numerical rating scale (0 no pain 10 severe pain) was 0.2 points every 2 weeks for controls and 1.04 points every 2 weeks for PEA ($P < 0.001$). Placebo accounted for 1% of pain variability over time, whereas PEA accounted for 35% of variability. Age, gender, and pain etiology did not influence responses. The average pain score at 60 days was <3/10 (0 no pain 10 severe pain) in 81.9% of PEA-treated individuals and 40.9% for those treated with placebo [161].

The second meta-analysis published in 2017 involved controlled trials of PEA for pain [142]. Randomized trials published up to May 1, 2015, were included. Trials were either with placebo, inactive, or active comparators. The primary outcome was the change in VAS. Random effects modeling was used for the primary outcome and fixed effect modeling for a sensitivity analysis. Publication bias was assessed by funnel plot and Egger's analysis. Trials were grouped by dose, duration of study, and trial characteristic. Meta-regression was used to assess the effects of dose on outcomes. Of 25 references, 10 randomized trials were included. Daily doses ranged from 300 to 800 mg with the majority receiving 600 mg daily. Of the 1298 patients in the meta-analysis, 786 received micronized PEA, while 46% of studies had an inactive control. PEA was superior to the inactive comparator with a (WMD = 2.03, 95% CI: 1.19–2.87, z = 4.75, $P < 0.001$). By fixed effect modeling, the weighted mean difference (WMD) = 2.20, 95% CI: 2.00–2.41, z = 21.4, $P < 0.001$), and there was no publication bias. Stratified subgroup analysis did not show differences based on trial design. There was no response difference between doses and no association of efficacy with duration of treatment. In regard to tolerability, all-cause dropouts were reduced in the PEA-treated groups relative to other treatment arms, but this was not statistically significant relative to placebo or the inactive comparator ($P = 0.11$). All-cause dropouts were 1.1% of patients on PEA and 4.3% in the inactive controls/placebo treated patients. Adverse effects reported with PEA were gastrointestinal upset in two patients, drowsiness in one, and heart palpitations in one individual.

In summary, based on two meta-analyses and a large clinical trial, micronized PEA is safe, tolerable, and efficacious. There are discrepancies in the two meta-analysis which are dose-response and efficacy over time which will need clarification in future studies.

3.5 Conclusion

Nutraceuticals such as PEA are clinically active endocannabinoid system modulators. PEA targets mainly PPAR-alpha and mast cells and exhibits complex pharmacodynamics. Animal models suggest that bioavailability increases with inflammation and several studies and meta-analyses suggest that PEA exhibits robust effects in treating pain with few side effects. Larger trials are needed to provide clear evidence of clinical benefits for PEA and other future endocannabinoid system modulators.

References (Synthetic Cannabinoids)

1. Abouchedid R, Ho JH, Hudson S, Dines A, Archer JR, Wood DM, Dargan PI. Acute toxicity associated with use of 5F-derivations of synthetic cannabinoid receptor agonists with analytical confirmation. J Med Toxicol. 2016;12:396–401.
2. Adamowicz P. Fatal intoxication with synthetic cannabinoid MDMB-CHMICA. Forensic Sci Int. 2016;261:e5–10.
3. Annuzzi G, Piscitelli F, Di Marino L, Patti L, Giacco R, Costabile G, Bozzetto L, Riccardi G, Verde R, Petrosino S, Rivellese AA, Di Marzo V. Differential alterations of the concentrations of endocannabinoids and related lipids in the subcutaneous adipose tissue of obese diabetic patients. Lipids Health Dis. 2010;9:43.
4. Alipour A, Patel PB, Shabbir Z, Gabrielson S. Review of the many faces of synthetic cannabinoid toxicities. Ment Health Clin. 2019;9:93–9.
5. Argamany JR, Reveles KR, Duhon B. Synthetic cannabinoid hyperemesis resulting in rhabdomyolysis and acute renal failure. Am J Emerg Med. 2016;34(765):e1–2.
6. Benford DM, Caplan JP. Psychiatric sequelae of Spice, K2, and synthetic cannabinoid receptor agonists. Psychosomatics. 2011;52:295.
7. Benowitz NL, Jones RT. Cardiovascular and metabolic considerations in prolonged cannabinoid administration in man. J Clin Pharmacol. 1981;21:214S–23S.
8. Bisogno T, Martire A, Petrosino S, Popoli P, Di Marzo V. Symptom-related changes of endocannabinoid and palmitoylethanolamide levels in brain areas of R6/2 mice, a transgenic model of Huntington's disease. Neurochem Int. 2008;52:307–13.
9. Bogdanovic V, Mrdjanovic J, Borisev I. A review of the therapeutic antitumor potential of cannabinoids. J Altern Complement Med. 2017;23:831–6.
10. Bonhaus DW, Chang LK, Kwan J, Martin GR. Dual activation and inhibition of adenylyl cyclase by cannabinoid receptor agonists: evidence for agonist-specific trafficking of intracellular responses. J Pharmacol Exp Ther. 1998;287:884–8.
11. Breivogel CS, Wells JR, Jonas A, Mistry AH, Gravley ML, Patel RM, Whithorn BE, Brenseke BM. Comparison of the neurotoxic and seizure-inducing effects of synthetic and endogenous cannabinoids with delta(9)-tetrahydrocannabinol. Cannabis Cannabinoid Res. 2020;5:32–41.
12. Brents LK, Gallus-Zawada A, Radominska-Pandya A, Vasiljevik T, Prisinzano TE, Fantegrossi WE, Moran JH, Prather PL. Monohydroxylated metabolites of the K2 synthetic cannabinoid JWH-073 retain intermediate to high cannabinoid 1 receptor (CB1R) affinity and exhibit neutral antagonist to partial agonist activity. Biochem Pharmacol. 2012;83:952–61.
13. Brents LK, Zimmerman SM, Saffell AR, Prather PL, Fantegrossi WE. Differential drug-drug interactions of the synthetic Cannabinoids JWH-018 and JWH-073: implications for drug abuse liability and pain therapy. J Pharmacol Exp Ther. 2013;346:350–61.
14. Burkey TH, Quock RM, Consroe P, Ehlert FJ, Hosohata Y, Roeske WR, Yamamura HI. Relative efficacies of cannabinoid CB1 receptor agonists in the mouse brain. Eur J Pharmacol. 1997;336:295–8.
15. Caballero FJ, Soler-Torronteras R, Lara-Chica M, Garcia V, Fiebich BL, Munoz E, Calzado MA. AM404 inhibits NFAT and NF-kappaB signaling pathways and impairs migration and invasiveness of neuroblastoma cells. Eur J Pharmacol. 2015;746:221–32.
16. Caffarel MM, Andradas C, Mira E, Perez-Gomez E, Cerutti C, Moreno-Bueno G, Flores JM, Garcia-Real I, Palacios J, Manes S, Guzman M, Sanchez C. Cannabinoids reduce ErbB2-driven breast cancer progression through Akt inhibition. Mol Cancer. 2010;9:196.

17. Canazza I, Ossato A, Trapella C, Fantinati A, De Luca MA, Margiani G, Vincenzi F, Rimondo C, Di Rosa F, Gregori A, Varani K, Borea PA, Serpelloni G, Marti M. Effect of the novel synthetic cannabinoids AKB48 and 5F-AKB48 on "tetrad", sensorimotor, neurological and neurochemical responses in mice. In vitro and in vivo pharmacological studies. Psychopharmacology. 2016;233:3685–709.
18. Castaneto MS, Gorelick DA, Desrosiers NA, Hartman RL, Pirard S, Huestis MA. Synthetic cannabinoids: epidemiology, pharmacodynamics, and clinical implications. Drug Alcohol Depend. 2014;144:12–41.
19. Castaneto MS, Wohlfarth A, Desrosiers NA, Hartman RL, Gorelick DA, Huestis MA. Synthetic cannabinoids pharmacokinetics and detection methods in biological matrices. Drug Metab Rev. 2015;47:124–74.
20. Chimalakonda KC, Bratton SM, Le VH, Yiew KH, Dineva A, Moran CL, James LP, Moran JH, Radominska-Pandya A. Conjugation of synthetic cannabinoids JWH-018 and JWH-073, metabolites by human UDP-glucuronosyltransferases. Drug Metab Dispos. 2011;39:1967–76.
21. Chimalakonda KC, Seely KA, Bratton SM, Brents LK, Moran CL, Endres GW, James LP, Hollenberg PF, Prather PL, Radominska-Pandya A, Moran JH. Cytochrome P450-mediated oxidative metabolism of abused synthetic cannabinoids found in K2/Spice: identification of novel cannabinoid receptor ligands. Drug Metab Dispos. 2012;40:2174–84.
22. Chung SC, Hammarsten P, Josefsson A, Stattin P, Granfors T, Egevad L, Mancini G, Lutz B, Bergh A, Fowler CJ. A high cannabinoid CB(1) receptor immunoreactivity is associated with disease severity and outcome in prostate cancer. Eur J Cancer. 2009;45:174–82.
23. Cohen K, Rosenzweig S, Rosca P, Pinhasov A, Weizman A, Weinstein A. Personality traits and psychotic proneness among chronic synthetic cannabinoid users. Front Psych. 2020;11:355.
24. Cohen K, Weinstein AM. Synthetic and non-synthetic cannabinoid drugs and their adverse effects-a review from public health prospective. Front Public Health. 2018;6:162.
25. Compton DR, Rice KC, De Costa BR, Razdan RK, Melvin LS, Johnson MR, Martin BR. Cannabinoid structure-activity relationships: correlation of receptor binding and in vivo activities. J Pharmacol Exp Ther. 1993;265:218–26.
26. Cooper ZD. Adverse effects of synthetic cannabinoids: management of acute toxicity and withdrawal. Curr Psychiatry Rep. 2016;18:52.
27. Costain WJ, Tauskela JS, Rasquinha I, Comas T, Hewitt M, Marleau V, Soo EC. Pharmacological characterization of emerging synthetic cannabinoids in HEK293T cells and hippocampal neurons. Eur J Pharmacol. 2016;786:234–45.
28. Courts J, Maskill V, Gray A, Glue P. Signs and symptoms associated with synthetic cannabinoid toxicity: systematic review. Australas Psychiatry. 2016;24:598–601.
29. Cusick E, Gupta V. Pimavanserin. In: StatPearls. Treasure Island (FL); 2020.
30. Daris B, Tancer Verboten M, Knez Z, Ferk P. Cannabinoids in cancer treatment: therapeutic potential and legislation. Bosn J Basic Med Sci. 2019;19:14–23.
31. Darke S, Duflou J, Farrell M, Peacock A, Lappin J. Characteristics and circumstances of synthetic cannabinoid-related death. Clin Toxicol (Phila). 2020;58:368–74.
32. Davis MP. Cannabinoids for symptom management and cancer therapy: the evidence. J Natl Compr Cancer Netw. 2016;14:915–22.
33. De Luca MA, Castelli MP, Loi B, Porcu A, Martorelli M, Miliano C, Kellett K, Davidson C, Stair JL, Schifano F, Di Chiara G. Native CB1 receptor affinity, intrinsic activity and accumbens shell dopamine stimulant properties of third generation SPICE/K2 cannabinoids: BB-22, 5F-PB-22, 5F-AKB-48 and STS-135. Neuropharmacology. 2016;105:630–8.
34. DeKarske D, Alva G, Aldred JL, Coate B, Cantillon M, Jacobi L, Nunez R, Norton JC, Abler V. An open-label, 8-week study of safety and efficacy of pimavanserin treatment in adults with Parkinson's disease and depression. J Parkinsons Dis. 2020;10:1751–61.
35. Demir R, Leuwer M, de la Roche J, Krampfl K, Foadi N, Karst M, Dengler R, Haeseler G, Ahrens J. Modulation of glycine receptor function by the synthetic cannabinoid HU210. Pharmacology. 2009;83:270–4.
36. Do Y, McKallip RJ, Nagarkatti M, Nagarkatti PS. Activation through cannabinoid receptors 1 and 2 on dendritic cells triggers NF-kappaB-dependent apoptosis: novel role for endogenous and exogenous cannabinoids in immunoregulation. J Immunol. 2004;173:2373–82.

37. Emery SM, Alotaibi MR, Tao Q, Selley DE, Lichtman AH, Gewirtz DA. Combined antiproliferative effects of the aminoalkylindole WIN55,212-2 and radiation in breast cancer cells. J Pharmacol Exp Ther. 2014;348:293–302.
38. Erratico C, Negreira N, Norouzizadeh H, Covaci A, Neels H, Maudens K, van Nuijs AL. In vitro and in vivo human metabolism of the synthetic cannabinoid AB-CHMINACA. Drug Test Anal. 2015;7:866–76.
39. Escelsior A, Belvederi Murri M, Corsini GP, Serafini G, Aguglia A, Zampogna D, Cattedra S, Nebbia J, Trabucco A, Prestia D, Olcese M, Barletta E, Pereira da Silva B, Amore M. Cannabinoid use and self-injurious behaviours: a systematic review and meta-analysis. J Affect Disord. 2020;278:85–98.
40. Fan F, Compton DR, Ward S, Melvin L, Martin BR. Development of cross-tolerance between delta 9-tetrahydrocannabinol, CP 55,940 and WIN 55,212. J Pharmacol Exp Ther. 1994;271:1383–90.
41. Fantegrossi WE, Moran JH, Radominska-Pandya A, Prather PL. Distinct pharmacology and metabolism of K2 synthetic cannabinoids compared to Delta(9)-THC: mechanism underlying greater toxicity? Life Sci. 2014;97:45–54.
42. Fantegrossi WE, Wilson CD, Berquist MD. Pro-psychotic effects of synthetic cannabinoids: interactions with central dopamine, serotonin, and glutamate systems. Drug Metab Rev. 2018;50:65–73.
43. Fattore L, Cossu G, Martellotta CM, Fratta W. Intravenous self-administration of the cannabinoid CB1 receptor agonist WIN 55,212-2 in rats. Psychopharmacology. 2001;156:410–6.
44. Fattore L, Fratta W. Beyond THC: the new generation of cannabinoid designer drugs. Front Behav Neurosci. 2011;5:60.
45. Felder CC, Joyce KE, Briley EM, Mansouri J, Mackie K, Blond O, Lai Y, Ma AL, Mitchell RL. Comparison of the pharmacology and signal transduction of the human cannabinoid CB1 and CB2 receptors. Mol Pharmacol. 1995;48:443–50.
46. Ferrari F, Ottani A, Giuliani D. Cannabimimetic activity in rats and pigeons of HU 210, a potent antiemetic drug. Pharmacol Biochem Behav. 1999;62:75–80.
47. Ford BM, Tai S, Fantegrossi WE, Prather PL. Synthetic pot: not your grandfather's marijuana. Trends Pharmacol Sci. 2017;38:257–76.
48. Ford RD, Balster RL, Dewey WL, Beckner JS. Delta 9-THC and 11-OH-delta 9-THC: behavioral effects and relationship to plasma and brain levels. Life Sci. 1977;20:1993–2003.
49. Foti F, Sica S, Alma E, De Cristofaro R, Mores N, Vetrugno G. Sudden nasal bleeding and brodifacoum: a case of accidental exposure or attempted homicide? Leg Med (Tokyo). 2020;47:101772.
50. Fraguas-Sanchez AI, Fernandez-Carballido A, Torres-Suarez AI. Phyto-, endo- and synthetic cannabinoids: promising chemotherapeutic agents in the treatment of breast and prostate carcinomas. Expert Opin Investig Drugs. 2016;25:1311–23.
51. Franklin A, Parmentier-Batteur S, Walter L, Greenberg DA, Stella N. Palmitoylethanolamide increases after focal cerebral ischemia and potentiates microglial cell motility. J Neurosci. 2003;23:7767–75.
52. Franklin AB, Carlson PC, Rex A, Rockweit JT, Garza D, Culhane E, Volker SF, Dusek RJ, Shearn-Bochsler VI, Gabriel MW, Horak KE. Grass is not always greener: rodenticide exposure of a threatened species near marijuana growing operations. BMC Res Notes. 2018;11:94.
53. Funada M, Takebayashi-Ohsawa M. Synthetic cannabinoid AM2201 induces seizures: involvement of cannabinoid CB1 receptors and glutamatergic transmission. Toxicol Appl Pharmacol. 2018;338:1–8.
54. Ghisleni G, Kazlauckas V, Both FL, Pagnussat N, Mioranzza S, Rocha JB, Souza DO, Porciuncula LO. Diphenyl diselenide exerts anxiolytic-like effect in Wistar rats: putative roles of GABAA and 5HT receptors. Prog Neuro-Psychopharmacol Biol Psychiatry. 2008;32:1508–15.
55. Greish K, Mathur A, Al Zahrani R, Elkaissi S, Al Jishi M, Nazzal O, Taha S, Pittala V, Taurin S. Synthetic cannabinoids nano-micelles for the management of triple negative breast cancer. J Control Release. 2018;291:184–95.

56. Griffiths P, Sedefov R, Gallegos A, Lopez D. How globalization and market innovation challenge how we think about and respond to drug use: 'Spice' a case study. Addiction. 2010;105:951–3.
57. Grim TW, Samano KL, Ignatowska-Jankowska B, Tao Q, Sim-Selly LJ, Selley DE, Wise LE, Poklis A, Lichtman AH. Pharmacological characterization of repeated administration of the first generation abused synthetic cannabinoid CP47,497. J Basic Clin Physiol Pharmacol. 2016;27:217–28.
58. Hancox JC, James AF. Refining insights into high-affinity drug binding to the human ether-a-go-go-related gene potassium channel. Mol Pharmacol. 2008;73:1592–5.
59. Hancox JC, McPate MJ, El Harchi A, Zhang YH. The hERG potassium channel and hERG screening for drug-induced torsades de pointes. Pharmacol Ther. 2008;119:118–32.
60. Hart S, Fischer OM, Ullrich A. Cannabinoids induce cancer cell proliferation via tumor necrosis factor alpha-converting enzyme (TACE/ADAM17)-mediated transactivation of the epidermal growth factor receptor. Cancer Res. 2004;64:1943–50.
61. Hess C, Schoeder CT, Pillaiyar T, Madea B, Muller CE. Pharmacological evaluation of synthetic cannabinoids identified as constituents of spice. Forensic Toxicol. 2016;34:329–43.
62. Hinz B, Ramer R. Anti-tumour actions of cannabinoids. Br J Pharmacol. 2019;176: 1384–94.
63. Hobbs M, Patel R, Morrison PD, Kalk N, Stone JM. Synthetic cannabinoid use in psychiatric patients and relationship to hospitalisation: a retrospective electronic case register study. J Psychopharmacol. 2020;34:648–53.
64. Hruba L, McMahon LR. The cannabinoid agonist HU-210: pseudo-irreversible discriminative stimulus effects in rhesus monkeys. Eur J Pharmacol. 2014;727:35–42.
65. Hruba L, McMahon LR. Apparent affinity estimates and reversal of the effects of synthetic cannabinoids AM-2201, CP-47,497, JWH-122, and JWH-250 by rimonabant in rhesus monkeys. J Pharmacol Exp Ther. 2017;362:278–86.
66. Hsieh C, Brown S, Derleth C, Mackie K. Internalization and recycling of the CB1 cannabinoid receptor. J Neurochem. 1999;73:493–501.
67. Hutchison RD, Ford BM, Franks LN, Wilson CD, Yarbrough AL, Fujiwara R, Su MK, Fernandez D, James LP, Moran JH, Patton AL, Fantegrossi WE, Radominska-Pandya A, Prather PL. Atypical pharmacodynamic properties and metabolic profile of the abused synthetic cannabinoid AB-PINACA: potential contribution to pronounced adverse effects relative to delta(9)-THC. Front Pharmacol. 2018;9:1084.
68. Jaenicke NJ, Pogoda W, Paulke A, Wunder C, Toennes SW. Retrospective analysis of synthetic cannabinoids in serum samples–epidemiology and consumption patterns. Forensic Sci Int. 2014;242:81–7.
69. Jin MJ, Lee J, In MK, Yoo HH. Characterization of in vitro metabolites of CP 47,497, a synthetic cannabinoid, in human liver microsomes by LC-MS/MS. J Forensic Sci. 2013;58:195–9.
70. Kaur R, Ambwani SR, Singh S. Endocannabinoid system: a multi-facet therapeutic target. Curr Clin Pharmacol. 2016;11:110–7.
71. Kazory A, Aiyer R. Synthetic marijuana and acute kidney injury: an unforeseen association. Clin Kidney J. 2013;6:330–3.
72. Keresztes A, Streicher JM. Synergistic interaction of the cannabinoid and death receptor systems – a potential target for future cancer therapies? FEBS Lett. 2017;591:3235–51.
73. Khan MI, Sobocinska AA, Brodaczewska KK, Zielniok K, Gajewska M, Kieda C, Czarnecka AM, Szczylik C. Involvement of the CB2 cannabinoid receptor in cell growth inhibition and G0/G1 cell cycle arrest via the cannabinoid agonist WIN 55,212-2 in renal cell carcinoma. BMC Cancer. 2018;18:583.
74. Kim JH, Kwon SS, Kong TY, Cheong JC, Kim HS, In MK, Lee HS. AM-2201 inhibits multiple cytochrome P450 and uridine 5'-diphospho-glucuronosyltransferase enzyme activities in human liver microsomes. Molecules. 2017;22
75. Kim S, Choi WG, Kwon M, Lee S, Cho YY, Lee JY, Kang HC, Song IS, Lee HS. In vitro inhibitory effects of APINACA on human major cytochrome P450, UDP-glucuronosyltransferase enzymes, and drug transporters. Molecules. 2019;24

76. Klein Nulent TJ, Van Diest PJ, van der Groep P, Leusink FK, Kruitwagen CL, Koole R, Van Cann EM. Cannabinoid receptor-2 immunoreactivity is associated with survival in squamous cell carcinoma of the head and neck. Br J Oral Maxillofac Surg. 2013;51:604–9.
77. Kong TY, Kim JH, Kim DK, Lee HS. Synthetic cannabinoids are substrates and inhibitors of multiple drug-metabolizing enzymes. Arch Pharm Res. 2018;41:691–710.
78. Kong TY, Kwon SS, Cheong JC, Kim HS, Kim JY, Lee HS. In vitro inhibitory effects of synthetic cannabinoid EAM-2201 on cytochrome P450 and UDP-glucuronosyltransferase enzyme activities in human liver microsomes. Molecules. 2018;23
79. Lapoint J, James LP, Moran CL, Nelson LS, Hoffman RS, Moran JH. Severe toxicity following synthetic cannabinoid ingestion. Clin Toxicol (Phila). 2011;49:760–4.
80. Macfarlane V, Christie G. Synthetic cannabinoid withdrawal: a new demand on detoxification services. Drug Alcohol Rev. 2015;34:147–53.
81. Maldonado R, Rodriguez de Fonseca F. Cannabinoid addiction: behavioral models and neural correlates. J Neurosci. 2002;22:3326–31.
82. Martellotta MC, Cossu G, Fattore L, Gessa GL, Fratta W. Self-administration of the cannabinoid receptor agonist WIN 55,212-2 in drug-naive mice. Neuroscience. 1998;85:327–30.
83. Martinez-Martinez E, Gomez I, Martin P, Sanchez A, Roman L, Tejerina E, Bonilla F, Merino AG, de Herreros AG, Provencio M, Garcia JM. Cannabinoids receptor type 2, CB2, expression correlates with human colon cancer progression and predicts patient survival. Onco Targets Ther. 2015;2:131–41.
84. Marusich JA, Wiley JL, Lefever TW, Patel PR, Thomas BF. Finding order in chemical chaos – continuing characterization of synthetic cannabinoid receptor agonists. Neuropharmacology. 2018;134:73–81.
85. Mercolini L, Protti M. Biosampling strategies for emerging drugs of abuse: towards the future of toxicological and forensic analysis. J Pharm Biomed Anal. 2016;130:202–19.
86. Michalski CW, Oti FE, Erkan M, Sauliunaite D, Bergmann F, Pacher P, Batkai S, Muller MW, Giese NA, Friess H, Kleeff J. Cannabinoids in pancreatic cancer: correlation with survival and pain. Int J Cancer. 2008;122:742–50.
87. Monte AA, Calello DP, Gerona RR, Hamad E, Campleman SL, Brent J, Wax P, Carlson RG, Acmt Toxicology Investigators Consortium. Characteristics and treatment of patients with clinical illness due to synthetic cannabinoid inhalation reported by medical toxicologists: a ToxIC database study. J Med Toxicol. 2017;13:146–52.
88. Morales P, Blasco-Benito S, Andradas C, Gomez-Canas M, Flores JM, Goya P, Fernandez-Ruiz J, Sanchez C, Jagerovic N. Selective, nontoxic CB(2) cannabinoid o-quinone with in vivo activity against triple-negative breast cancer. J Med Chem. 2015;58:2256–64.
89. Morgan D, Kondabolu K, Kuipers A, Sakhuja R, Robertson KL, Rowland NE, Booth RG. Molecular and behavioral pharmacology of two novel orally-active 5HT2 modulators: potential utility as antipsychotic medications. Neuropharmacology. 2013;72:274–81.
90. Muller H, Sperling W, Kohrmann M, Huttner HB, Kornhuber J, Maler JM. The synthetic cannabinoid spice as a trigger for an acute exacerbation of cannabis induced recurrent psychotic episodes. Schizophr Res. 2010;118:309–10.
91. Muller L, Radtke A, Decker J, Koch M, Belge G. The synthetic cannabinoid WIN 55,212-2 elicits death in human cancer cell lines. Anticancer Res. 2017;37:6341–5.
92. Muneta-Arrate I, Diez-Alarcia R, Horrillo I, Meana JJ. Pimavanserin exhibits serotonin 5-HT2A receptor inverse agonism for Galphai1- and neutral antagonism for Galphaq/11-proteins in human brain cortex. Eur Neuropsychopharmacol. 2020;36:83–9.
93. Nacca N, Vatti D, Sullivan R, Sud P, Su M, Marraffa J. The synthetic cannabinoid withdrawal syndrome. J Addict Med. 2013;7:296–8.
94. Naccarato M, Pizzuti D, Petrosino S, Simonetto M, Ferigo L, Grandi FC, Pizzolato G, Di Marzo V. Possible anandamide and palmitoylethanolamide involvement in human stroke. Lipids Health Dis. 2010;9:47. https://doi.org/10.1186/1476-511X-9-47.
95. Nithipatikom K, Isbell MA, Endsley MP, Woodliff JE, Campbell WB. Anti-proliferative effect of a putative endocannabinoid, 2-arachidonylglyceryl ether in prostate carcinoma cells. Prostaglandins Other Lipid Mediat. 2011;94:34–43.

96. Oh JH, Lee JY, Baeg MK, Han KH, Choi MG, Park JM. Antineoplastic effect of WIN 55,212-2, a cannabinoid agonist, in a murine xenograft model of gastric cancer. Chemotherapy. 2013;59:200–6.
97. Olea-Herrero N, Vara D, Malagarie-Cazenave S, Diaz-Laviada I. Inhibition of human tumour prostate PC-3 cell growth by cannabinoids R(+)-Methanandamide and JWH-015: involvement of CB2. Br J Cancer. 2009;101:940–50.
98. Ortega A, Garcia-Hernandez VM, Ruiz-Garcia E, Meneses-Garcia A, Herrera-Gomez A, Aguilar-Ponce JL, Montes-Servin E, Prospero-Garcia O, Del Angel SA. Comparing the effects of endogenous and synthetic cannabinoid receptor agonists on survival of gastric cancer cells. Life Sci. 2016;165:56–62.
99. Ossato A, Vigolo A, Trapella C, Seri C, Rimondo C, Serpelloni G, Marti M. JWH-018 impairs sensorimotor functions in mice. Neuroscience. 2015;300:174–88.
100. Pant S, Deshmukh A, Dholaria B, Kaur V, Ramavaram S, Ukor M, Teran GA. Spicy seizure. Am J Med Sci. 2012;344:67–8.
101. Patel KD, Davison JS, Pittman QJ, Sharkey KA. Cannabinoid CB(2) receptors in health and disease. Curr Med Chem. 2010;17:1393–410.
102. Patsos HA, Hicks DJ, Greenhough A, Williams AC, Paraskeva C. Cannabinoids and cancer: potential for colorectal cancer therapy. Biochem Soc Trans. 2005;33:712–4.
103. Patton AL, Seely KA, Chimalakonda KC, Tran JP, Trass M, Miranda A, Fantegrossi WE, Kennedy PD, Dobrowolski P, Radominska-Pandya A, McCain KR, James LP, Endres GW, Moran JH. Targeted metabolomic approach for assessing human synthetic cannabinoid exposure and pharmacology. Anal Chem. 2013;85:9390–9.
104. Patton AL, Seely KA, Yarbrough AL, Fantegrossi W, James LP, McCain KR, Fujiwara R, Prather PL, Moran JH, Radominska-Pandya A. Altered metabolism of synthetic cannabinoid JWH-018 by human cytochrome P450 2C9 and variants. Biochem Biophys Res Commun. 2018;498:597–602.
105. Paul ABM, Simms L, Amini S, Paul AE. Teens and spice: a review of adolescent fatalities associated with synthetic cannabinoid use. J Forensic Sci. 2018;63:1321–4.
106. Petrosino S, Ménard B, Zsürger N, Di Marzo V, Chabry J. Alteration of the endocannabinoid system in mouse brain during prion disease. Neuroscience. 2011;177:292–7.
107. Petrosino S, Palazzo E, de Novellis V, Bisogno T, Rossi F, Maione S, Di Marzo V. Changes in spinal and supraspinal endocannabinoid levels in neuropathic rats. Neuropharmacology. 2007;52:415–22.
108. Petrosino S, Di Marzo V. The pharmacology of palmitoylethanolamide and first data on the therapeutic efficacy of some of its new formulations. Br J Pharmacol. 2017;174:1349–65.
109. Presley BC, Jansen-Varnum SA, Logan BK. Analysis of synthetic cannabinoids in botanical material: a review of analytical methods and findings. Forensic Sci Rev. 2013;25:27–46.
110. Qamri Z, Preet A, Nasser MW, Bass CE, Leone G, Barsky SH, Ganju RK. Synthetic cannabinoid receptor agonists inhibit tumor growth and metastasis of breast cancer. Mol Cancer Ther. 2009;8:3117–29.
111. Ramer R, Hinz B. Cannabinoids as anticancer drugs. Adv Pharmacol. 2017;80:397–436.
112. Ramos JA, Bianco FJ. The role of cannabinoids in prostate cancer: basic science perspective and potential clinical applications. Indian J Urol. 2012;28:9–14.
113. Roberto D, Klotz LH, Venkateswaran V. Cannabinoid WIN 55,212-2 induces cell cycle arrest and apoptosis, and inhibits proliferation, migration, invasion, and tumor growth in prostate cancer in a cannabinoid-receptor 2 dependent manner. Prostate. 2019;79:151–9.
114. Robson H, Braund R, Glass M, Ashton J, Tatley M. Synthetic cannabis: adverse events reported to the New Zealand Pharmacovigilance Centre. Clin Toxicol (Phila). 2020:1–8.
115. Ross CH, Singh P, Simon EL. Hemorrhagic soft tissue upper airway obstruction from brodifacoum-contaminated synthetic cannabinoid. J Emerg Med. 2019;57:47–50.
116. Sanchez C, Galve-Roperh I, Canova C, Brachet P, Guzman M. Delta9-tetrahydrocannabinol induces apoptosis in C6 glioma cells. FEBS Lett. 1998;436:6–10.

117. Sarfaraz S, Afaq F, Adhami VM, Malik A, Mukhtar H. Cannabinoid receptor agonist-induced apoptosis of human prostate cancer cells LNCaP proceeds through sustained activation of ERK1/2 leading to G1 cell cycle arrest. J Biol Chem. 2006;281:39480–91.
118. Seely KA, Brents LK, Radominska-Pandya A, Endres GW, Keyes GS, Moran JH, Prather PL. A major glucuronidated metabolite of JWH-018 is a neutral antagonist at CB1 receptors. Chem Res Toxicol. 2012;25:825–7.
119. Seely KA, Patton AL, Moran CL, Womack ML, Prather PL, Fantegrossi WE, Radominska-Pandya A, Endres GW, Channell KB, Smith NH, McCain KR, James LP, Moran JH. Forensic investigation of K2, Spice, and "bath salt" commercial preparations: a three-year study of new designer drug products containing synthetic cannabinoid, stimulant, and hallucinogenic compounds. Forensic Sci Int. 2013;233:416–22.
120. Seely KA, Prather PL, James LP, Moran JH. Marijuana-based drugs: innovative therapeutics or designer drugs of abuse? Mol Interv. 2011;11:36–51.
121. Showalter VM, Compton DR, Martin BR, Abood ME. Evaluation of binding in a transfected cell line expressing a peripheral cannabinoid receptor (CB2): identification of cannabinoid receptor subtype selective ligands. J Pharmacol Exp Ther. 1996;278:989–99.
122. Skryabin VY, Vinnikova MA. Psychotic disorders in patients who use synthetic cannabinoids. J Psychiatr Pract. 2019;25:485–90.
123. Sugiura T, Oka S, Gokoh M, Kishimoto S, Waku K. New perspectives in the studies on endocannabinoid and cannabis: 2-arachidonoylglycerol as a possible novel mediator of inflammation. J Pharmacol Sci. 2004;96:367–75.
124. Sweeney B, Talebi S, Toro D, Gonzalez K, Menoscal JP, Shaw R, Hassen GW. Hyperthermia and severe rhabdomyolysis from synthetic cannabinoids. Am J Emerg Med. 2016;34(121):e1–2.
125. Tai S, Fantegrossi WE. Pharmacological and toxicological effects of synthetic cannabinoids and their metabolites. Curr Top Behav Neurosci. 2017;32:249–62.
126. Tai S, Hyatt WS, Gu C, Franks LN, Vasiljevik T, Brents LK, Prather PL, Fantegrossi WE. Repeated administration of phytocannabinoid Delta(9)-THC or synthetic cannabinoids JWH-018 and JWH-073 induces tolerance to hypothermia but not locomotor suppression in mice, and reduces CB1 receptor expression and function in a brain region-specific manner. Pharmacol Res. 2015;102:22–32.
127. Thakur GA, Nikas SP, Makriyannis A. CB1 cannabinoid receptor ligands. Mini Rev Med Chem. 2005;5:631–40.
128. Thapa D, Lee JS, Heo SW, Lee YR, Kang KW, Kwak MK, Choi HG, Kim JA. Novel hexahydrocannabinol analogs as potential anti-cancer agents inhibit cell proliferation and tumor angiogenesis. Eur J Pharmacol. 2011;650:64–71.
129. Toennes SW, Geraths A, Pogoda W, Paulke A, Wunder C, Theunissen EL, Ramaekers JG. Pharmacokinetic properties of the synthetic cannabinoid JWH-018 in oral fluid after inhalation. Drug Test Anal. 2018;10:644–50.
130. Vigolo A, Ossato A, Trapella C, Vincenzi F, Rimondo C, Seri C, Varani K, Serpelloni G, Marti M. Novel halogenated derivates of JWH-018: behavioral and binding studies in mice. Neuropharmacology. 2015;95:68–82.
131. Vincenzi F, Targa M, Corciulo C, Tabrizi MA, Merighi S, Gessi S, Saponaro G, Baraldi PG, Borea PA, Varani K. Antinociceptive effects of the selective CB2 agonist MT178 in inflammatory and chronic rodent pain models. Pain. 2013;154:864–73.
132. Wiley JL, Lefever TW, Marusich JA, Grabenauer M, Moore KN, Huffman JW, Thomas BF. Evaluation of first generation synthetic cannabinoids on binding at non-cannabinoid receptors and in a battery of in vivo assays in mice. Neuropharmacology. 2016;110:143–53.
133. Wiley JL, Marusich JA, Lefever TW, Antonazzo KR, Wallgren MT, Cortes RA, Patel PR, Grabenauer M, Moore KN, Thomas BF. AB-CHMINACA, AB-PINACA, and FUBIMINA: affinity and potency of novel synthetic cannabinoids in producing delta9-tetrahydrocannabinol-like effects in mice. J Pharmacol Exp Ther. 2015;354:328–39.

134. Xian S, Parayath NN, Nehoff H, Giles NM, Greish K. The use of styrene maleic acid nanomicelles encapsulating the synthetic cannabinoid analog WIN55,212-2 for the treatment of cancer. Anticancer Res. 2015;35:4707–12.
135. Xian XS, Park H, Cho YK, Lee IS, Kim SW, Choi MG, Chung IS, Han KH, Park JM. Effect of a synthetic cannabinoid agonist on the proliferation and invasion of gastric cancer cells. J Cell Biochem. 2010;110:321–32.
136. Xu D, Wang J, Zhou Z, He Z, Zhao Q. Cannabinoid WIN55, 212-2 induces cell cycle arrest and inhibits the proliferation and migration of human BEL7402 hepatocellular carcinoma cells. Mol Med Rep. 2015;12:7963–70.
137. Yeruva RR, Mekala HM, Sidhu M, Lippmann S. Synthetic cannabinoids-"spice" can induce a psychosis: a brief review. Innov Clin Neurosci. 2019;16:31–2.
138. You Y, Proctor RM, Vasilko ED, Robinson MA. Doping control analysis of four JWH-250 metabolites in equine urine by liquid chromatography-tandem mass spectrometry. Drug Test Anal. 2019;11:649–58.
139. Zimmermann US, Winkelmann PR, Pilhatsch M, Nees JA, Spanagel R, Schulz K. Withdrawal phenomena and dependence syndrome after the consumption of "spice gold". Dtsch Arztebl Int. 2009;106:464–7.
140. Zogopoulos P, Korkolopoulou P, Patsouris E, Theocharis S. The antitumor action of cannabinoids on glioma tumorigenesis. Histol Histopathol. 2015;30:629–45.
141. Zuba D, Byrska B, Maciow M. Comparison of "herbal highs" composition. Anal Bioanal Chem. 2011;400:119–26.

References (Palmitoylethanolamide Pharmacology Efficacy and Safety)

142. Artukoglu BB, Beyer C, Zuloff-Shani A, Brener E, Bloch MH. Efficacy of palmitoylethanolamide for pain: a meta-analysis. Pain Physician. 2017;20:353–62.
143. Cantarella G, Scollo M, Lempereur L, Saccani-Jotti G, Basile F, Bernardini R. Endocannabinoids inhibit release of nerve growth factor by inflammation-activated mast cells. Biochem Pharmacol. 2011;82:380–8.
144. Chiurchiu V, Leuti A, Smoum R, Mechoulam R, Maccarrone M. Bioactive lipids ALIAmides differentially modulate inflammatory responses of distinct subsets of primary human T lymphocytes. FASEB J. 2018;32:5716–23.
145. Cruccu G, Stefano GD, Marchettini P, Truini A. Micronized palmitoylethanolamide: a post hoc analysis of a controlled study in patients with low back pain – sciatica. CNS Neurol Disord Drug Targets. 2019;18:491–5.
146. D'Amico R, Impellizzeri D, Cuzzocrea S, Di Paola R. ALIAmides update: palmitoylethanolamide and its formulations on management of peripheral neuropathic pain. Int J Mol Sci. 2020;21
147. De Filippis D, Negro L, Vaia M, Cinelli MP, Iuvone T. New insights in mast cell modulation by palmitoylethanolamide. CNS Neurol Disord Drug Targets. 2013;12:78–83.
148. De Petrocellis L, Davis JB, Di Marzo V. Palmitoylethanolamide enhances anandamide stimulation of human vanilloid VR1 receptors. FEBS Lett. 2001;506:253–6.
149. di Marzo V, Skaper SD. Palmitoylethanolamide: biochemistry, pharmacology and therapeutic use of a pleiotropic anti-inflammatory lipid mediator. CNS Neurol Disord Drug Targets. 2013;12:4–6.
150. Gabrielsson L, Mattsson S, Fowler CJ. Palmitoylethanolamide for the treatment of pain: pharmacokinetics, safety and efficacy. Br J Clin Pharmacol. 2016;82:932–42.

151. Grillo SL, Keereetaweep J, Grillo MA, Chapman KD, Koulen P. N-Palmitoylethanolamine depot injection increased its tissue levels and those of other acylethanolamide lipids. Drug Des Devel Ther. 2013;7:747–52.
152. Guida F, Luongo L, Boccella S, Giordano ME, Romano R, Bellini G, Manzo I, Furiano A, Rizzo A, Imperatore R, Iannotti FA, D'Aniello E, Piscitelli F, Sca Rossi F, Cristino L, Di Marzo V, de Novellis V, Maione S. Palmitoylethanolamide induces microglia changes associated with increased migration and phagocytic activity: involvement of the CB2 receptor. Sci Rep. 2017;7:375.
153. Hesselink JM. Evolution in pharmacologic thinking around the natural analgesic palmitoylethanolamide: from nonspecific resistance to PPAR-alpha agonist and effective nutraceutical. J Pain Res. 2013;6:625–34.
154. Hesselink JM, Hekker TA. Therapeutic utility of palmitoylethanolamide in the treatment of neuropathic pain associated with various pathological conditions: a case series. J Pain Res. 2012;5:437–42.
155. Ho WS, Barrett DA, Randall MD. Entourage' effects of N-palmitoylethanolamide and N-oleoylethanolamide on vasorelaxation to anandamide occur through TRPV1 receptors. Br J Pharmacol. 2008;155:837–46.
156. Impellizzeri D, Bruschetta G, Cordaro M, Crupi R, Siracusa R, Esposito E, Cuzzocrea S. Micronized/ultramicronized palmitoylethanolamide displays superior oral efficacy compared to nonmicronized palmitoylethanolamide in a rat model of inflammatory pain. J Neuroinflammation. 2014;11:136.
157. Ji RR, Chamessian A, Zhang YQ. Pain regulation by non-neuronal cells and inflammation. Science. 2016;354:572–7.
158. Leleux J, Williams RO 3rd. Recent advancements in mechanical reduction methods: particulate systems. Drug Dev Ind Pharm. 2014;40:289–300.
159. Morsanuto V, Galla R, Molinari C, Uberti F. A new palmitoylethanolamide form combined with antioxidant molecules to improve its effectivess on neuronal aging. Brain Sci. 2020;10
160. Nestmann ER. Safety of micronized palmitoylethanolamide (microPEA): lack of toxicity and genotoxic potential. Food Sci Nutr. 2017;5:292–309.
161. Paladini A, Fusco M, Cenacchi T, Schievano C, Piroli A, Varrassi G. Palmitoylethanolamide, a special food for medical purposes, in the treatment of chronic pain: a pooled data meta-analysis. Pain Physician. 2016;19:11–24.
162. Petrosino S, Cordaro M, Verde R, Schiano Moriello A, Marcolongo G, Schievano C, Siracusa R, Piscitelli F, Peritore AF, Crupi R, Impellizzeri D, Esposito E, Cuzzocrea S, Di Marzo V. Oral ultramicronized palmitoylethanolamide: plasma and tissue levels and spinal anti-hyperalgesic effect. Front Pharmacol. 2018;9:249.
163. Petrosino S, Schiano Moriello A, Cerrato S, Fusco M, Puigdemont A, De Petrocellis L, Di Marzo V. The anti-inflammatory mediator palmitoylethanolamide enhances the levels of 2-arachidonoyl-glycerol and potentiates its actions at TRPV1 cation channels. Br J Pharmacol. 2016;173:1154–62.
164. Petrosino S, Schiano Moriello A, Verde R, Allara M, Imperatore R, Ligresti A, Mahmoud AM, Peritore AF, Iannotti FA, Di Marzo V. Palmitoylethanolamide counteracts substance P-induced mast cell activation in vitro by stimulating diacylglycerol lipase activity. J Neuroinflammation. 2019;16:274.
165. Ribeiro A, Pontis S, Mengatto L, Armirotti A, Chiurchiu V, Capurro V, Fiasella A, Nuzzi A, Romeo E, Moreno-Sanz G, Maccarrone M, Reggiani A, Tarzia G, Mor M, Bertozzi F, Bandiera T, Piomelli D. A potent systemically active N-acylethanolamine acid amidase inhibitor that suppresses inflammation and human macrophage activation. ACS Chem Biol. 2015;10:1838–46.
166. Schmid PC, Krebsbach RJ, Perry SR, Dettmer TM, Maasson JL, Schmid HH. Occurrence and postmortem generation of anandamide and other long-chain N-acylethanolamines in mammalian brain. FEBS Lett. 1995;375:117–20.

167. Scuderi C, Esposito G, Blasio A, Valenza M, Arietti P, Steardo L Jr, Carnuccio R, De Filippis D, Petrosino S, Iuvone T, Di Marzo V, Steardo L. Palmitoylethanolamide counteracts reactive astrogliosis induced by beta-amyloid peptide. J Cell Mol Med. 2011;15:2664–74.
168. Siracusa R, Impellizzeri D, Cordaro M, Crupi R, Esposito E, Petrosino S, Cuzzocrea S. Anti-inflammatory and neuroprotective effects of co-UltraPEALut in a mouse model of vascular dementia. Front Neurol. 2017;8:233.
169. Skaper SD, Facci L, Barbierato M, Zusso M, Bruschetta G, Impellizzeri D, Cuzzocrea S, Giusti P. N-palmitoylethanolamine and neuroinflammation: a novel therapeutic strategy of resolution. Mol Neurobiol. 2015;52:1034–42.
170. Smart D, Jonsson KO, Vandevoorde S, Lambert DM, Fowler CJ. 'Entourage' effects of N-acyl ethanolamines at human vanilloid receptors. Comparison of effects upon anandamide-induced vanilloid receptor activation and upon anandamide metabolism. Br J Pharmacol. 2002;136:452–8.
171. Vacondio F, Bassi M, Silva C, Castelli R, Carmi C, Scalvini L, Lodola A, Vivo V, Flammini L, Barocelli E, Mor M, Rivara S. Amino acid derivatives as palmitoylethanolamide pro-drugs: synthesis, in vitro metabolism and In vivo plasma profile in rats. PLoS One. 2015;10:e0128699.
172. Wang J, Zheng J, Kulkarni A, Wang W, Garg S, Prather PL, Hauer-Jensen M. Palmitoylethanolamide regulates development of intestinal radiation injury in a mast cell-dependent manner. Dig Dis Sci. 2014;59:2693–703.
173. Wellner N, Diep TA, Janfelt C, Hansen HS. N-acylation of phosphatidylethanolamine and its biological functions in mammals. Biochim Biophys Acta. 2013;1831:652–62.
174. Xanthos DN, Pungel I, Wunderbaldinger G, Sandkuhler J. Effects of peripheral inflammation on the blood-spinal cord barrier. Mol Pain. 2012;8:44.

Chapter 4
Cannabinoid-Based Medicines as Cancer Therapy

Contents

4.1 Introduction 117
4.2 Terminology 118
4.3 Antineoplastic Activity of Different Cannabis Formulations 119
4.4 Cannabinoids and Graft Versus Host Disease 122
4.5 Cannabinoids and Immune Checkpoint Inhibitors 123
4.6 Using High-Dose Cannabinoids to Treat Cancer (Phoenix Tears/Rick Simpson Oil) .. 124
4.7 Hail Mary Pass 124
4.8 Conclusion 124
References 125

4.1 Introduction

Cannabinoid-based medicines (CBM) have a demonstrated benefit for patients with cancer-related or chemotherapy-related symptoms (see Chap. 5). These compounds may also have an emerging role in the treatment of malignancies. The first published report of cannabinoids (THC-predominant cannabis extracts) demonstrated antitumour effects on the growth of lung adenocarcinoma cells in vitro; an in vivo model using mice fed with the same extracts showed similar findings [34].

Since then, many other malignancies demonstrating expression of CB1 and CB2 receptors (lung, glioma, thyroid, lymphoma, skin, pancreas, endometrial, breast, prostate) have been investigated using cannabinoids and cannabinoid receptor antagonists in pre-clinical studies [2, 12, 43]. The effects observed include anti-proliferation, prevention of cell transport, anti-angiogenesis, and pro-apoptosis [58]. Aggressive cancers demonstrate increased expression of the CB1 and CB2 receptors (e.g., ovarian, colorectal cancers) [54]. Likewise, aggressive breast cancers (termed triple-negative relating to the lack of expression of actionable receptors) express CB2 receptors on their surface [11, 25]. The G-protein receptor 55 (GPR55) is also expressed in multiple cancer sites (e.g., glioblastoma, astrocytoma,

C. Cyr et al., *Cannabis and Cannabinoid-Based Medicines in Cancer Care*,
https://doi.org/10.1007/978-3-030-89918-9_4

breast carcinoma, melanoma, cervical and ovarian carcinomas, prostate carcinoma, and B-cell myelomas), and reduced expression of this receptor reflects a reduction in malignant potential of these cells [40]. Gliomas have been shown to have upregulated CB1 and CB2 receptors, with an associated reduction of FAAH, a degradative enzyme for the naturally occurring anandamide. This reflects the role of the endocannabinoid system in disorders of cellular regulation and malignancy [58].

There are several proposed pathways to explain the effects of cannabinoids on cancer cells, based on work done in several disease sites, including breast cancer, gliomas, melanoma, and pancreatic cancer [3, 16, 25, 46]. Simply put, activation of the CB1 or CB2 receptors leads to several downstream actions that can result in cell death. The mechanisms involve different signaling cascades inhibiting cell survival, stimulating apoptosis, preventing angiogenesis, and reducing the cells' ability to proliferate and metastasize, a key factor in the development of malignant tumors [13]. While an exhaustive review of the multiple mechanisms involved is beyond the scope of this chapter, several are seen in Fig. 4.1 with explanations in Table 4.1.

Oncologists are always looking for improved treatments for all sites of malignancy. Clinical trials in oncology are most often evaluating and adding newer agents to established protocols to improve patient outcomes. Supportive therapies also must be at least neutral in their effects upon the cancer. Investigators have combined cannabis extracts with a number of chemotherapy agents *in vitro* and *in vivo* animal models, generally demonstrating reduction in cell numbers and viability, and no negative impact upon the antineoplastic activity, at least with traditional chemotherapeutic agents. Pancreatic, glioma, gastric, lung, and colon cell cultures have been investigated associating cannabinoids with common and frequently used antineoplastic agents, including gemcitabine, nab-paclitaxel, paclitaxel, temozolomide, and 5-fluorouracil [15, 20, 28, 32, 37, 56]. Synergism inducing cancer cell death is a common finding, which bodes well for future human clinical trials of cannabinoids [58]. Anecdotal reports of patients who used cannabinoids with chemotherapy resulting in prolonged survival may be an observational signal of future "clinical proof" of this concept [17, 50].

4.2 Terminology

The term "endocannabinoidome" is still not widely used by clinicians and researchers, and in order to avoid confusion, its use to describe the *expanded* endocannabinoid system (ECS) will be restricted to the first chapter of this book. For the present chapter, the more commonly used term "endocannabinoid system (ECS)" will be used to describe most concepts relating to both the more specific canonical receptors and enzymes and the larger system of molecular targets and ligands. The "endocannabinoidome" will only be mentioned in order to point out a clinically relevant difference between these two related concepts.

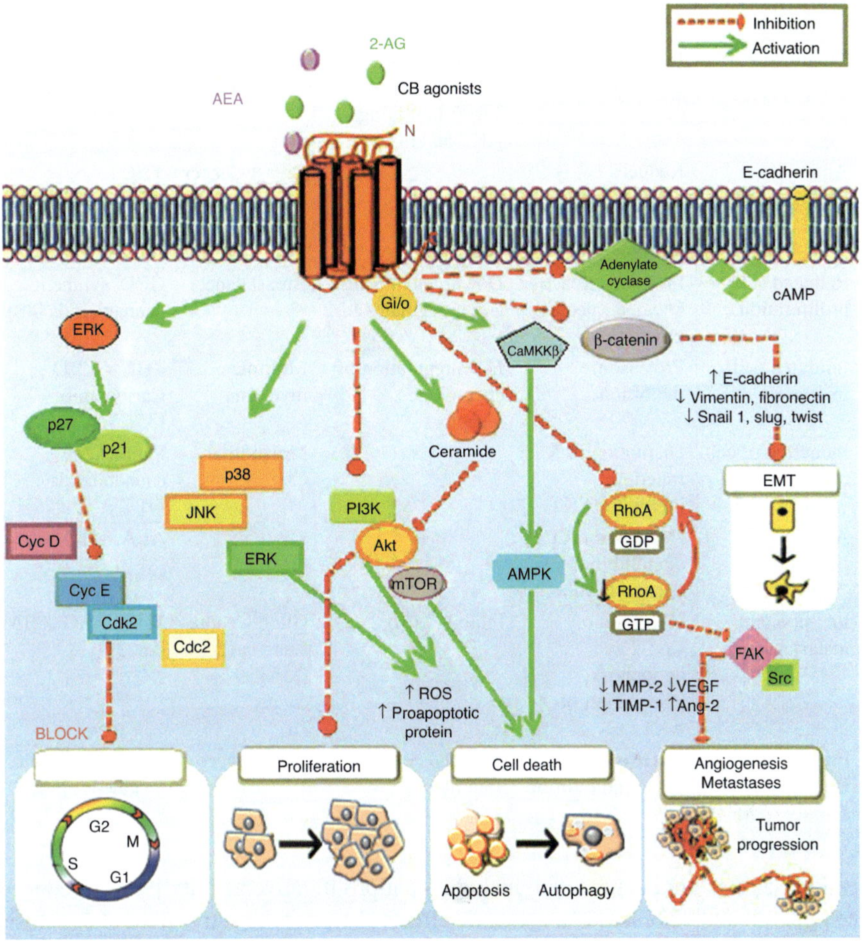

Fig. 4.1 Schematic representation of the main signaling cascades highlighting the downstream CB receptor activation by cannabinoids which impact all the hallmark processes of cancer such as proliferation, apoptosis, migration, invasion, angiogenesis and EMT (epithelial-mesenchymal transition). (Reference: Das et al. [13]. (Springer publication))

4.3 Antineoplastic Activity of Different Cannabis Formulations

Several other cannabinoids have been studied in the lab for possible anti-neoplastic activity. These include cannabigerol (CBG), cannabichromene (CBC), cannabidivarin (CBDV), cannabinol (CBN), and tetrahydrocannabivarin (THCV) [54]. As of the date of writing, these studies are lab-based using a variety of cancer cell cultures (e.g., breast, glioma, prostate, and colon) and for CBG in vivo animal models [9]. Several

Table 4.1 Preclinical evidence of cannabinoid antitumor activity

Antineoplastic activity	Mechanism	Downstream effect	Cancer type	Involved cannabinoid
Stimulation of autophagy	Increase in ceramide by cell	ER stress leading to upregulation of TRB3 inhibiting AKT and mTOR	Glioblastoma	THC, CBD [27, 41]
Anti-angiogenesis	Reduces expression of VEGF and its receptor		Breast Cancer	THC microparticles
Reduced cell proliferation	Promotes Reactive Oxygen Species production	Downregulates Id-1 and upregulates Id-2	Breast cancer	CBD, synthetic cannabinoids [48]
Inhibited cell migration	Proteasome inhibition	Downregulation of chemokine receptors	Multiple myeloma	THC + CBD + Carfilzomib [35]
Induction of cell cycle arrest	Disruption of Rb function, inhibiting AKT		Melanoma	Synthetic cannabinoids [4]
Apoptosis	Decreased cAMP via inhibition of adenylyl cyclase		Thyroid, prostate	AEA, THC [8]
Invasion and metastasis	Inhibition of Cox-2 and hypophos-phorylation of AKT	Inhibits MMP2	Glioblastoma, Lung cancer Cervical cancer	THC, 2-AG, AEA [23, 39]
FAAH blockade Decreases activity of MMP	Overexpression of tissue inhibitor of MMP	Reduced cell viability	Lung cancer	FAAH inhibitors (synthetic) [60]

cellular effects are documented, including antiproliferative activity [9, 51], reduced cell growth and viability [14], cytotoxic effects [14], and the stimulation of apoptosis [26]. Combinations of these minor cannabinoids with THC and CBD have shown some promise in several neoplastic cell lines. For example, a combination consisting of THC, CBD, CBG, and cannabinol displayed the most cytotoxicity against human breast cell lines (MCF-7) inducing apoptosis [44]. Most recently, Lah and colleagues paired CBG with THC and CBD to treat glioma cell cultures. Their findings showed some synergy for the CBG-CBD combination, with little additive benefit with the addition of THC. Both CBG and CBD inhibited glioblastoma invasion in a similar fashion as temozolomide [26]. Their findings suggest that adding THC may not be of value in the combined treatment of glioblastoma and that CBG may in fact play a larger role. Although these and other studies hold promise and support this concept of the use of whole cannabis extracts, no studies in humans have as yet made it to print.

Despite the emerging evidence of antineoplastic activity, some older in vitro studies demonstrated cancer cell stimulation in the form of increased proliferation and loss of immune-mediated cancer suppressor activity when treated with cannabinoid extracts [34, 36]. Details of these findings are seen in Table 4.2. Mckallip

Table 4.2 Effects of THC and CBD on specific cancer cell lines

	Glioma	Lung cancer	Breast cancer
THC	Stimulated cell growth Increased EGFR expression Increased tumor cell proliferation[1]	Cell survival unaffected[2] Increased tumor growth[1 6] Increased cell proliferation[1] Inhibited immune response[5 6], reduced killing of tumor cells[5]	Increased tumor growth[3] Increased tumor proliferation[4] Inhibited immune response[3] Increased metastatic potential[3]
CBD	Nil		

1. Hart et al. [22], 2. Baram et al. [5], 3. Mckallip et al. [29], 4. Takeda et al. [53], 5. Burnette-Curley and Cabral [10], 6. Zhu et al. [63]

et al. [29], based on their results with in vitro breast cancer cells, hypothesized "the degree of sensitivity of a tumor to delta-9-THC may be directly related to the level of CB1 and CB2 expression" of the cells. Most often, these effects resulted from treatment with varying doses of THC. In these studies, higher concentrations of administered cannabinoid caused inhibitory and anti-neoplastic activity effects, whereas low doses stimulated growth and proliferation of the malignant cells [32]. There is little evidence in the literature showing that CBD stimulates malignant cells or induces neoplastic potential. Recent investigations support the possibility of CBD as a protective agent [18].

Thus, conflicting evidence points to the need for sober second thought before outright recommending cannabinoids for any and all cancer patients. To quote Dr. Donald Abrams:

> "But again, mice and rats are not people, and what is observed *in vitro* does not necessarily translate into clinical medicine. The preclinical evidence that cannabinoids might have direct anticancer activity is provocative as well, but more research is warranted." [1]

Cannabis as a whole plant product has not been studied clinically as a treatment for malignancy. Unfortunately, many claims of the "curative" benefits of cannabis (fresh buds, dried cannabis, or "oil" products) can be found in the lay press, especially on the Internet and social media. These reports (mostly anonymously authored), extrapolate the results of preclinical work (employing cell culture or animal models) to humans without any basis in fact [47]. There have been a handful of published case reports [17, 50] documenting either prolongation of survival or reduction of cancer burden using cannabinoid products (no objective review of the products used) and, curiously, in children.

There are only two peer-reviewed and published clinical studies (as of the date of writing) using cannabinoids in human cancer patients. The earlier study enrolled those with glioblastoma multiforme, based on extensive preclinical work done by the same group of investigators [21]. This small study (9 patients) demonstrated the safety of daily intracranial administration of delta-9 THC (range of 10–64 days) with total doses ranging from 0.8 mg to 3.29 mg THC. Biopsies of the treated tumors were obtained, and antiproliferative effects were demonstrated in some of the patients. All patients eventually progressed and died from their tumor, none due to the effects of the extract. These investigators are actively continuing their clinical and research work, spearheading the focus on CNS tumors [58].

The second, recently published study described the combined use of nabiximols (cannabis extract containing 2.5 mg CBD and 2.7 mg THC per 0.1 ml delivered via oromucosal spray) with dose-intense temozolomide in patients with recurrent, previously treated glioblastoma multiforme. Twenty-one patients were enrolled (12 in the active arm, 9 in placebo) using an individualized dosing formula (up to 12 sprays or 30 mg CBD/32.4 mg THC) in addition to the standard dose dense temozolomide (85 mg/m^2 daily) for up to 1 year duration. The mean duration of treatment was similar for both groups (24.9 weeks for the nabiximols group versus 23.6 weeks for the placebo group), with discontinuation rates nearly equal in both groups (16.7% nabiximols compared with 22.2% in the placebo group). At the 12-month point, a majority of the nabiximols-treated patients were alive (10/12 or 83%) versus 4/9 or 44% of the placebo group, a statistically significant survival increase ($p = 0.042$). Overall survival benefit was seen in the nabiximols group (median OS 21.8 months) compared with only 12.1 months for the placebo group. Combined treatment-related toxicities reported were generally mild with dizziness (11/18 patients) and nausea (7/18 patients) being most common [57].

4.4 Cannabinoids and Graft Versus Host Disease

Graft-versus-host disease (GvHD) is a condition related to treatment of cancers, but not directly caused by chemotherapy. When a patient with a hematologic malignancy (leukemia, lymphoma, and myeloma are the most common) undergoes intensive chemotherapy, the bone marrow is often targeted with ablation to destroy the cancer stem cells and provide prolonged progression free survival or indeed, cure. The use of donor stem cells (allogeneic stem cell transplantation or SCT) to provide marrow support/salvage may produce an intense immune-mediated reaction ("graft") that can cause widespread effects to several organs, such as skin, liver, lungs, etc. [45]. This clinical syndrome is caused by the response of the donated cells to histocompatibility antigens found on the tissues of the recipient and is one of the most difficult posttreatment conditions to treat [42]. Several preclinical studies have demonstrated the involvement of the CB2 receptor in the regulation of T cell function [31, 33, 62], which can be targeted to minimize the potential disability of GvHD.

Employing these findings, a group out of Israel completed a clinical phase II trial using cannabidiol for adjunctive therapy of GvHD [61]. Forty-eight adult patients at risk of developing GVHD after allogeneic stem cell transplantation for acute leukemia or myelodysplasia were evaluated using CBD at doses of 200–300 mg per day. Those patients who were given the standard treatment for GvHD prophylaxis as well as CBD had a lower incidence of acute Grade 2–4 GVHD compared to those using only the standard therapy. They also had a lower incidence of chronic GvHD and improved quality of life. These findings resulted in a longer and larger controlled trial that is not yet published in the literature [24]. A recent case report in abstract form [49] supported this work, detailing the striking benefits to a young woman (allogeneic SCT for T-cell ALL) of using a CBD-rich product to treat an otherwise drug-resistant case of skin GvHD. The doses of cannabinoids were very similar to those used by Yeshurun et al. (285 mg CBD −15 mg THC), and the results were persistent 8 months after initiation [49]. Further research in this area is expected, as GvHD continues to be a major cause of morbidity and mortality for those undergoing allogeneic transplants [62].

4.5 Cannabinoids and Immune Checkpoint Inhibitors

The introduction and now widespread use of immunotherapy for malignancies has resulted in patients experiencing reduction in tumor burden and, in some cases, durable remissions in otherwise advanced and metastatic disease [38, 55, 59]. The use of immune checkpoint inhibitors is being touted as the next great leap in treatment of malignancies and has engendered hope for cure in otherwise incurable situations [19, 55].

A recent report from Israel documented reduction in tumor response in several cases of patients using cannabis while undergoing immunotherapy with nivolumab for advanced lung, renal cell, and melanoma carcinomas [52]. Over the period of a year, 140 patients were identified (51 using cannabis in addition to nivolumab and 89 who were not using cannabis). Of the 116 cases living more than 2 months, 44 using cannabis had a reduced rate of response (33.3% vs 17.6% for NSCLC; 43.3% vs 10% for RCC and melanoma). Multivariate analysis supported the contention that cannabis use alone was associated with reduced rate of response to nivolumab. This did not translate to a change in overall survival in this cohort, although univariate analysis did show weak significance. The same researchers reported on a different cohort of patients principally treated with nivolumab or pembrolizumab for advanced cancers (NSCLC, melanoma, RCC, and others) and using cannabis (oral and inhaled formats) [6]. The patient group using cannabis (34 patients) were again found to have a statistically significant reduction in the rate of response to the immunotherapy agents and also a significantly shorter time to progression ($p = 0.0025$) and reduced overall survival ($p = 0.00094$) when compared to the group of non-cannabis users (68 patients). Interestingly, the cannabis user group also experienced significantly less treatment-related adverse events when compared to the non-using patients ($p = 0.057$). These findings are supported by a recent abstract published in the *Journal of Clinical Oncology* [7]. The authors found a significant reduction in overall survival of patients using cannabis (5 patients using inhalation and 23 using oral pharmaceutical formats) compared with non-users (76 patients) in the order of 16 vs 40 months ($p = 0.004$).

4.6 Using High-Dose Cannabinoids to Treat Cancer (Phoenix Tears/Rick Simpson Oil)

Rick Simpson is a Canadian engineer and cannabis activist who claims that using high potency cannabis extracts have helped "cure" a skin condition that was purportedly cancer in 2003. He has since advocated for the use of the concentrated oil extract which now bears his name. Rick Simpson Oil (RSO), also known as "Phoenix tears" is not a branded product, and Rick Simpson himself provides an online resource for patients to produce it themselves.

Followers have recommended using Rick Simpson Oil for other conditions as well, including asthma, epilepsy, and opioid withdrawal. However, cancer patients are especially at risk as some misinformed advocates have even suggested that patients reduce or stop their treatments in favor of this approach. Patients should be reminded that there is no conclusive evidence to suggest using such large doses of THC, CBD, or other cannabinoids will affect the outcome of any form of cancer [30]. Furthermore, it may in fact increase their risk of involuntary intoxication, reduce the efficacy of certain anticancer treatments, and may possibly promote the growth of certain types of cancer cells. Although research has clearly shown that cannabinoids play a major role in cancer pathology, it is too early to promote the use of high potency cannabinoids as a primary treatment regimen.

4.7 Hail Mary Pass

A "Hail Mary pass" is a sports term in American football dating back to the 1920s and describes a play that has a very small chance of being successful. In cancer care, there often comes a moment when standard and accepted treatment options run out and where the disease continues to progress. This is one situation where a trial of RSO might be chosen by certain patients. After having completed every treatment regimen for their cancer, and as a last, desperate attempt to halt the illness, patients may require supervision during their use of high potency cannabinoids to identify and intervene if toxicity occurs. See Chap. 7 for more details on patient counseling on the use of these products.

4.8 Conclusion

The endocannabinoid system was originally thought to display a wide range of physiological effects via the CB1 and CB2 receptors. However, recent discoveries have expanded our knowledge of this complex system, which is now considered to play a major role in tumor pathology via an expanded network of orphan receptors and secondary ligands known as the endocannabinoidome. Preclinical findings suggest a potential role for several cannabinoids as antineoplastic agents and for the prevention of GvHD, although the precise formulation to be used and further therapeutic window may vary depending on many factors, including tumor biology. These and other variables need to be determined before safely introducing these compounds as adjuncts to standard therapeutics. Until further data provides a clearer picture, there are certain clinical settings where cancer patients should avoid using cannabinoids, such as when receiving immune checkpoint inhibitors. Furthermore, the use of high-dose cannabinoids as stand-alone agents intended for disease modifying effects cannot be recommended at this time.

References

1. Abrams DI. Integrating cannabis into clinical cancer care. Curr Oncol. 2016;23(S2):S8–S14. https://doi.org/10.3747/co.23.3099.
2. Alexander A, Smith PF, Rosengren RJ. Cannabinoids in the treatment of cancer. Cancer Lett. 2009;285:6–12.
3. Bachari A, Piva TJ, Alireza Salami S, Jamshidi N, Mantri N. Roles of cannabinoids in melanoma: evidence from in vivo studies. Int J Mol Sci. 2020;21:6040. https://doi.org/10.3390/ijms21176040.
4. Blázquez C, Carracedo A, Barrado L, et al. Cannabinoid receptors as novel targets for the treatment of melanoma. FASEB J. 2006;20:2633–5.
5. Baram L, Peled E, Berman P, et al. The heterogeneity and complexity of Cannabis extracts as antitumor agents. Oncotarget. 2019;10:4091–106.
6. Bar-Sela G, Cohen I, Campisi-Pinto S, et al. Cannabis consumption used by cancer patients during immunotherapy correlates with poor clinical outcome. Cancers. 2020;12:2447–65. https://doi.org/10.3390/cancers12092447.
7. Biedny A, Szpunar S, Abdalla A, Kafri Z, Hadid TH. The effect of concomitant cannabinoids during immune checkpoint inhibitor treatment of advanced stage malignancy. J Clin Oncol. 2020;38(15 suppl). https://doi.org/10.1200/JCO.2020.38.15_suppl.e15064.
8. Bifulco M, Malfitano AM, Pisanti S, Laezza C. Endocannabinoids in endocrine andrelated tumours. Endocr Relat Cancer. 2008;15:391–408.
9. Borrelli F, Pagano E, Romano B, et al. Colon carcinogenesis is inhibited by the TRPM8 antagonist cannabigerol, a Cannabis-derived non-psychotropic cannabinoid. Carcinogenesis. 2014;35:2787–97.
10. Burnette-Curley D, Cabral GA. Differential inhibition of RAW264.7 macrophage tumoricidal activity by delta 9tetrahydrocannabinol. Proc Soc Exp Biol Med. 1995;210:64–76.
11. Caffarel MM, Andradas C, Mira E, et al. Cannabinoids reduce ErbB2-driven breast cancer progression through Akt inhibition. Mol Cancer. 2010;9:196.
12. Carracedo A, Gironella M, Lorente M, et al. Cannabinoids induce apoptosis of pancreatic tumor cells via endoplasmic reticulum stress-related genes. Cancer Res. 2006;66:6748–55.
13. Das S, Kaul K, Mishra S, Charan M, Ganju RK. Cannabinoid signaling in cancer. In: Bukiya A, editor. Recent advances in cannabinoid physiology and pathology. Advances in experimental medicine and biology, vol. 1162. Cham: Springer; 2019. https://doi.org/10.1007/978-3-030-21737-2_4.
14. De Petrocellis L, Ligresti A, Schiano Moriello A, et al. Non-THC cannabinoids inhibit prostate carcinoma growth in vitro and in vivo: pro-apoptotic effects and underlying mechanisms. Br J Pharmacol. 2013;168:79–102.

15. Donadelli M, Dando I, Zaniboni T, et al. Gemcitabine/cannabinoid combination triggers autophagy in pancreatic cancer cells through a ROS-mediated mechanism. Cell Death Dis. 2011;2:e152.
16. Ellert-Miklaszewska A, Ciechomska IA, Kaminska B. Cannabinoid signaling in glioma cells – Chapter 11. In: Barańska J, editor. Glioma signaling, Advances in experimental medicine and biology, vol. 1202; 2020. https://doi.org/10.1007/978-3-030-30651-9_11.
17. Foroughi M, Hendson G, Sargent MA, Steinbok P. Spontaneous regression of septum pellucidum/forniceal pilocytic astrocytomas—possible role of Cannabis inhalation. Childs Nerv Syst. 2011;27:671–9. https://doi.org/10.1007/s00381-011-1410-4.
18. García-Morales L, Castillo AM, Ramírez JT, Zamudio-Meza H, Domínguez-Robles MC, Meza I. CBD reverts the mesenchymal invasive phenotype of breast cancer cells induced by the inflammatory cytokine IL-1_β. Int J Mol Sci. 2020;21:2429. https://doi.org/10.3390/ijms21072429.
19. Gettinger S, Horn L, Jackman D, et al. Five-year follow-up of nivolumab in previously treated advanced non–small-cell lung cancer: results from the CA209-003 study. J Clin Oncol. 2018;36:1675–84.
20. Gustafsson SB, Lindgren T, Jonsson M, et al. Cannabinoid receptor-independent cytotoxic effects of cannabinoids in human colorectal carcinoma cells: synergism with 5-fluorouracil. Cancer Chemother Pharmacol. 2009;63:691–701.
21. Guzman M, Duarte MJ, Blazquez C, et al. A pilot clinical study of delta 9-tetrahydrocannabinol in patients with recurrent glioblastoma multiforme. Br J Cancer. 2006;95:197–203.
22. Hart S, Fischer OM, Ullrich A. Cannabinoids induce cancer cell proliferation via tumor necrosis factor-converting enzyme (TACE/ADAM17)-mediated transactivation of the epidermal growth factor receptor. Cancer Res. 2004;64:1943–50.
23. Hermanson DJ, Marnett LJ. Cannabinoids, endocannabinoids, and cancer. Cancer Metastasis Rev. 2011;30:599–612.
24. Kalytera Reports Data for First Cohort in Phase 2 Clinical Study Evaluating CBD in Prevention of Acute GVHD. Kalytera press release, March 22, 2019. https://kalytera.co/news/kalytera-reports-data-for-first-cohort-in-phase-2-clinical-study-evaluating-cbd-in-prevention-of-acute-gvhd/.
25. Kisková T, Mungenast F, Suváková M, Jäger W, Thalhammer T. Future aspects for cannabinoids in breast cancer therapy. Int J Mol Sci. 2019;20:1673. https://doi.org/10.3390/ijms20071673.
26. Lah TT, Novak M, Pena Almidon MA, et al. Cannabigerol is a potential therapeutic agent in a novel combined therapy for glioblastoma. Cell. 2021;10:340–61. https://doi.org/10.3390/cells10020340.
27. Lee XC, Werner E, Falasca M. Molecular mechanism of autophagy and its regulation by cannabinoids in cancer. Cancers. 2021;13:1211. https://doi.org/10.3390/cancers13061211.
28. Mangal N, Lawrence P, Ragulan C, Desai K, Pacchetti B, Reebye V, Sadanandam A, Sodergren MH. Therapeutic effects of cannabidiol in combination with chemotherapy in pancreatic ductal adenocarcinoma. Abstract P3–23 International Cannabinoid Research Society 31st Annual Symposium 2021.
29. McKallip RJ, Nagarkatti M, Nagarkatti PS. Delta-9-tetrahydrocannabinol enhances breast cancer growth and metastasis by suppression of the antitumor immune response. J Immunol. 2005;174:3281–9. https://doi.org/10.4049/jimmunol.174.6.3281.
30. McSweeney LJ, McEneaney P, O'Reilly S. Cannabis versus combination chemotherapy; n = 1 trial in Hodgkin's lymphoma. Irish J Med Sci. 2019;188:1085–6. https://doi.org/10.1007/s11845-018-1914-y.
31. Mechoulam R. Cannabis – the Israeli perspective. J Basic Clin Physiol Pharmacol. 2016;27:181–7. https://doi.org/10.1515/jbcpp-2015-0091.
32. Miyato H, Kitayama J, Yamashita H, et al. Pharmacological synergism between cannabinoids and paclitaxel in gastric cancer cell lines. J Surg Res. 2009;155:40–7.

33. Moe A, Sauber G, Zhou V, Lapitz A, Hillard C, Drobyski WR. Recipient signaling through the cannabinoid type 2 receptor regulates IL-6 independent neuroinflammation during graft versus host disease. Blood. 2019;134(Supplement_1):195. https://doi.org/10.1182/blood-2019-122746.
34. Munson AE, Harris LA, Friedman MA, Dewey WL, Carchman RA. Antineoplastic activity of cannabinoids. J Natl Cancer Inst. 1975;55:597–602.
35. Nabissi M, Morelli MB, Offdani M, et al. Cannabinoids synergize with carfilzomib, reducing multiple myeloma cells viability and migration. Oncotarget. 2016;7:77543–57.
36. Preet A, Ganju RK, Groopman JE. D(9)-Tetrahydrocannabinol inhibits epithelial growth factor-induced lung cancer cell migration *in vitro* as well as its growth and metastasis *in vivo*. Oncogene. 2008;27:339–46.
37. Preet A, Qamri Z, Nasser MW, et al. Cannabinoid receptors, CB1 and CB2, as novel targets for inhibition of non–small cell lung cancer growth and metastasis. Cancer Prev Res. 2010;4:65–75. https://doi.org/10.1158/1940-6207.CAPR-10-0181.
38. Postow MA, Callahan MK, Wolchok JD. Immune checkpoint blockade in cancer therapy. J Clin Oncol. 2015;33:1974–82.
39. Ramer R, Hinz B. Inhibition of cancer cell invasion by cannabinoids via increased expression of tissue inhibitor of matrix metalloproteinases-1. J Natl Cancer Inst. 2008;100:59–69.
40. Ross RA. L-α-lysophosphatidylinositol meets GPR55: a deadly relationship. Trends Pharmacol Sci. 2011;32:265–9. https://doi.org/10.1016/j.tips.2011.01.005.
41. Salazar M, Carracedo A, Salanueva IJ, et al. TRB3 links ER stress to autophagy in cannabinoid anti-tumoral action. Autophagy. 2009;5:1048–9.
42. Sarantopoulos S, Cardones AR, Sullivan KM. How I treat refractory chronic graft-versus-host disease. Blood. 2019;133:1191–200. https://doi.org/10.1182/blood-2018-04-785899.
43. Sarfaraz S, Adhami VM, Syed DN, Afaq F, Mukhtar H. Cannabinoids for cancer treatment: progress and promise. Cancer Res. 2008;68:339–42.
44. Schoeman R, Beukes N, Frost C. Cannabinoid combination induces cytoplasmic vacuolation in MCF-7 breast cancer cells. Molecules. 2020;25:4682–903. https://doi.org/10.3390/molecules25204682.
45. Schoemans HM, Lee SJ, Ferrara JL, et al. EBMT−NIH−CIBMTR Task Force position statement on standardized terminology & guidance for graft-versus-host disease assessment. Bone Marrow Transplant. 2018;53:1401–15. https://doi.org/10.1038/s41409-018-0204-7.
46. Sharafi G, He H, Nikfarjam M. Potential use of cannabinoids for treatment of pancreatic cancer. J Pancreatic Cancer. 2019;5:1. http://online.liebertpub.com/doi/10.1089/pancan.2018.0019
47. Shi S, Brant AR, Sabolch A, et al. False news of a cannabis cancer cure. Cureus. 2019;11(1):e3918. https://doi.org/10.7759/cureus.3918.
48. Shrivastava A, Kuzontkoski PM, Groopman JE, Prasad A. Cannabidiol induces programmed cell death in breast cancer cells by coordinating the cross-talk between apoptosis and autophagy. Mol Cancer Ther. 2011;10:1161–72.
49. Shore TB, Ryan JB, Samuel MB. A case report of the benefit of Cannabidiol (Cannabidiol (CBD)-predominant medical cannabis preparation) in the Management of Refractory Skin Graft vs Host Disease (GVHD). Biol Blood Marrow Transplant. 2020;3(Supplement):S177–8. https://doi.org/10.1016/j.bbmt.2019.12.736.
50. Singh Y, Bali C. Cannabis extract treatment for terminal acute lymphoblastic leukemia with a Philadelphia Chromosome mutation. Case Rep Oncol. 2013;6:585–92. https://doi.org/10.1159/000356446.
51. Snell A. Meta-analysis of cannabigerol effects on breast cancer tissue cells. Undergraduate Honors Theses. 2021;42. https://digscholarship.unco.edu/honors/42.
52. Taha T, Meiri D, Talhamy S, et al. Cannabis impacts tumor response rate to nivolumab in patients with advanced malignancies. Oncologist. 2019;24:549–54.
53. Takeda S, Yamaori S, Motoya E, et al. Delta(9)-tetrahydrocannabinol enhances MCF-7 cell proliferation via cannabinoid receptor-independent signaling. Toxicology. 2008;245:141–6.

54. Tomko AM, Whynot EG, Ellis LD, Dupré DJ. Anti-Cancer Potential of Cannabinoids, Terpenes, and Flavonoids Present in Cannabis Cancers 2020, 12, 1985; https://doi.org/10.3390/cancers12071985.
55. Topalian SL, Hodi FS, Brahmer JR, et al. Five-year survival and correlates among patients with advanced melanoma, renal cell carcinoma, or non-small cell lung cancer treated with nivolumab. JAMA Oncol. 2019;5:1411–20.
56. Torres S, Lorente M, Rodriguez-Fornes F, et al. A combined preclinical therapy of cannabinoids and temozolomide against glioma. Mol Cancer Ther. 2011;10:90–103.
57. Twelves C, Sabel M, Checketts D, et al. A phase 1b randomised, placebo-controlled trial of nabiximols cannabinoid oromucosal spray with temozolomide in patients with recurrent glioblastoma. Br J Cancer. 2021;124:1379–87. https://doi.org/10.1038/s41416-021-01259-3.
58. Velasco G, Sanchez C, Guzman M. Anticancer mechanisms of cannabinoids. Curr Oncol. 2016;23(S2):S23–32.
59. Wei SC, Duffy CR, Allison JP. Fundamental mechanisms of immune checkpoint blockade therapy. Cancer Discov. 2018;8:1069–86.
60. Winkler K, Ramer R, Dithmer S, Ivanov I, Merkord J, Hinz B. Fatty acid amide hydrolase inhibitors confer anti-invasive and antimetastatic effects on lung cancer cells. Oncotarget. 2016;7:15047–64.
61. Yeshurun M, Shpilberg O, Herscovici C, et al. Cannabidiol for the prevention of graft-versus-host-disease after allogeneic hematopoietic cell transplantation: results of a phase II study. Biol Blood Marrow Transplant. 2015;21:1770–5. https://doi.org/10.1016/j.bbmt.2015.05.018.
62. Yuan C-Y, Zhou V, Sauber G. Signaling through the type 2 cannabinoid receptor regulates the severity of acute and chronic graft versus host disease. Blood. 2021;137:1241–55. https://doi.org/10.1182/blood.2020004871.
63. Zhu LX, Sharma S, Stolina M, et al. Delta-9-tetrahydrocannabinol inhibits antitumor immunity by a CB2 receptor-mediated, cytokine-dependent pathway. J Immunol. 2000;165:373–80.

Chapter 5
Cannabinoid-Based Medicines and Cancer Symptom Management

Contents

5.1 Introduction.......... 129
5.2 Terminology.......... 132
5.3 Chemotherapy-Induced Nausea and Vomiting.......... 133
5.4 Appetite Stimulation.......... 136
5.5 Pain.......... 137
5.6 Sleep.......... 140
5.7 Drug-Sparing Effects.......... 141
5.8 Topical Applications for Wound Healing and Analgesia.......... 142
5.9 Multimodal Symptom Treatment in Advanced Cancer.......... 143
5.10 Conclusion.......... 144
References.......... 145

5.1 Introduction

Cannabis use among cancer patients is not uncommon, although the data on the actual prevalence is conflicting. Smaller surveys seem to indicate higher rates of use, while larger population-based surveys seem to indicate that the opposite is true.

In a survey of cancer patients presenting to a Canadian cancer center published in 2018, 43% of respondents reported any lifetime use; however, only 18% of respondents sufficiently completed the surveys. Of the 356 patients who reported cannabis use within the 6 months preceding the survey, 36% were new users. Their reasons for use included cancer-related pain (46%), nausea (34%), other cancer symptoms (31%), and noncancer-related reasons (56%) [62]. In another survey, more than half of cancer patients had used cannabis at some point [41]. In a larger survey aimed at adult cancer patients treated in the USA conducted by the National

C. Cyr et al., *Cannabis and Cannabinoid-Based Medicines in Cancer Care*,
https://doi.org/10.1007/978-3-030-89918-9_5

Cancer Institute, 926 of 2737 (34%) completed the survey, and 27% used cannabis in the last year [74].

However, in the National Survey on Drug Use and Health, which was carried out from 2015 to 2019, data was gathered from 214,505 participants, and results differed from the preceding surveys. In all, 4741 (3.8%) of individuals with past (>1 year ago) cancer diagnosis and 1518 (1.2%) with recent cancer answered the survey. Results indicated that cannabis use was lower for individuals with past (8.9%) or current (9.9%) diagnosis of cancer, when compared to individuals without a history of cancer (15.9%) [25].

Another recent survey of American cancer patients performed during the COVID pandemic compared cannabis use among cancer patients to that of individuals without cancer. Cancer survivors were more likely to report use of cannabis as a way of managing nausea/vomiting (40.5% versus 20.3%, $p = 0.006$), headaches or migraines (35.4% versus 19.0%, $p = 0.020$), seizures (8.9% versus 1.3%, $p = 0.029$), and sleep problems (70.9% versus 54.4%, $p = 0.033$) or as an appetite stimulant (39.2% versus 17.7%, $p = 0.003$) [16]. The diverging results in the prevalence of cannabis use among cancer patients are certainly intriguing and warrant further investigation.

Cannabis has been used for thousands of years in the treatment of various medical ailments in many different cultures [78]. Its medicinal use is documented in the papyri of ancient Egypt and even earlier in Chinese herbals [78]. Regarded as a beneficial form of pharmacotherapy, it remained as such until 1941 when it was removed from the US Pharmacopeia and National Formulary (USP-NF) due to changes in the political environment [78]. Over the next 40 years, the pharmacological properties of cannabis went largely unstudied except for a handful of researchers [78]. We are now uncovering what earlier cultures had already defined in terms of the efficacy of cannabinoid-based medicines. We will look at their properties as they pertain to:

- Chemotherapy-induced nausea and vomiting (CINV), Appetite stimulation, Pain, Sleep and Drug sparing effects
- Topical application for wound healing and analgesia
- Multimodal symptom management in advanced cancer and palliative care patients

The science surrounding the use of cannabis for medical purposes is still in its infancy. Of the few available randomized controlled trials, many suffer from an increased risk of bias and false results.

Although observational studies using cannabis in symptom management appear to indicate promising results, history has shown that many if not most associations identified in observational investigations will likely turn out to be falsely positive when tested in randomized trials [45]. There are six characteristics of studies which increase the risk of false discovery, reducing the likelihood that the findings are true, or increase the risk of bias [44]:

- Smaller studies
- Studies with a greater number of outcome measures and less selective tests of the association

- Smaller effect size
- Studies with a greater flexibility in design, definitions, outcomes, and analytic tests
- Greater financial interest and prejudice in the scientific field
- The "hotter" the field is, scientifically and sociopolitically

Many cannabis trials suffer from these characteristics. The contradictory findings between observational studies and meta-analysis may reflect the non-replicability of observational studies either due to hidden confounders, robust placebo effects, patient selection, or investigator and patient convictions that cannabis is beneficial. Accordingly, conclusions drawn from observational studies require a very cautious interpretation of nominally statistically significant findings despite political and social pressures to put forth such studies as truth.

Randomized clinical trials examining the use of cannabis are still few in number, and fewer still are considered of high quality. The early studies, most of which have been carried out in the last 20 years, remain difficult to reproduce. Reproducibility is a necessary step to validate initial findings, and the ability to replicate a study requires transparency where the set of procedures are detailed, and the methods permit readers to visualize the entire trial process from data collection to analysis [34]. However, cannabis trials to date have for the most part used non-standardized cannabis products and derivatives, examined different delivery methods and populations, and used different designs, analysis, outcome measures, and timeframes. As a result, the inconsistencies of clinical studies are still not focused on reliability and replicability [66].

Evidence on medical uses of cannabis and other Cannabinoid-Based Medicines (CBM) is therefore highly variable due to these methodological limitations, and conclusions are weak, contradictory, or largely inconsistent in most of the comparisons. Furthermore, most trials present other design flaws, including proper titration and longer trial periods, both considered important for tolerability and efficacy when introducing cannabis to inexperienced individuals. This may explain in part the high rate of adverse events and dropout rates found in short-term studies carried out over a few days or weeks compared to longer-term observational studies. For example, an Israeli study collected data from 2970 cancer patients treated with medical cannabis between 2015 and 2017. After 6 months of follow-up, 902 patients (24.9%) died, and 682 (18.8%) stopped the cannabis (less than 5% due to adverse events, however); 1211 (60.6%) responded, of which 95.9% reported an improvement in their condition [91].

The dose-response curve of THC, leading to progressive subjective effects, often requires a prolonged period of acclimatization. For many cannabis clinicians, this is a guiding principle when introducing any CBM. However, many studies used in systematic reviews rapidly titrate cannabinoids which may explain the increased reporting of adverse events. Clinicians with cannabis experience often recommend trial periods of careful experimentation over the course of several weeks or months, which may be necessary in many individuals before arriving at a steady state of tolerability and perceived efficacy. This is particularly the case when using unregulated products of varying potency, where accidental intoxications are common and require close monitoring. More on these subjects can be found in Chaps. 6 and 7.

Furthermore, cannabis research remains an arduous and politically delicate scientific endeavor. In Canada, where cannabis for medical and recreational use has been legalized and regulated, its status as an unrecognized medication plays a significant role in explaining the long delays in approval of study design by health regulators. Along with a highly speculative return on investment (ROI), many licensed cannabis producers feel reluctant to invest in costly research. Hence, these are some of the factors which explain why evidence for efficacy will fall short of present-day standards, at least until patentable formulations enter the market and permit larger, more expensive trials.

Fortunately, new standardized formulations in the form of capsules, softgels, and precise metered inhalers are helping to reduce much of the unpredictability of cannabis effects. Patients living in jurisdictions where regulated cannabis products are found can now adjust dosages more precisely and, when counseled appropriately, safely find a therapeutic window which works best for them [76, 77].

The role of each delivery method, whether inhaled or overly administered, varies according to symptom characteristics. Shorter-duration symptoms such as spasms, nausea, and initial insomnia may respond more favorably to quick acting inhalation, particularly if the patient does not want to be burdened with psychoactivity for an extended period. However, the available inhaled formulations are outdated, for the most part. Smoking or vaping raw dried flower or diluted extracts with presently available technology still produces a very wide pharmacokinetic range. Using higher-dose THC products may inadvertently produce intoxication with only a few inhalations with any significant breath hold. This issue of other unconventional delivery methods such as inhalation by smoking will be dealt with in more detail in Chap. 7.

In summary, conflicting results from small trials will require further long-term studies in order to determine efficacy of cannabinoids in cancer symptom management. Meanwhile, presently available data suggests that THC and other CB1 receptor agonists may be more effective in treating neuropathic pain than other forms of cancer pain.

5.2 Terminology

The term “endocannabinoidome” is still not widely used by clinicians and researchers, and in order to avoid confusion, its use to describe the *expanded* endocannabinoid system (ECS) will be restricted to the first chapter of this book. For the present chapter, the more commonly used term “endocannabinoid system (ECS)” will be used to describe most concepts relating to both the more specific canonical receptors and enzymes and the larger system of molecular targets and ligands. The "endocannabinoidome" will only be mentioned in order to point out a clinically relevant difference between these two related concepts.

"Cannabinoid-Based Medicines" will be used preferentially as a general umbrella term to describe all compounds containing either approved or non-approved cannabinoids derived from either natural cannabis or synthetically produced. The term "cannabis" and "medical cannabis" will only be used contextually when discussing the use of plant-based products specifically.

5.3 Chemotherapy-Induced Nausea and Vomiting

Nausea and vomiting are very common symptoms encountered in cancer care. They can arise from chemotherapy, radiotherapy (RINV), or other causes such as brain metastasis, bowel obstruction, gastroparesis, constipation, hypercalcemia, or the use of drugs (opioids, NSAIDs, antibiotics, or antidepressants). Although vomiting can be a more unpleasant experience, it can often relieve nausea temporarily and is usually easier to treat. Persistent nausea without vomiting is often more difficult to manage and may have a greater impact on patient quality of life [12]. In some cases, protracted and uncontrolled nausea may be an indication for palliative sedation [20]. Adequate control of vomiting is therefore not a good measure of treatment success.

The use of CBM to treat nausea and vomiting has been mostly studied in the context of chemotherapy-induced nausea and vomiting (CINV). These debilitating symptoms are experienced by up to 75 percent of patients undergoing chemotherapy treatments [97], and despite the use of prophylactic antiemetics, the prevalence of breakthrough nausea or vomiting can affect up to 40% of cancer patients. Not only does the physical act of eating become difficult due to nausea, but the intrinsic emotional value of food is decreased due to changes in olfactory sense receptors. Foods that once were enjoyable now become intolerable for the patient by either smell or visual presentation; and for some patients, even the mention of food can induce nausea.

Effective control of nausea and vomiting is therefore important for several reasons. In the short term, adequate control of CINV does indeed increase the quality of life. However, the long-term control of nausea and vomiting can play a role in a patient's ability to continue on with treatment and ultimately increase their chances of survival [95].

Nausea and vomiting attributable to chemotherapy can be divided into five categories [92]:

1. *Acute CINV* – occurs within the first 24 h after receiving chemotherapy with peak reaction occurring around 5–6 h.
2. *Delayed CINV* – occurs anywhere after 24 h to 1 week following chemotherapy with peak reactions occurring between 48 and 72 h

3. *Breakthrough CINV* – occurs within 5 days of receiving chemotherapy even while on antiemetic therapy. This may require additional treatment with a subsequent antiemetic
4. *Refractory CINV* – occurs in additional chemotherapy cycles in spite of optimal antiemetic therapy
5. *Anticipatory CINV* – a conditioned patient response due to poorly controlled CINV from a previous chemotherapy session wherein a previous unconditioned stimulus (taste, smell) now triggers nausea/vomiting in the patient

The advent of 5-hydroxytryptamine (5HT3) receptor antagonists (e.g., ondansetron, palonosetron, granisetron) and NK1 receptor antagonists (aprepitant, rolapitant, casopitant, fosaprepitant, netupitant) has brought about increasing relief from CINV previously not completely controlled with standard neuroleptic agents like metoclopramide, haloperidol, and prochlorperazine and corticosteroids [29]. Drugs that block several receptors (e.g., mirtazapine or olanzapine) may be advantageous if symptoms seem refractory [111]. With advancing disease, the choice of a palliative antiemetic is often empirical. Usually, a first medication is titrated to efficacy, maximum recommended, or tolerated dose. Subsequent agents are then added in a stepwise manner [111].

While combinations with these two to three medication protocols are the current standard of care [43], many patients experience some element of nausea and vomiting during their cancer treatment [95]. In addition, several of the antiemetics come with their own side effects that may make them intolerable to the patient, including constipation, headache, and sleep disturbance [111]. The combination of CINV and medication side effects may contribute to explain why up to 20% of chemotherapy patients discontinue their treatments [42].

Cannabinoid-Based Medicines have been shown to provide benefits for CINV [97]. The endocannabinoid system plays an important role in the pathogenesis of nausea and vomiting, demonstrated by the fact that blocking the CB1 and CB2 receptors produces emesis [93]. The proposed mechanism for the control of nausea and vomiting by Δ9-tetrahydrocannabinol (THC) therefore lies in the regulation of brainstem activity via activation of the CB1 and CB2 endocannabinoid receptors [29]. In addition, these medicines also have a role in the regulation of vagal reflexes involving enterochromaffin cells of the gastrointestinal tract managing nausea and vomiting similar to that of 5HT3 antagonists [95]. THC has been shown to improve CINV in studies that go back several decades [90]. The isolation and synthesis of the THC molecule in the 1960s, 1970s, and 1980s allowed for the production of the currently used pharmaceutical cannabinoids [85]. Dronabinol was first approved in 1986 as treatment for CINV followed by the synthetic THC analogue nabilone, both of which act as CB1 receptor agonists [85, 109].

The evidence is convincing for their efficacy. In a systematic review of 30 randomized comparisons including dronabinol, nabilone, and levonantradol (unavailable synthetic analog of dronabinol) vs placebo, it was found that these medical cannabinoids were more clinically effective for nausea control than the current standard antiemetics [58]. In addition, CBM were the preferred treatment of choice by the patient for CINV

[58]. A recent systematic review and meta-analysis by Whiting et al. included 28 randomized control trials (RCTs) pertaining to CINV and assessed a variety of medical cannabis products including nabilone, dronabinol, nabiximols, and cannabis extracts of THC [110]. These showed superior management of CINV compared to placebo or current standard-of-care comparator [110]. A Cochrane Review also showed patients reported an absence of CINV with Cannabinoid-Based Medicines more often than placebo and that there was no difference in CINV than with other antiemetics [97]. This evidence points to the usefulness of Cannabinoid-Based Medicines as an auxiliary antiemetic for management of nausea and vomiting in chemotherapy patients. Given that a large proportion of patients terminate chemotherapy due to unregulated nausea or vomiting, it is important that consideration be given to these medications when thinking about adjusting dosing or adding a supplementary medication [49].

Although the evidence supporting the use of pharmaceutical grade cannabinoids for CINV is clear, the evidence for either inhaled or orally administered cannabis or cannabis extracts is less strong. One needs to be reminded that many of the older studies looking to assess the tolerability of cannabinoids for CINV often overlook the issue of tolerance and in some cases used potentially toxic initial doses of THC (up to 15 mg). Moreover, few comparative studies exist.

Only dronabinol has been compared with ondansetron and demonstrated equal efficacy, though the combination of both these agents did not result in a synergistic response [64]. Few large-scale RCTs have used raw/dried cannabis or its extracts for CINV, and none have directly compared these to current standards of therapy (5HT3 antagonists, NK1 antagonists, atypical antipsychotic meds). A phase II trial has shown promise being the first to have a CBM in an oral mucosal spray with both CBD and THC (1:1) [29]. Compared to placebo, it provided more effective control for delayed CINV. That was followed by a phase II/III crossover trial of an oral cannabis extract of CBD/THC (1:1) which demonstrated greater patient preference over placebo but with an increased side effect profile [36]. The trial used nabiximols with a 5HT3 (serotonin) and NK1 receptor inhibitor to prevent chemotherapy-induced nausea and vomiting in patients receiving high-emetogenic medications and who had significant nausea with the first cycle [36]. The cannabis extract produced a modest 10% difference in nausea and vomiting relative to 5HT3/NK1 receptor blocker double drug prophylaxis. In this study, 41% of patients had prior cannabis experience, and patient preference for nabiximols far exceeded objective improvement in nausea and vomiting. The question remains whether nabiximols may have reduced anxiety or the perceived unpleasantness of nausea rather than the symptom itself. Furthermore, only three of the participants were also given olanzapine which is standard for or high-risk emetogenic chemotherapy [21–23, 112]. A further phase III study may provide further answers [36].

While 5HT3 receptor antagonists and NK1 antagonists have for the most part provided effective relief for acute CINV, anticipatory nausea remains problematic in up to 25–59% of chemotherapy patients [84]. For patients dealing with CINV, this condition can be equally disabling or worse [95]. Currently, the only recommended pharmacologic therapy for anticipatory nausea is benzodiazepines such as lorazepam [83]. Recent studies in animal models using exogenous cannabinoids and stimulation of endogenous cannabinoids to reduce anticipatory nausea have shown promising results [83, 86]. Preclinical results also suggest that increased levels of 2-arachidonoylglycerol (2-AG) and anandamide (AEA) can improve nausea immediately following chemotherapy and anticipatory CINV [84].

5.4 Appetite Stimulation

Cachexia is a multifactorial process seen in many chronic diseases including Alzheimer's, human immunodeficiency virus (HIV)/AIDS, multiple sclerosis, and some forms of diabetes [9, 104, 108]. Cancer-related cachexia anorexia syndrome (CACS) is a disease-specific dysregulation of the normal appetite and metabolism processes by malignant factors, with some contribution from common chemo- and immunotherapy regimens [87]. CACS is defined by reduced dietary intake, lipolysis, and muscle wasting/sarcopenia [8]. Managing CACS can present many challenges for the patient, family, and the healthcare team. Finding an effective treatment has also been proven to be a challenge. Despite many clinical trials, the most recent clinical practice guideline from ASCO for CACS can only advise evidence-supported benefits such as dietary counseling and short-term course of corticosteroids (e.g., dexamethasone or prednisone) or progesterone analogues [87].

The endocannabinoid system plays a complex role in the regulation of appetite and metabolism as seen from preclinical work in animal models [32]. A recent study in humans showed that various forms of cannabis by oral ingestion and inhalation produced a decrease in insulin sensitivity [32]. This is in line with previous research where cannabis users are prone to weight gain and insulin resistance and merits further investigation into its use as an appetite stimulant [32]. While current human trials still show that evidence is lacking for therapeutic approval, there is a pressing demand from patients and their care teams for phase III clinical trials to establish its efficacy [81]. It is also important to explore the pharmacokinetics of CBM in the CACS patient population due to the challenges in dosing and possible drug interactions [81].

Cannabinoid-Based Medicines, which include cannabis, have long been known as potential appetite stimulants [8]. Anecdotal reports from recreational users often relate stories of increased hunger and the need for salty and sweet foods ("the munchies") post-cannabis use [82]. Only recently have we started to elucidate the science behind what may be the cause of this powerful appetite stimulation. Most currently available formulations of cannabinoids have been studied for appetite stimulation, including synthetic cannabinoids such as dronabinol and nabilone, dried cannabis flower, and oral-mucosal extracts. Results remain conflicting, and further long-term studies will be needed to determine efficacy.

However, several small reports have shown that both the smoking of cannabis and the oral intake of cannabis-based extracts may stimulate appetite in cancer patients [63], although significant weight gain was not shown to occur in this patient population. CB1 receptor agonists (dronabinol, nabilone) are approved in Canada and other jurisdictions to treat cachexia in patients with HIV and have also been used for patients with cancer [63, 89]. As an appetite stimulant, nabilone has been stated to have a moderately effective benefit in relieving patients of anorexia. In a randomized, double-blind, placebo-controlled clinical trial, the effect of nabilone vs placebo was studied to determine efficacy on appetite, nutritional status, and quality of life in patients diagnosed with advanced non-small cell lung cancer. A total of 65 outpatients were assessed for eligibility, and 47 were randomized to receive nabilone (0.5 mg/2 weeks followed by 1.0 mg/6 weeks) or placebo. After 8 weeks, patients on nabilone increased caloric intake by an average of 342 kcal compared to patients on placebo. Quality of life significantly improved on nabilone, particularly role functioning, but also emotional and social functioning. Pain and insomnia were also noted by patients to be improved [103].

In other clinical settings, cannabinoids have been shown to be effective for appetite stimulation. One pilot study has demonstrated weight gain benefits in Alzheimer patients given oral dronabinol [104]. However, larger randomized controlled trials (RCTs) did not report the same outcomes. RCTs carried out during the early 2000s in advanced cancer patients involved dronabinol and cannabis extracts [99]. The endpoints of the study comparing cannabis extracts and THC to placebo in patients with CACS included change in appetite and quality-of-life measures. These showed no significant differences in appetite (use of cannabis extracts (73%) versus placebo (69%)) nor quality of life [99]. An earlier RCT using dronabinol versus megestrol acetate for appetite stimulation and weight gain demonstrated that megestrol was superior for appetite stimulation and that adding dronabinol to megestrol did not confer any further benefit [46]. These results point to the possibility that the use of whole cannabis plant preparations (dried or fresh flower, whole plant extracts), as opposed to purified or synthetic analogues, may have further orexigenic properties which may have not been fully elucidated by these study designs [46, 99].

A recent systematic review examining the role of cannabinoids on cancer cachexia further confirms the findings that cannabinoids have a potential role in increasing appetite [108]. However, the authors also concluded that quality of life was not shown to be improved in the three eligible studies. It is important to point out that the follow-up period of the trials used in this review were of less than 6 weeks. The role of cannabinoids in the modulation of appetite and cachexia awaits the results from long-term studies.

5.5 Pain

Pain associated with cancer is a common symptom. Studies have shown that between 70 and 90% of people with advanced cancer experience substantial pain [48]. Cancer pain can be grouped into three categories [19]:

1. *Somatic pain – invasion of tumor cells into connective tissues*
2. *Visceral pain – invasion of tumor cells into visceral organs*

3. *Neuropathic pain – pain elicited from damage to the central and peripheral nervous systems*

While opiates remain the mainstay of therapy, they can also be ineffective or intolerable due to the complex and individualized nature of cancer pain [26]. There is therefore an urgent need to provide patients with adjunctive therapies when pain is not well managed. In these cases, cannabis may be effective, particularly in patients with neuropathic cancer-related pain.

Cannabis and hemp have been used for thousands of years in many cultures to ameliorate pain with the oldest specimen being discovered in the Yanghai Tombs in China dating back to 2700 years ago [47]. From Aruvedic practitioners of India to the Egyptian papyrus, cannabis was used as an analgesic. In the nineteenth century, cannabis was researched by neurologist Sir William Gowers for its potential in treating migraines. In some cultures, these traditional teachings have been handed down to future generations where indigenous communities throughout the world still use cannabis for pain and other medicinal purposes [14].

Animal studies have shown that both exogenous and endogenous cannabinoid pathways are implicated in pain perception and analgesia [63]. They exert their action through attenuation of hyperalgesia and altering behavior to painful stimuli []. Murine models have shown attenuation of mechanical hyperalgesia via the CB1 receptor [26]. Stimulation of CB2 receptors in the spinal cord and dorsal root ganglion is shown to provide analgesia to bone tumors in similar models [26]. In addition, studies have shown that selective CB2 agonism not only attenuates spontaneous and evoked pain both acutely and chronically in mice with bone cancer but also prevents bone loss and fracture [55]. This provides promise for future clinical trials as bone pain resulting from breast, prostate, myeloma, and lung cancers bring about chronic pain that is often difficult to control and greatly impacts quality of life and function for patients [26, 55]. The fact that CB2 receptor agonists do not impact the respiratory centers and reward pathways like opiates makes them potentially promising in the use of pain related to bone cancer.

Cannabinoid-Based Medicines primarily act via THC agonism on the CB1 receptors in the central and peripheral nervous systems and the CB2 receptors on immune cells and peripheral nervous cells [55]. In addition to traditionally acting on the CB1 and CB2 receptors to produce their analgesic effect, they may also act via cannabinoid G protein-coupled receptors (GPR55 and GPR 18) and other nuclear receptors [105]. Studies today have shown analgesic benefit in the use of cannabinoids in rheumatoid arthritis, fibromyalgia, and multiple sclerosis [105]. However, the question regarding the clinical benefits of CBM in cancer pain specifically remains unresolved.

Of the different types of pain syndromes encountered, neuropathic pain continues to be one of the most difficult ongoing conditions to manage for oncology patients. Meta-analyses and clinical trials suggest that the analgesic benefits of CBM and cannabinoids may be more pronounced in neuropathic pain than for other types of noncancer pain [96, 105]. This has warranted The Canadian Pain Society into changing their recommendation and adding cannabinoids as a definitive third-line option for pain management in treating chronic neuropathic pain [68].

A rapid qualitative systematic review suggested that cannabinoids may have a modest analgesic effect for chronic neuropathic pain conditions and that the use of cannabinoids is relatively safe, with few severe adverse events [54]. A meta-analysis of randomized trials consisting of 16 studies which included 1750 patients who were treated either with synthetic or plant-based cannabis for at least 2 weeks raised more concerns over tolerability [70]. Those reaching a 50% reduction in pain intensity were found in 21% of cannabis users versus 17% with placebo (*P* equal 0.05; 95% confidence interval 0–0.9). The number needed to treat to benefit a single patient (NNTB) was 20. The NNTB for a 30% reduction in pain was 11. The number needed to harm (NNTH) determined by withdrawal from study was 25, the NNTH for CNS effects was 3, and the NNTH for psychiatric events was 10. The Cohen D for a 50% reduction in pain was 0.16 which would fall below even a small improvement. A Bayesian probability of superiority was 54%, which is almost a flip of a coin. The Cohen D for a 30% reduction in pain was 0.28 which would be a small benefit with a Bayesian probability of superiority of 58%, again almost a flip of a coin. In a systematic review and meta-analysis of cannabis adverse effects involving 79 randomized trials, the relative risk of harm with cannabis was 1.86. The relative risk of harm with oromucosal THC was 1.88 and for oral THC 2.18 [65]. However, the evaluation of nabiximol spray for chemotherapy-induced neuropathic pain (CINP) has shown potential for future RCTs [57].

The evidence for efficacy of CBM in non-neuropathic cancer pain is less solid. Despite a multitude of animal studies showing the attenuation of non-neuropathic pain by cannabinoids, there have been few clinical trials proving its efficacy [4]. The preponderance of available randomized trials suggest that there is insufficient evidence for the *singular* use of cannabis in treating other forms of cancer pain [31, 33, 40, 48, 53, 69, 79]. One study did note that advanced cancer patients whose pain was uncontrolled by opioids achieved a reduction in pain scores with the use of THC/CBD extract (nabiximols) as an adjunctive therapy [48]. Additional studies show support for further research into the use of nabiximol spray as an adjunctive therapy to opioids due to their analgesic effects in those with advanced cancer [79]. Current meta-analyses and systematic reviews also tend to suggest that cannabinoids have limited benefits in cancer-related pain [13, 40, 70]. The review by Boland et al. further concluded that in adults with advanced cancer, the addition of cannabinoids to opioids did not improve cancer pain. This analysis may have been limited by the high mortality rate among participants and the lack of alteration in dosing to limit adverse effects including dizziness and nausea [13].

However, a great number of cancer patients are using cannabis for pain, despite the lack of evidence. An anonymous survey in Canada showed that 18% of patients reported using cannabis in the past 6 months, and of those, 46% used it for cancer-related pain [13]. Similar studies were also carried out in the USA in states where cannabis has been legalized showing patients were using cannabis for cancer pain [13]. Furthermore, in a survey of 426 palliative care providers, 70% believe that cannabis not only could improve nausea and appetite but also was effective in reducing cancer pain. Only 26% stated that they were unsure of the benefits [56].

A review in The Lancet on the use of cannabis to treat mental health conditions pointed out that cannabis may be more beneficial if a pain comorbidity is present. Thus, when anxiety is associated with chronic pain, a therapeutic trial may provide better outcomes than treating anxiety as an isolated symptom [11].

5.6 Sleep

Sleep disturbance is a common concern among oncology patients. The onset of disruptions in sleep is likely related to chemotherapy, acute or chronic pain, and anxiety [3]. Other medications used for supportive purposes (corticosteroids, anti-nauseants) can also impact sleep patterns. Patients relate lying awake in bed either unable to get to sleep or wake up 2–3 h after falling asleep. Sleep disturbance due to pain often exists in a bidirectional relationship, where patients wake up in pain and are unable to fall back asleep, or because of accumulated lack of sleep, patients experience decreased pain thresholds [38].

The studies surrounding exogenous cannabinoids and sleep are still preliminary [38]. Inhaled cannabis has long been known for its hypnotic and relaxing effects with ancient texts and pharmacopeia documenting preparations used as anesthetics in surgery or sedatives during childbirth []. Research on cannabis and its effects on sleep date back to the 1970s, showing decreases in sleep onset latency, reductions in waking after sleep onset, and increases in slow wave sleep [5, 50]. Most of the research suggested cannabis use over the short term could improve sleep disturbances, but none of this work was done using cancer patients. At the molecular level, CB1 cannabinoid receptors and other components of the ECS interact with multiple systems that may affect sleep – wake cycles including serotonergic, GABAergic, glutamic, and dopaminergic receptors [17]. Sleep disruptions due to chronic pain conditions such as fibromyalgia and multiple sclerosis have significantly improved with the use of cannabis, often as a secondary outcome [5, 10, 71]. Again, the use of cannabis for sleep disturbances in cancer patients has not been examined in any greater detail.

Several systematic reviews have examined the role of cannabis and CBM in sleep disorders. A recently published critical review of clinical trials highlighted 18 studies that looked at the effect of synthetic preparations of THC (nabilone and dronabinol) on sleep [52]. Exclusively reported as a secondary outcome, quality of sleep improved as subjectively recorded by the majority of subjects [52]. An additional review by Suraev et al. examined the effects of cannabis on sleep disorders in 14 preclinical studies and 12 clinical studies. Although some preliminary therapeutic benefits were found, the authors concluded there is currently not enough objective, large-scale research available and too much bias in the existing literature to recommend cannabis as a treatment for sleep disorder [100]. The review also highlighted some promising studies which warrant further investigation [100].

Preclinical animal studies demonstrate that the serotonin-related pathways of sleep apnea could be suppressed through the exogenous cannabinoid system via THC. It may also be suppressed via stimulation of the endogenous cannabinoid pathway by oleamide, a naturally occurring fatty acid derived from oleic acid which may have sleep-inducing properties [18]. An additional pilot study further demonstrated improved self-reported sleep outcomes for people with obstructive sleep apnea with use of dronabinol [17]. Other cross-sectional studies have looked at the effects of whole plant medical cannabis and insomnia in elderly patients with chronic pain [101]. Preliminary findings point to a positive impact from whole plant use where participants were waking less frequently at night [101]. Given some of these initial findings, further randomized control trials are necessary to determine efficacy [101].

Whiting et al. showed a positive association between cannabis use and improved sleep outcome in a meta-analysis review. In 19 placebo-controlled studies where sleep was a secondary outcome, positive results were noted in sleep quality and sleep disturbance with cannabis use [110].

Even though THC is primarily known for its sleep-inducing effects, CBD is now being further researched to elucidate its effects on sleep [50]. For those with normal sleep patterns, CBD does not seem to affect sleep outcomes, but for those with insomnia, high doses of CBD do increase the amount of time the person stays asleep and decreases the number of awakenings [38]. It is important to note that several studies have shown that sleep can also be disrupted due to abrupt withdrawal after discontinuation of long-term use of cannabis [50].

While the effects of CBM in oncology patients who suffer sleep disturbance have not yet been researched, this is an area yet to be explored given the preliminary research being done in areas such as sleep apnea and other sleep disorders [67].

5.7 Drug-Sparing Effects

Preclinical studies have demonstrated robust evidence for the opioid-sparing effects of cannabinoids, and a recent review suggests that cannabinoids help patients reduce their use of opioids [72]. However, retrospective and observational studies, including randomized trials, have given mixed results.

A retrospective cohort study of patients gaged morphine equivalent daily dose (MEDD) from baseline to day 84 in patients on cannabis plus opioids compared with an opioid-only group. A total of 83 patients were included: 61 in the opioid monotherapy group and 22 in the cannabis plus opioid group. An increase in MEDD from the baseline to 84 days was seen in both the opioid monotherapy and opioid plus cannabis groups (28.8 vs 10.8). The study lacked power to detect a statistical difference, however [80]. A 2017 randomized trial suggested that inhaled cannabis provides a synergistic analgesic effect when associated with oxycodone [24]. Another small, randomized trial using dronabinol and oxycodone failed to show a synergistic effect [6] although a more recent RCT has shown that small doses of

Table 5.1 Adapted from the Consensus-Based Recommendations for Titrating Cannabinoids and Tapering of Opioids [94]

Step 1	CBD initiation	Start with 5 mg bid and titrate to 20–40 mg bid
Step 2	THC nighttime initiation	0.5–1 mg THC and titrate to 3 mg
Step 3	THC daytime initiation	0.5–1 mg THC and titrate max 30–40 mg/d
Step 4	Opioid tapering	5–10% MEDD every 1–4 weeks

dronabinol (2.5 mg) increased the analgesic effects of hydromorphone in a human laboratory pain model [28]. The evidence for opioid-sparing effects are inconsistent and will require larger randomized trials comparing different cannabinoid formulations, dosages, and routes of administration. Considering the relative safety of cannabis compared to opioids, a trial may be warranted for patients wishing to reduce their opioid use.

An international group of cannabis clinicians recently published a series of consensus-based recommendations for titrating cannabinoids and tapering of opioids [94]. The group arrived at a consensus on several issues using a modified Delphi process and based their decisions on clinical experience while recognizing the paucity of data to support this type of preliminary guidance. Recommendations include starting most, if not all, patients with CBD-rich products and titrating to a range of 5–20 mg of CBD bid. After an initial trial period, patients are reevaluated in order to determine if introducing small doses of THC is necessary. If this is the case, starting doses of THC in the range of 0.5–1 mg HS are given and gradually titrated to a maximum of 30–40 mg/d divided in two or three doses. If benefits occur, a gradual decrease of MEDD of 5–10% every 1–4 weeks is then undertaken (Table 5.1).

5.8 Topical Applications for Wound Healing and Analgesia

Topical application of cannabis for wound healing was documented in ancient times for treatment of burns in the first century CE and tumors in the late second century CE [75]. It is interesting and important to note that these benefits were derived using the whole raw plant [75]. Recent evidence supports that cannabinoid receptors exist on human endothelial and epidermal cells including skin nerve fibers, mast cells, and keratinocytes via immunofluorescence studies [98]. Such findings provide support for topical application of a cannabinoid receptor agonist that can provide analgesia in animal models [88]. Given the analgesic properties of cannabis and the location of the CB1 and CB2 receptors in the skin, research using human subjects is needed to show how these are activated in wound healing [60]. As the hydrophobic protective barrier of the skin is eroded by the wound, the absorption properties of a

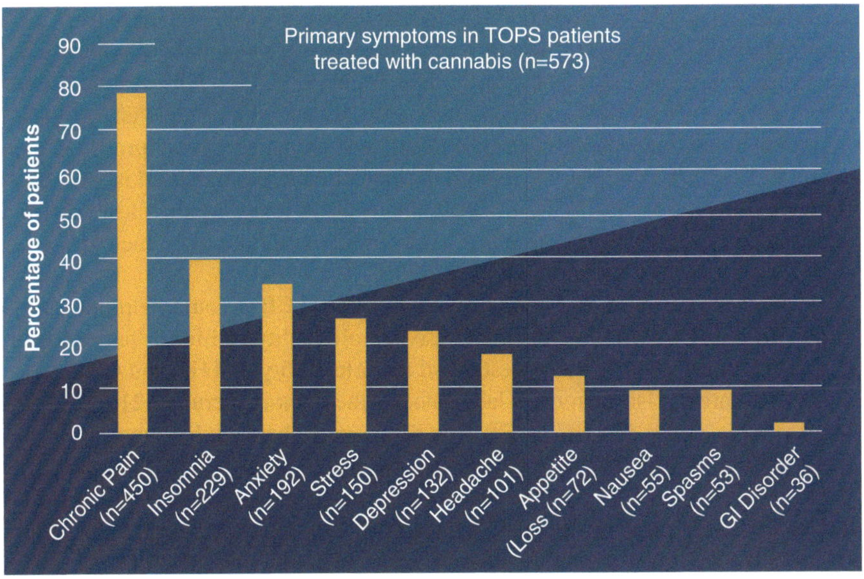

Fig. 5.1 Longitudinal study of >1600 Tilray patients at 20 medical clinics in 5 provinces, the largest Canadian national longitudinal cannabis study to date. This preliminary data is based on 573 patients enrolled before December 1, 2017

topical oil agent may be increased due to the increased lipophilic properties of the skin [60]. Two recently published case studies demonstrated benefit in reduction of pain and improved healing derived from topical cannabis application to a malignant wound [59] and for ulcers related to pyoderma gangrenosum [60].

5.9 Multimodal Symptom Treatment in Advanced Cancer

Trials examining the effects of cannabis to treat specific symptoms often fall short of providing conclusive benefits. However, subjects from several observational studies have reported that cannabis was felt to be more often beneficial in relieving multiple symptoms [91, 1]. A survey of medical cannabis patients from Canada has also corroborated these results (Fig. 5.1).

It is well known that patients with advanced cancers may have multiple symptoms, due to the cancer or the treatments or both [102, 107]. This can lead to the use of several medications targeted to the individual symptoms, which in turn may lead to problematic side effects, drug-drug interactions, and significant impact to the patient's quality of life. Cannabinoid-based medications, with the benefit of broader receptor activity and impact on several key symptoms may be beneficial for patients at this stage of their cancer journey [3, 27, 30]. The use of CBM has also been shown to reduce the use of other medications, including opioids and benzodiazepines, which can be problematic for those at the end of their lives [7, 61]. Some authors also support the use of CBM as an alternative method of reducing the distress patients experience as they near their death [2, 27, 51]. Observational studies of patients using CBM for symptoms have obtained similar results: individual symptoms improve, medication use is reduced, and patients report improvements in quality of life [3, 7, 61, 106]. In general, the cannabinoid product used is well tolerated by study participants, with dizziness and drowsiness being the most common findings. Few patients dropped out due to adverse events, but rather due to progression of disease or lack of benefit [3, 7, 91, 106].

A recent pivotal pilot study sought to determine if CBM could help reduce the burden of multiple symptoms and increase overall quality of life for patients with advanced cancers [35]. It also investigated the tolerability of THC and CBD doses in this population. Using an open label model, the authors recruited 21 patients to use escalating doses of THC or CBD and measured their total symptom distress scores at days 14 and 28. All patients had advanced cancer treated by a palliative and supportive care service, with a median survival of approximately 5 months. Eighteen of twenty-one (86%) completed the primary outcome measure (ESAS) on day 14, and nearly 40% completed the measures at the second time point (day 21). Response (reduction of 6 or more points on the distress score) was recorded in 9 of the 21 patients (43%). Individual symptoms showing the greatest improvement were anxiety, depression, and appetite. The study also determined median tolerated dosing of THC (10 mg/day) and CBD (300 mg/day) in this group, which had not been published previously. The authors plan for a larger, placebo-controlled trial using CBM (THC and CBD) in a fixed dose 1:1 ratio [39].

5.10 Conclusion

Introducing CBM as part of a multimodal symptom management approach may yield better outcomes than treating a single symptom. Hence, advanced cancer and palliative care patients are often ideal candidates for a medical trial of CBM, and recognizing the need to treat a cluster of symptoms may help narrow the choice to a more appropriate clinical setting. Symptom clusters may include of course the main targets for which CBM have been studied: pain, chemotherapy-induced nausea and vomiting, and insomnia. However, if these symptoms are considered mild, searching for other clues, such as anxiety, restlessness, sadness, anhedonia, social isolation, fatigue, and loss of appetite, may provide evidence for an endocannabinoidome in need of supplementation.

Fortunately, the probabilities of having absolute contraindications to using low doses of CBM remain very small, even in frail cancer patients. Observational data studying clinically monitored cannabis use in large cancer populations have indicated that the vast majority of patients claim that cannabis improves their overall quality of life and that it is rarely discontinued due to adverse effects. Educating patients on dosage, use of different administration routes, and formulations and types of cannabis products can be time-consuming and require an efficient workflow and ideally the assistance of a knowledgeable pharmacist or trusted staff.

References

1. Abuhasira R, Schleider LB-L, Mechoulam R, Novack V. Epidemiological characteristics, safety and efficacy of medical cannabis in the elderly. Eur J Intern Med. 2018;49:44–50. https://doi.org/10.1016/j.ejim.2018.01.019.
2. Aggarwal SK. Use of cannabinoids in cancer care: palliative care. Curr Oncol. 2016;23:S33–6. https://doi.org/10.3747/co.23.2962.
3. Aviram J, Lewitus GM, Vysotski Y, Uribayev A, Procaccia S, Cohen I, Leibovici A, Abo-Amna M, Akria L, Goncharov D, Mativ N, Kauffman A, Shai A, Hazan O, Bar-Sela G, Meiri D. Short-term medical cannabis treatment regimens produced beneficial effects among palliative cancer patients. Pharmaceuticals (Basel). 2020;13:E435. https://doi.org/10.3390/ph13120435.
4. Aviram J, Pud D, Gershoni T, Schiff-Keren B, Ogintz M, Vulfsons S, Yashar T, Adahan H-M, Brill S, Amital H, Goor-Aryeh I, Robinson D, Green L, Segal R, Fogelman Y, Tsvieli O, Yellin B, Vysotski Y, Morag O, Tashlykov V, Sheinfeld R, Goor R, Meiri D, Eisenberg E. Medical cannabis treatment for chronic pain: outcomes and prediction of response. Eur J Pain. 2021;25:359–74. https://doi.org/10.1002/ejp.1675.
5. Babson KA, Sottile J, Morabito D. Cannabis, cannabinoids, and sleep: a review of the literature. Curr Psychiatry Rep. 2017;19:23. https://doi.org/10.1007/s11920-017-0775-9.
6. Babalonis S, Lofwall MR, Sloan PA, Nuzzo PA, Fanucchi LC, Walsh SL. Cannabinoid modulation of opioid analgesia and subjective drug effects in healthy humans. Psychopharmacology. https://doi.org/10.1007/s00213-019-05293-1.
7. Bar-Sela G, Vorobeichik M, Drawsheh S, Omer A, Goldberg V, Muller E. The medical necessity for medicinal cannabis: prospective, observational study evaluating the treatment in cancer patients on supportive or palliative care. Evid Based Complement Alternat Med. 2013;2013:510392. https://doi.org/10.1155/2013/510392.
8. Bar-Sela G, Zalman D, Semenysty V, Ballan E. The effects of dosage-controlled cannabis capsules on cancer-related cachexia and anorexia syndrome in advanced cancer patients: pilot study. Integr Cancer Ther. 2019;18:1534735419881498. https://doi.org/10.1177/1534735419881498.
9. Beal JE, Olson R, Laubenstein L, Morales JO, Bellman P, Yangco B, Lefkowitz L, Plasse TF, Shepard KV. Dronabinol as a treatment for anorexia associated with weight loss in patients with AIDS. J Pain Symptom Manag. 1995;10:89–97. https://doi.org/10.1016/0885-3924(94)00117-4.
10. Beaulieu P, Boulanger A, Desroches J, Clark AJ. Medical cannabis: considerations for the anesthesiologist and pain physician. Can J Anaesth. 2016;63:608–24. https://doi.org/10.1007/s12630-016-0598-x.
11. Black N, Stockings E, Campbell G, Tran LT, Zagic D, Hall WD, Farrell M, Degenhardt L. Cannabinoids for the treatment of mental disorders and symptoms of mental disorders: a systematic review and meta-analysis. Lancet Psychiatry. 2019; https://doi.org/10.1016/S2215-0366(19)30401-8.
12. Bloechl-Daum B, Deuson RR, Mavros P, Hansen M, Herrstedt J. Delayed nausea and vomiting continue to reduce patients' quality of life after highly and moderately emetogenic chemotherapy despite antiemetic treatment. J Clin Oncol. 2006;24:4472–8. https://doi.org/10.1200/JCO.2006.05.6382.
13. Boland EG, Bennett MI, Allgar V, Boland JW. Cannabinoids for adult cancer-related pain: systematic review and meta-analysis. BMJ Support Palliat Care. 2020;10:14–24. https://doi.org/10.1136/bmjspcare-2019-002032.

14. Bonini SA, Premoli M, Tambaro S, Kumar A, Maccarinelli G, Memo M, Mastinu A. Cannabis sativa: a comprehensive ethnopharmacological review of a medicinal plant with a long history. J Ethnopharmacol. 2018;227:300–15. https://doi.org/10.1016/j.jep.2018.09.004.
15. Bonnie RJ. The marijuana conviction: a history of marijuana prohibition in the United States. Lindesmith Center; 1974.
16. Camacho-Rivera M, Islam JY, Rodriguez DL, Vidot DC. Cannabis use among cancer survivors amid the COVID-19 pandemic: results from the COVID-19 cannabis health study. Cancers (Basel). 2021;13:3495. https://doi.org/10.3390/cancers13143495.
17. Carley DW, Prasad B, Reid KJ, Malkani R, Attarian H, Abbott SM, Vern B, Xie H, Yuan C, Zee PC. Pharmacotherapy of apnea by cannabimimetic enhancement, the PACE clinical trial: effects of dronabinol in obstructive sleep apnea. Sleep. 2017;41:zsx184. https://doi.org/10.1093/sleep/zsx184.
18. Carley DW, Radulovacki M. Pharmacology of vagal afferent influences on disordered breathing during sleep. Respir Physiol Neurobiol. 2008;164:197–203. https://doi.org/10.1016/j.resp.2008.06.021.
19. Carver AC, Foley KM. Therapeutic approaches to cancer pain. In: Holland-Frei cancer medicine. 6th ed. BC Decker; 2003.
20. Cherny N. Oxford textbook of palliative medicine, Oxford textbook of palliative medicine. Oxford University Press; 2015.
21. Chiu L, Chow R, DeAngelis C, Lock M, Simone CB. Secondary and cumulative meta-analysis of olanzapine for antiemetic prophylaxis for chemotherapy-induced nausea and vomiting: do we still need to study its effectiveness? Ann Palliat Med. 2021;10:2540–7. https://doi.org/10.21037/apm-20-1462.
22. Chiu L, Chow R, Popovic M, Navari RM, Shumway NM, Chiu N, Lam H, Milakovic M, Pasetka M, Vuong S, Chow E, DeAngelis C. Efficacy of olanzapine for the prophylaxis and rescue of chemotherapy-induced nausea and vomiting (CINV): a systematic review and meta-analysis. Support Care Cancer. 2016;24:2381–92. https://doi.org/10.1007/s00520-016-3075-8.
23. Chow R, Herrstedt J, Aapro M, Chiu L, Lam H, Prsic E, Lock M, DeAngelis C, Navari RM. Olanzapine for the prophylaxis and rescue of chemotherapy-induced nausea and vomiting: a systematic review, meta-analysis, cumulative meta-analysis and fragility assessment of the literature. Support Care Cancer. 2021:1–21. https://doi.org/10.1007/s00520-020-05935-7.
24. Cooper ZD, Bedi G, Ramesh D, Balter R, Comer SD, Haney M. Impact of co-administration of oxycodone and smoked cannabis on analgesia and abuse liability. Neuropsychopharmacology. 2018;43:2046–55. https://doi.org/10.1038/s41386-018-0011-2.
25. Cousins MM, Jannausch ML, Coughlin LN, Jagsi R, Ilgen MA. Prevalence of cannabis use among individuals with a history of cancer in the United States. Cancer. 2021; https://doi.org/10.1002/cncr.33646.
26. Curto-Reyes V, Llames S, Hidalgo A, Menéndez L, Baamonde A. Spinal and peripheral analgesic effects of the CB2 cannabinoid receptor agonist AM1241 in two models of bone cancer-induced pain. Br J Pharmacol. 2010;160:561–73. https://doi.org/10.1111/j.1476-5381.2009.00629.x.
27. Cyr C, Arboleda MF, Aggarwal SK, Balneaves LG, Daeninck P, Néron A, Prosk E, Vigano A. Cannabis in palliative care: current challenges and practical recommendations. Ann Palliat Med. 2018;7:463–77. https://doi.org/10.21037/apm.2018.06.04.
28. Dunn KE, Bergeria CL, Huhn AS, Speed TJ, Mun CJ, Vandrey R, Campbell CM. Within-subject, double-blinded, randomized, and placebo-controlled evaluation of the combined effects of the cannabinoid dronabinol and the opioid hydromorphone in a human laboratory pain model. Neuropsychopharmacology. 2021;46:1451–9. https://doi.org/10.1038/s41386-021-01007-4.
29. Duran M, Pérez E, Abanades S, Vidal X, Saura C, Majem M, Arriola E, Rabanal M, Pastor A, Farré M, Rams N, Laporte J-R, Capellà D. Preliminary efficacy and safety of an oromucosal standardized cannabis extract in chemotherapy-induced nausea and vomiting. Br J Clin Pharmacol. 2010a;70:656–63. https://doi.org/10.1111/j.1365-2125.2010.03743.x.

30. Dzierżanowski T. Prospects for the use of cannabinoids in oncology and palliative care practice: a review of the evidence. Cancers (Basel). 2019;11:E129. https://doi.org/10.3390/cancers11020129.
31. Fallon MT, Albert Lux E, McQuade R, Rossetti S, Sanchez R, Sun W, Wright S, Lichtman AH, Kornyeyeva E. Sativex oromucosal spray as adjunctive therapy in advanced cancer patients with chronic pain unalleviated by optimized opioid therapy: two double-blind, randomized, placebo-controlled phase 3 studies. Br J Pain. 2017;11:119–33. https://doi.org/10.1177/2049463717710042.
32. Farokhnia M, McDiarmid GR, Newmeyer MN, Munjal V, Abulseoud OA, Huestis MA, Leggio L. Effects of oral, smoked, and vaporized cannabis on endocrine pathways related to appetite and metabolism: a randomized, double-blind, placebo-controlled, human laboratory study. Transl Psychiatry. 2020;10:1–11. https://doi.org/10.1038/s41398-020-0756-3.
33. Fisher E, Moore RA, Fogarty AE, Finn DP, Finnerup NB, Gilron I, Haroutounian S, Krane E, Rice ASC, Rowbotham M, Wallace M, Eccleston C. Cannabinoids, cannabis, and cannabis-based medicine for pain management: a systematic review of randomised controlled trials. Pain. 2021;162:S45–66. https://doi.org/10.1097/j.pain.0000000000001929.
34. Goodman SN, Fanelli D, Ioannidis JPA. What does research reproducibility mean? Sci Transl Med. 2016;8:341ps12.
35. Good PD, Greer RM, Huggett GE, Hardy JR. An open-label pilot study testing the feasibility of assessing total symptom burden in trials of cannabinoid medications in palliative care. J Palliat Med. 2020;23:650–5. https://doi.org/10.1089/jpm.2019.0540.
36. Grimison P, Mersiades A, Kirby A, Lintzeris N, Morton R, Haber P, Olver I, Walsh A, McGregor I, Cheung Y, Tognela A, Hahn C, Briscoe K, Aghmesheh M, Fox P, Abdi E, Clarke S, Della-Fiorentina S, Shannon J, Gedye C, Begbie S, Simes J, Stockler M. Oral THC:CBD cannabis extract for refractory chemotherapy-induced nausea and vomiting: a randomised, placebo-controlled, phase II crossover trial. Ann Oncol. 2020;31:1553–60. https://doi.org/10.1016/j.annonc.2020.07.020.
37. Guerrero AV, Quang P, Dekker N, Jordan RCK, Schmidt BL. Peripheral cannabinoids attenuate carcinoma induced nociception in mice. Neurosci Lett. 2008;433:77–81. https://doi.org/10.1016/j.neulet.2007.12.053.
38. Haack M, Simpson N, Sethna N, Kaur S, Mullington J. Sleep deficiency and chronic pain: potential underlying mechanisms and clinical implications. Neuropsychopharmacology. 2020;45:205–16. https://doi.org/10.1038/s41386-019-0439-z.
39. Hardy J, Haywood A, Gogna G, Martin J, Yates P, Greer R, Good P. Oral medicinal cannabinoids to relieve symptom burden in the palliative care of patients with advanced cancer: a double-blind, placebo-controlled, randomised clinical trial of efficacy and safety of 1:1 delta-9-tetrahydrocannabinol (THC) and cannabidiol (CBD). Trials. 2020;21:611. https://doi.org/10.1186/s13063-020-04541-6.
40. Häuser W, Welsch P, Klose P, Radbruch L, Fitzcharles M-A. Efficacy, tolerability and safety of cannabinoid based medicines for cancer pain: a systematic review with meta-analysis of randomised controlled trials. Schmerz. 2019;33:424–36. https://doi.org/10.1007/s00482-019-0373-3.
41. Hawley P, Gobbo M. Cannabis use in cancer: a survey of the current state at BC cancer before recreational legalization in Canada. Curr Oncol. 2019;26:e425–32. https://doi.org/10.3747/co.26.4743.
42. Hernandez Torres C, Mazzarello S, Ng T, Dranitsaris G, Hutton B, Smith S, Munro A, Jacobs C, Clemons M. Defining optimal control of chemotherapy-induced nausea and vomiting-based on patients' experience. Support Care Cancer. 2015;23:3341–59. https://doi.org/10.1007/s00520-015-2801-y.
43. Hesketh PJ, Kris MG, Basch E, Bohlke K, Barbour SY, Clark-Snow RA, Danso MA, Dennis K, Dupuis LL, Dusetzina SB, Eng C, Feyer PC, Jordan K, Noonan K, Sparacio D, Lyman GH. Antiemetics: ASCO guideline update. JCO. 2020;38:2782–97. https://doi.org/10.1200/JCO.20.01296.

44. Ioannidis JPA. Why most published research findings are false. PLoS Med. 2005;2(8):e124. https://doi.org/10.1371/journal.pmed.0020124.
45. Ioannidis JPA. Effect of formal statistical significance on the credibility of observational associations. Am J Epidemiol. 2008;168:374–83.; discussion 384-390. https://doi.org/10.1093/aje/kwn156.
46. Jatoi A, Windschitl HE, Loprinzi CL, Sloan JA, Dakhil SR, Mailliard JA, Pundaleeka S, Kardinal CG, Fitch TR, Krook JE, Novotny PJ, Christensen B. Dronabinol versus megestrol acetate versus combination therapy for cancer-associated anorexia: a North Central Cancer Treatment Group study. J Clin Oncol. 2002;20:567–73. https://doi.org/10.1200/JCO.2002.20.2.567.
47. Jiang H, Li X, Zhao Y-X, Ferguson D, Hueber F, Bera S, Wang Y-F, Zhao L-C, Liu C-J, Li C-S. A new insight into Cannabis sativa (Cannabaceae) utilization from 2500-year-old Yanghai Tombs, Xinjiang, China. J Ethnopharmacol. 2007;108:414–22. https://doi.org/10.1016/j.jep.2006.05.034.
48. Johnson JR, Burnell-Nugent M, Lossignol D, Ganae-Motan ED, Potts R, Fallon MT. Multicenter, double-blind, randomized, placebo-controlled, parallel-group study of the efficacy, safety, and tolerability of THC:CBD extract and THC extract in patients with intractable cancer-related pain. J Pain Symptom Manag. 2010;39:167–79. https://doi.org/10.1016/j.jpainsymman.2009.06.008.
49. Jordan K, Kasper C, Schmoll H-J. Chemotherapy-induced nausea and vomiting: current and new standards in the antiemetic prophylaxis and treatment. Eur J Cancer. 2005;41:199–205. https://doi.org/10.1016/j.ejca.2004.09.026.
50. Kesner AJ, Lovinger DM. Cannabinoids, endocannabinoids and sleep. Front Mol Neurosci. 2020;13:125. https://doi.org/10.3389/fnmol.2020.00125.
51. Kleckner AS, Kleckner IR, Kamen CS, Tejani MA, Janelsins MC, Morrow GR, Peppone LJ. Opportunities for cannabis in supportive care in cancer. Ther Adv Med Oncol. 2019;11:1758835919866362. https://doi.org/10.1177/1758835919866362.
52. Kuhathasan N, Dufort A, MacKillop J, Gottschalk R, Minuzzi L, Frey BN. The use of cannabinoids for sleep: a critical review on clinical trials. Exp Clin Psychopharmacol. 2019;27:383–401. https://doi.org/10.1037/pha0000285.
53. Lichtman AH, Lux EA, McQuade R, Rossetti S, Sanchez R, Sun W, Wright S, Kornyeyeva E, Fallon MT. Results of a double-blind, randomized, placebo-controlled study of nabiximols oromucosal spray as an adjunctive therapy in advanced cancer patients with chronic uncontrolled pain. J Pain Symptom Manag. 2018;55:179–188.e1. https://doi.org/10.1016/j.jpainsymman.2017.09.001.
54. Longo R, Oudshoorn A, Befus D. Cannabis for chronic pain: a rapid systematic review of randomized control trials. Pain Manag Nurs. 2021;22:141–9. https://doi.org/10.1016/j.pmn.2020.11.006.
55. Lozano-Ondoua AN, Wright C, Vardanyan A, King T, Largent-Milnes TM, Nelson M, Jimenez-Andrade JM, Mantyh PW, Vanderah TW. A cannabinoid 2 receptor agonist attenuates bone cancer-induced pain and bone loss. Life Sci. 2010;86:646–53. https://doi.org/10.1016/j.lfs.2010.02.014.
56. Luba R, Earleywine M, Farmer S, Slavin M. Cannabis in end-of-life care: examining attitudes and practices of palliative care providers. J Psychoactive Drugs. 2018;50:348–54. https://doi.org/10.1080/02791072.2018.1462543.
57. Lynch ME, Cesar-Rittenberg P, Hohmann AG. A double-blind, placebo-controlled, crossover pilot trial with extension using an oral mucosal cannabinoid extract for treatment of chemotherapy-induced neuropathic pain. J Pain Symptom Manag. 2014;47:166–73. https://doi.org/10.1016/j.jpainsymman.2013.02.018.
58. Machado Rocha FC, Stéfano SC, De Cássia Haiek R, Rosa Oliveira LMQ, Da Silveira DX. Therapeutic use of Cannabis sativa on chemotherapy-induced nausea and vomiting among cancer patients: systematic review and meta-analysis. Eur J Cancer Care (Engl). 2008;17:431–43. https://doi.org/10.1111/j.1365-2354.2008.00917.x.

59. Maida V. Medical cannabis in the palliation of malignant wounds-a case report. J Pain Symptom Manag. 2017;53:e4–6. https://doi.org/10.1016/j.jpainsymman.2016.09.003.
60. Maida V, Corban J. Topical medical cannabis: a new treatment for wound pain-three cases of pyoderma gangrenosum. J Pain Symptom Manag. 2017;54:732–6. https://doi.org/10.1016/j.jpainsymman.2017.06.005.
61. Maida V, Ennis M, Irani S, Corbo M, Dolzhykov M. Adjunctive nabilone in cancer pain and symptom management: a prospective observational study using propensity scoring. J Support Oncol. 2008;6:119–24.
62. Martell K, Fairchild A, LeGerrier B, Sinha R, Baker S, Liu H, Ghose A, Olivotto IA, Kerba M. Rates of cannabis use in patients with cancer. Curr Oncol. 2018;25:219–25. https://doi.org/10.3747/co.25.3983.
63. Martin BR, Wiley JL. Mechanism of action of cannabinoids: how it may lead to treatment of cachexia, emesis, and pain. J Support Oncol. 2004;2:305–14; discussion 314-316.
64. Meiri E, Jhangiani H, Vredenburgh JJ, Barbato LM, Carter FJ, Yang H-M, Baranowski V. Efficacy of dronabinol alone and in combination with ondansetron versus ondansetron alone for delayed chemotherapy-induced nausea and vomiting. Curr Med Res Opin. 2007;23:533–43. https://doi.org/10.1185/030079907x167525.
65. Mohiuddin M, Blyth FM, Degenhardt L, Di Forti M, Eccleston C, Haroutounian S, Moore A, Rice ASC, Wallace M, Park R, Gilron I. General risks of harm with cannabinoids, cannabis, and cannabis-based medicine possibly relevant to patients receiving these for pain management: an overview of systematic reviews. Pain. 2021;162:S80–96. https://doi.org/10.1097/j.pain.0000000000002000.
66. Montero-Oleas N, Arevalo-Rodriguez I, Nuñez-González S, Viteri-García A, Simancas-Racines D. Therapeutic use of cannabis and cannabinoids: an evidence mapping and appraisal of systematic reviews. BMC Complement Med Ther. 2020;20:12. https://doi.org/10.1186/s12906-019-2803-2.
67. Monti JM, et al., editors. Cannabinoids and sleep, advances in experimental medicine and biology; 2021. p. 1297. https://doi.org/10.1007/978-3-030-61663-2_1.
68. Moulin D, Boulanger A, Clark AJ, Clarke H, Dao T, Finley GA, Furlan A, Gilron I, Gordon A, Morley-Forster PK, Sessle BJ, Squire P, Stinson J, Taenzer P, Velly A, Ware MA, Weinberg EL, Williamson OD, Canadian Pain Society. Pharmacological management of chronic neuropathic pain: revised consensus statement from the Canadian Pain Society. Pain Res Manag. 2014;19:328–35. https://doi.org/10.1155/2014/754693.
69. Mücke M, Carter C, Cuhls H, Prüß M, Radbruch L, Häuser W. Cannabinoids in palliative care: systematic review and meta-analysis of efficacy, tolerability and safety. Schmerz. 2016;30:25–36. https://doi.org/10.1007/s00482-015-0085-2.
70. Mücke M, Phillips T, Radbruch L, Petzke F, Häuser W. Cannabis-based medicines for chronic neuropathic pain in adults. Cochrane Database Syst Rev. 2018;3:CD012182. https://doi.org/10.1002/14651858.CD012182.pub2.
71. National Academies of Sciences, Engineering, and Medicine. Therapeutic effects of cannabis and cannabinoids. In: The health effects of cannabis and cannabinoids: the current state of evidence and recommendations for research. National Academies Press; 2017.
72. Nielsen S, Sabioni P, Trigo JM, Ware MA, et al. Opioid-sparing effect of cannabinoids: a systematic review and meta-analysis. Neuropsychopharmacology. 2017;42;1752–65. https://doi.org/10.1038/npp.2017.51.
73. Pain S. A potted history. Nature. 2015;525:S10–1. https://doi.org/10.1038/525S10a.
74. Pergam SA, Woodfield MC, Lee CM, Cheng G-S, Baker KK, Marquis SR, Fann JR. Cannabis use among patients at a comprehensive cancer center in a state with legalized medicinal and recreational use. Cancer. 2017;123:4488–97. https://doi.org/10.1002/cncr.30879.
75. Pertwee R, editor. Handbook of cannabis. Oxford: Oxford University Press; 2014. https://doi.org/10.1093/acprof:oso/9780199662685.001.0001.
76. Peters EN, Mosesova I, MacNair L, Vandrey R, Land MH, Ware MA, Turcotte C, Bonn-Miller MO. Safety, pharmacokinetics and pharmacodynamics of Spectrum yellow oil in healthy participants. J Analytical Toxicol. 2021a;00:1–15. https://doi.org/10.1093/jat/bkab026.

77. Peters EN, Mosesova I, MacNair L, Vandrey R, Land MH, Ware MA, Turcotte C, Bonn-Miller MO. Safety, pharmacokinetics and pharmacodynamics of Spectrum Red softgels in healthy participants. Poster P4-17, 31st Annual ICRS Symposium on the Cannabinoids 2021b.
78. Pisanti S, Bifulco M. Medical cannabis: a plurimillennial history of an evergreen. J Cell Physiol. 2019;234:8342–51. https://doi.org/10.1002/jcp.27725.
79. Portenoy RK, Ganae-Motan ED, Allende S, Yanagihara R, Shaiova L, Weinstein S, McQuade R, Wright S, Fallon MT. Nabiximols for opioid-treated cancer patients with poorly-controlled chronic pain: a randomized, placebo-controlled, graded-dose trial. J Pain. 2012;13:438–49. https://doi.org/10.1016/j.jpain.2012.01.003.
80. Pritchard ER, Dayer L, Belz J, Forseth B, Harrington SE, Painter JT. Effect of cannabis on opioid use in patients with cancer receiving palliative care. J Am Pharm Assoc. 2020;60; 244e247.
81. Reuter SE, Martin JH. Pharmacokinetics of cannabis in cancer cachexia-anorexia syndrome. Clin Pharmacokinet. 2016;55:807–12. https://doi.org/10.1007/s40262-015-0363-2.
82. Roberts CA, Jager G, Christiansen P, Kirkham TC. Exploring the munchies: an online survey of users' experiences of cannabis effects on appetite and the development of a Cannabinoid Eating Experience Questionnaire. J Psychopharmacol. 2019;33:1149–59. https://doi.org/10.1177/0269881119862526.
83. Rock EM, Limebeer CL, Parker LA. Anticipatory nausea in animal models: a review of potential novel therapeutic treatments. Exp Brain Res. 2014;232:2511–34. https://doi.org/10.1007/s00221-014-3942-9.
84. Rock EM, Parker LA. Cannabinoids as potential treatment for chemotherapy-induced nausea and vomiting. Front Pharmacol. 2016;7:221. https://doi.org/10.3389/fphar.2016.00221.
85. Rock EM, Sticht MA, Limebeer CL, Parker LA. Cannabinoid regulation of acute and anticipatory nausea. Cannabis Cannabinoid Res. 2016;1:113–21. https://doi.org/10.1089/can.2016.0006.
86. Rock EM, Limebeer CL, Pertwee RG, Mechoulam R, Parker LA. Therapeutic potential of cannabidiol, cannabidiolic acid, and cannabidiolic acid methyl ester as treatments for nausea and vomiting. Cannabis Cannabinoid Res. 2021;6(4):266–74. https://doi.org/10.1089/can.2021.0041.
87. Roeland EJ, Bohlke K, Baracos VE, Bruera E, del Fabbro E, Dixon S, Fallon M, Herrstedt J, Lau H, Platek M, Rugo HS, Schnipper HH, Smith TJ, Tan W, Loprinzi CL. Management of cancer cachexia: ASCO guideline. JCO. 2020;38:2438–53. https://doi.org/10.1200/JCO.20.00611.
88. Rukwied R, Watkinson A, McGlone F, Dvorak M. Cannabinoid agonists attenuate capsaicin-induced responses in human skin. Pain. 2003;102:283–8. https://doi.org/10.1016/S0304-3959(02)00401-3.
89. Salamone JD, McLaughlin PJ, Sink K, Makriyannis A, Parker LA. Cannabinoid CB1 receptor inverse agonists and neutral antagonists: effects on food intake, food-reinforced behavior and food aversions. Physiol Behav. 2007;91:383–8. https://doi.org/10.1016/j.physbeh.2007.04.013.
90. Sallan SE, Zinberg NE, Frei E. Antiemetic effect of delta-9-tetrahydrocannabinol in patients receiving cancer chemotherapy. N Engl J Med. 1975;293:795–7. https://doi.org/10.1056/NEJM197510162931603.
91. Schleider LB-L, Mechoulam R, Lederman V, Hilou M, Lencovsky O, Betzalel O, Shbiro L, Novack V. Prospective analysis of safety and efficacy of medical cannabis in large unselected population of patients with cancer. Eur J Intern Med. 2018;49:37–43. https://doi.org/10.1016/j.ejim.2018.01.023.
92. Schwartzberg LS. Chemotherapy-induced nausea and vomiting: which antiemetic for which therapy? Oncology. 2007;21:946–53; discussion 954, 959, 962 passim.
93. Sharkey KA, Darmani NA, Parker LA. Regulation of nausea and vomiting by cannabinoids and the endocannabinoid system. Eur J Pharmacol. 2014;722 https://doi.org/10.1016/j.ejphar.2013.09.068.

94. Sihota A, Smith BK, Ahmed S-A, Bell A, Blain A, Clarke H, Cooper ZD, Cyr C, Daeninck P, Deshpande A, Ethans K, Flusk D, Le Foll B, Milloy M-J, Moulin DE, Naidoo V, Ong M, Perez J, Rod K, Sealey R, Sulak D, Walsh Z, O'Connell C. Consensus-based recommendations for titrating cannabinoids and tapering opioids for chronic pain control. Int J Clin Pract. 2021:e13871. https://doi.org/10.1111/ijcp.13871.
95. Slatkin NE. Cannabinoids in the treatment of chemotherapy-induced nausea and vomiting: beyond prevention of acute emesis. J Support Oncol. 2007;5:1–9.
96. Smetana GW, Tetrault JM, Hill KP, Burns RB. Should you recommend cannabinoids for this patient with painful neuropathy? Grand rounds discussion from Beth Israel Deaconess Medical Center. Ann Intern Med. 2021;174:237–46. https://doi.org/10.7326/M20-7945.
97. Smith LA, Azariah F, Lavender VT, Stoner NS, Bettiol S. Cannabinoids for nausea and vomiting in adults with cancer receiving chemotherapy. Cochrane Database Syst Rev. 2015; https://doi.org/10.1002/14651858.CD009464.pub2.
98. Ständer S, Schmelz M, Metze D, Luger T, Rukwied R. Distribution of cannabinoid receptor 1 (CB1) and 2 (CB2) on sensory nerve fibers and adnexal structures in human skin. J Dermatol Sci. 2005;38:177–88. https://doi.org/10.1016/j.jdermsci.2005.01.007.
99. Strasser F, Luftner D, Luftner D, Possinger K, Ernst G, Ruhstaller T, Meissner W, Ko Y-D, Schnelle M, Reif M, Cerny T. Comparison of orally administered cannabis extract and delta-9-tetrahydrocannabinol in treating patients with cancer-related anorexia-cachexia syndrome: a multicenter, phase III, randomized, double-blind, placebo-controlled clinical trial from the Cannabis-In-Cachexia-Study-Group. J Clin Oncol. 2006;24:3394–400. https://doi.org/10.1200/JCO.2005.05.1847.
100. Suraev AS, Marshall NS, Vandrey R, McCartney D, Benson MJ, McGregor IS, Grunstein RR, Hoyos CM. Cannabinoid therapies in the management of sleep disorders: a systematic review of preclinical and clinical studies. Sleep Med Rev. 2020;53:101339. https://doi.org/10.1016/j.smrv.2020.101339.
101. Sznitman SR, Vulfsons S, Meiri D, Weinstein G. Medical cannabis and insomnia in older adults with chronic pain: a cross-sectional study. BMJ Support Palliat Care. 2020a;10:415–20. https://doi.org/10.1136/bmjspcare-2019-001938.
102. Teunissen SCCM, Wesker W, Kruitwagen C, de Haes HCJM, Voest EE, de Graeff A. Symptom prevalence in patients with incurable cancer: a systematic review. J Pain Symptom Manag. 2007;34:94–104. https://doi.org/10.1016/j.jpainsymman.2006.10.015.
103. Turcott JG, Núñez MD, Flores-Estrada D, Oñate-Ocaña LF, Zatarain-Barrón ZL, Barrón F, Arrieta O. The effect of nabilone on appetite, nutritional status, and quality of life in lung cancer patients: a randomized, double-blind clinical trial. Support Care Cancer. 2018;26:3029–38. https://doi.org/10.1007/s00520-018-4154-9.
104. Volicer L, Stelly M, Morris J, McLaughlin J, Volicer BJ. Effects of dronabinol on anorexia and disturbed behavior in patients with Alzheimer's disease. Int J Geriatr Psychiatry. 1997;12:913–9.
105. Vučković S, Srebro D, Vujović KS, Vučetić Č, Prostran M. Cannabinoids and pain: new insights from old molecules. Front Pharmacol. 2018;9:1259. https://doi.org/10.3389/fphar.2018.01259.
106. Waissengrin B, Urban D, Leshem Y, Garty M, Wolf I. Patterns of use of medical cannabis among Israeli cancer patients: a single institution experience. J Pain Symptom Manag. 2015;49:223–30. https://doi.org/10.1016/j.jpainsymman.2014.05.018.
107. Walsh D, Donnelly S, Rybicki L. The symptoms of advanced cancer: relationship to age, gender, and performance status in 1,000 patients. Support Care Cancer. 2000;8:175–9. https://doi.org/10.1007/s005200050281.
108. Wang J, Wang Y, Tong M, Pan H, Li D. Medical cannabinoids for cancer cachexia: a systematic review and meta-analysis. Biomed Res Int. 2019;2019:e2864384. https://doi.org/10.1155/2019/2864384.
109. Ware MA, Daeninck P, Maida V. A review of nabilone in the treatment of chemotherapy-induced nausea and vomiting. Ther Clin Risk Manag. 2008;4:99–107.

110. Whiting PF, Wolff RF, Deshpande S, Di Nisio M, Duffy S, Hernandez AV, Keurentjes JC, Lang S, Misso K, Ryder S, Schmidlkofer S, Westwood M, Kleijnen J. Cannabinoids for medical use: a systematic review and meta-analysis. JAMA. 2015;313:2456–73. https://doi.org/10.1001/jama.2015.6358.
111. Wickham RJ. Nausea and vomiting not related to cancer therapy: intractable problem or clinical challenge? J Adv Pract Oncol. 2020;11:476–88. https://doi.org/10.6004/jadpro.2020.11.5.4.
112. Yanai T, Iwasa S, Hashimoto H, Ohyanagi F, Takiguchi T, Takeda K, Nakao M, Sakai H, Nakayama T, Minato K, Arai T, Suzuki K, Shimada Y, Nagashima K, Terakado H, Yamamoto N. A double-blind randomized phase II dose-finding study of olanzapine 10 mg or 5 mg for the prophylaxis of emesis induced by highly emetogenic cisplatin-based chemotherapy. Int J Clin Oncol. 2018;23:382–8. https://doi.org/10.1007/s10147-017-1200-4.

Chapter 6
Patient Evaluation: Precautions and Managing Expectations

Contents

6.1 Introduction 154
6.2 Terminology 155
6.3 General Considerations 155
6.4 Risks of Cannabis Use 157
6.5 Potential Increased Cancer Risk with Cannabis Use 159
6.6 Contraindications and Precautions 160
6.7 Managing Physician Expectations 162
6.8 Managing Patient Expectations 163
6.9 Patient Evaluation 164
6.10 The Initial Interview: Key Clinical Questions and Commentary 165
6.11 Detailed Medical History 168
6.11.1 Neurological Effects and Driving Performance 168
6.11.2 Cardiovascular Effects 170
6.11.3 Pulmonary Effects 171
6.11.4 Gastrointestinal Effects 172
6.11.5 Immune System Modulatory Effects 173
6.12 Detailed Psychiatric History 173
6.12.1 Screening for Clinical High Risk for Psychosis (CHR) 174
6.12.2 Possible Protective Effects of CBD in THC-Induced Psychotic-Like Symptoms 175
6.12.3 Anxiety and Depression 176
6.12.4 Bipolar Disease 176
6.12.5 Post-traumatic Stress Disorder 176
6.12.6 Addiction Issues 177
6.12.7 Tolerance 177
6.12.8 Use of Cannabis in Mild Cognitive Impairment or Dementia 177
6.13 Dealing with Trauma-Sensitive Patients 178
6.14 Medication History 179
6.15 Cannabis History 180
6.16 Conclusion 181
References 183

C. Cyr et al., *Cannabis and Cannabinoid-Based Medicines in Cancer Care*,
https://doi.org/10.1007/978-3-030-89918-9_6

6.1 Introduction

Prior to initiating cannabis for medical purposes, an appropriate evaluation is required to determine suitability. Subsequent close monitoring is also an essential aspect intended to increase the likelihood of benefits and reduce potential harms. This is particularly important in frail or immunocompromised cancer patients on polypharmacy and who are at increased risk of functional impairment, delirium, or falls. According to a recent survey, however, only 32% of patients using cannabis for medical reasons received support from their doctor [13]. The use of recreational cannabis has been known to produce unpredictable side effects and increases the risk of several mental health illnesses, dependency, and abuse. This, along with the fact that the diversity and quality of products remain non-standardized and untested in many jurisdictions, has, at least for the time being, provided most healthcare providers with ample justification to wait until the level of evidence reaches a comfortable threshold before suggesting this class of medication. Cannabis is indeed a complex substance and one that does not follow the current "one molecule-one receptor" paradigm. However, understanding how to initiate and monitor its most active compounds, THC and CBD, in most clinical settings is relatively simple to master.

Cannabis can either improve or deteriorate the level of global functioning of individuals, and this should serve as the basis of patient evaluation prior to introduction of treatment. Use of SMART (Specific, Measurable, Achievable, Realistic and anchored within a Time frame) goals is a convenient way of fixing a clear objective with patients and caregivers to determine whether cannabis treatment has indeed achieved its desired intention.

Patient risk stratification prior to the use of cannabis is focused mainly on the specific side effects of THC and CBD, which are the most abundant cannabinoids found in the cannabis plant. However, the majority of the acute and chronic risks of cannabis use can be attributed almost exclusively to THC. Consequently, the use of high-THC cannabis products in the general patient population requires careful evaluation prior to initiation and ongoing monitoring, particularly if long-term use is to be considered. In advanced cancer or palliative care situations, however, where cannabis might be used for a shorter time period, certain chronic risks may not be as relevant, and more attention can be focused on preventing acute side effects, drug interactions, and improving tolerability.

Family physicians and other first-line healthcare workers are ideally placed to manage expectations and monitor global functioning targets in patients who decide to use cannabis. The decision to introduce this class of medication, including pharmaceutical cannabinoid products such as nabilone, dronabinol, and nabiximols, must only be taken after a careful and thorough medical assessment and ideally carried out by a dedicated interdisciplinary team. The pivotal role of pharmacists with a solid understanding of cannabis pharmacology cannot be understated as the evaluation of complex patients who are often frail and on polypharmacy can be especially challenging for the limited training received by *bud tenders* and *cannabis counselors*. However, only a few states, such as Connecticut, have enacted cannabis legislation requiring pharmacists to supervise cannabis distribution and patient counseling. Certain countries where legislation has been enacted, such as Germany, have also required that medical cannabis products may only be supplied through pharmacies on presentation of a special prescription.

This chapter will therefore provide a systematic approach to patient evaluation, provide a series of practical recommendations on how to assess and counsel patients before authorizing medical cannabis, and will broach other important topics before considering any Cannabinoid-Based Medicine in advanced cancer and palliative care patients. Initial assessment will aim to determine the necessary precautions which need to be taken for reducing potential harms, with a specific focus on recognizing and mitigating risk factors for psychotic-like or dissociative reactions which may occur even with moderate doses of THC in sensitive or frail individuals. The second part of this chapter will provide an overview on managing expectations and preconceived ideas about the potential benefits of cannabis. This can be challenging, particularly since unfounded or exaggerated information is widely disseminated which requires counseling and realignment with more evidence-based data.

For administration and dosing recommendations in specific patient populations and conditions, these will be addressed in chapter seven.

6.2 Terminology

The term "Endocannabinoidome" is still not widely used by clinicians and researchers, and in order to avoid confusion, its use to describe the *expanded* endocannabinoid system (ECS) will be restricted to the first chapter of this book. For the present chapter, the more commonly used term "endocannabinoid system (ECS)" will be used to describe most concepts relating to both the more specific canonical receptors and enzymes and the larger system of molecular targets and ligands. The "endocannabinoidome" will only be mentioned in order to point out a clinically relevant difference between these two related concepts.

"Cannabinoid-Based Medicines" will be used preferentially as a general umbrella term to describe all compounds containing either approved or non-approved cannabinoids derived from either natural or synthetically produced cannabis. The term "cannabis" and "medical cannabis" will only be used contextually when discussing the use of plant-based products specifically.

6.3 General Considerations

1. Official guidelines

   At the present time, cannabis is not approved as a first-line medication in any clinical setting. However, in the spring 2018 edition of the *Information for Health Care Professionals* document, Health Canada has determined that the "evidence thus far from some observational studies and clinical studies suggests that cannabis (limited evidence) and prescription cannabinoids (e.g. dronabinol, nabilone, or nabiximols) may be useful in alleviating a wide variety of single or co-occurring symptoms often encountered in the palliative care setting. These symptoms may include, but are not limited to, intractable nausea and vomiting associated with chemotherapy or radiotherapy, anorexia/cachexia, severe intractable pain, severe depressed mood and anxiety, and insomnia. A limited number of observational studies suggest that the use of cannabinoids for palliative care may also potentially be associated with a decrease in the number of some medications used by this patient population" [33]. The Canadian Medical Association has also come forward in "acknowledging the unique requirements of patients suffering from a terminal illness or chronic disease for which conventional therapies have not been effective and for whom cannabis may provide relief" [32].

2. Timing

   This is a key factor to take into consideration when considering the introduction of medical cannabis, particularly in chronic and life-threatening illnesses. End-of-life trajectories tend to differ according to diagnosis, and in general, neurodegenerative and most chronic diseases will exhibit a slow gradual decline in health status. However, cancer patients tend to maintain a good level of functioning until the later stages of the disease which is followed by a rapid decline (Fig. 6.1). Cannabis is a complex blend of compounds which must interact with a person's individual endocannabinoid system. Since it may take some time to adjust to several of the unique effects of cannabis, and particularly THC, early introduction may be advisable in cancer and palliative care settings before health status may not allow for slow titration to an effective dose and further experimentation with higher therapeutic windows. This highly variable features of cannabis effects often requires several weeks or months in order to limit potential physical and psychoactive side effects before beginning to explore the benefits of higher dose psychoactivity.

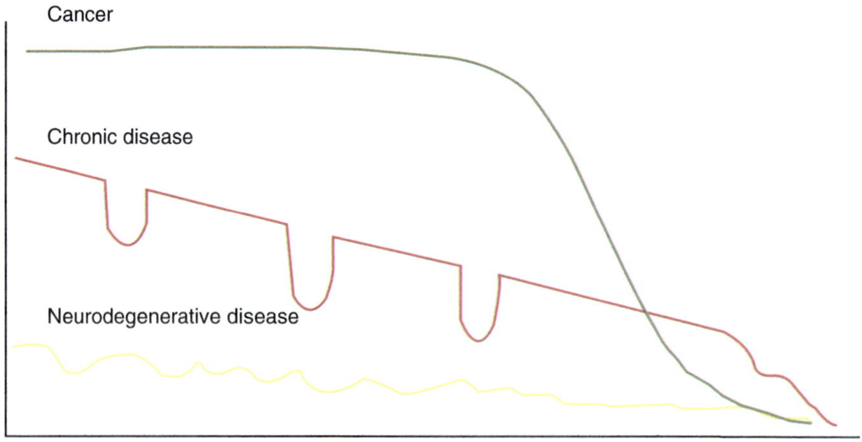

Fig. 6.1 End of life trajectories. (Adapted from [67])

3. Prior experience
   Many patients believe they are already "self-medicating" with cannabis, but in our experience this often leads to inappropriate use (either subtherapeutic dosing of CBD or supratherapeutic dosing of THC). This does not mean they will not eventually be suitable candidates for medical cannabis, but this underlies the necessity of having clinical oversight and guidance. These situations often require appropriate counseling in order to provide accurate information about the benefits and harms of cannabis use for their condition and to ensure patients receive the maximum benefit from this treatment option.
4. Cannabis use in elderly or dementia patients
   A trial of cannabis for medical use in advanced cancer and palliative care often occurs in older populations. Although there is little data examining cannabis use in the elderly, studies have shown that the greatest increase in the prevalence of cannabis use between 2013 and 2016 was observed in older populations, increasing by 71.4% in this age group, and they are more likely to report cannabis use for medical versus recreational purposes [66]. More than 50% of adults above 50 who consume cannabis are probably long-term users. According to a national survey, the reported medical use of cannabis in patients over 50 years of age varied from 34.6% to 50.9% [112]. Luckily, the available studies suggest that sub-psychoactive oral doses of THC below 2 mg do not increase the risk of psychotic-like reactions in elderly patients [1, 52]. However, doses in the range of 10 mg may induce psychotic-like reactions in many cannabis-naive individuals [22]. The addition of CBD may help reduce some of these effects, although the benefits and exact dosage (or ratio) remain uncertain [76]. Risks of falls due to medications are also a concern in the elderly, and THC has been known to affect balance and coordination. However, a double-blind, crossover RCT examining the effects of THC on balance and gait in 18 patients with dementia demonstrated that a 1.5 mg dose of THC given twice daily was well tolerated and did not significantly increase the risk of falls [113]. See section on psychiatric assessment for further explanations and Chap. 7 for more information on choosing products, dosage, and titration.

6.4 Risks of Cannabis Use

Cannabis is a complex blend of different active compounds that each carry their own specific risk/benefit profiles. Although they were isolated only recently, the risks associated with the use of cannabis have been described in the medical literature for nearly two centuries. It was in 1838 that Dr. William O'Shaughnessy introduced cannabis to Western medicine on his return from the Bengal region in India. He witnessed the role of cannabis as a means to relieve suffering in the last days and hours of life. He also was keenly aware of the long-term harms associated with chronic use in the local population and in the British troops stationed there at the time [85].

To avoid such consequences, the introduction of medical cannabis requires a rigorous evaluation before deciding if it is an appropriate therapeutic option for a patient, at a given point in their disease course, and whether it is congruous with their expectations. This begins with addressing basic safety issues.

Cannabis has long been considered a relatively safe drug. There has not been any documented evidence of death attributable to (natural) cannabis overdose, thanks in part to the relatively low number of CB1 receptors in the brain stem and respiratory centers. Rodent models of LD50 values have been extrapolated at more than 15,000 mg [83], which represents more than ten times the average daily THC intake from very heavy users [60]. The theoretical lethal dose of dried cannabis (with a THC potency of 20%) would be in the order of approximately 75 kg. The same is not true for illicit synthetic cannabinoids which have been linked with fatalities (see Chap. 3).

However, the endocannabinoid system's conflicting role, providing either anti-tumor effects or potentially increasing the growth and spread of cancer cells, combined with the recent arrival of immune modulators in oncology, has alerted us to the fact that cannabis use in cancer care may prove to be a dangerous combination in some patients [105]. Cannabis can also have an impact on global patient functioning and lead to several short- and long-term harms. The endocannabinoid system modulates neurotransmitter release in the CNS via activation of the CB1 receptor and can either improve or worsen mood, sleep, appetite, and memory. It can produce several distressing physical and psychological symptoms, such as tachycardia, hypotension, syncope, panic attacks, and psychotic-like reactions, which can usually be mitigated with careful initial dosing and slow titration. The addition of CBD has been reported to reduce certain physical and psychological symptoms, but there still remain unanswered questions relating to the ratio or dose of CBD required to achieve this effect [76]. One study seemed to demonstrate a reduction in psychotic-like symptoms when doses of CBD of 400 mg were added to an 8 mg dose of THC, although an increase in psychoactivity was noted when a smaller 4 mg dose of CBD was given [101]. Although no method has been established that will accurately predict or prevent psychotic-like reactions in all individuals consuming cannabis, there are several key elements that can be addressed which will reduce this risk significantly.

Table 6.1 Major adverse effects associated with cannabis use

Acute[a]	Chronic
Dizziness, sedation	Impaired learning and cognitive development
Impaired working memory and attention	Mental health issues
Impaired motor coordination	Cannabis use disorder (CUD)
Dry mouth	Respiratory illness (smoking)
Orthostatic hypotension	Pregnancy outcomes
Supine hypertension	Treatment failure with checkpoint inhibitors
Tachycardia	Increased risk of testicular cancer
Acute psychosis and paranoia (high THC)	Possible increased risk of HPV-associated HNSCC[b]
Altered judgment and increased risk-taking behavior	

[a]Acute side effects are due to THC administration in a dose-dependent manner
[b]In vitro study has shown that CB1 receptor agonists can promote progression of HPV-positive HNSCC through p38 MAPK pathway activation. Case control studies have also suggested an association [65]

Major adverse events associated with cannabis use are almost exclusively related to THC, which can produce several dose-dependent psychological and physical side effects (Table 6.1). These can usually be prevented or mitigated with careful titration. Doses of THC required to produce mild psychoactive effects are generally well tolerated, not unlike other common medications (36). As the dose increases, psychoactivity becomes more pronounced and may be accompanied with greater adverse mental and physical effects. These risks remain low, however. Beyond a further dose threshold, THC will eventually produce psycholytic and psychedelic effects (see Chap. 8). In an unprepared set and setting, in trauma-sensitive individuals or those at clinical high risk for psychosis (CHR), this can often lead to symptoms of unpleasant intoxication and brief psychotic-like reactions or anxiety attacks (Table 6.2).

6.5 Potential Increased Cancer Risk with Cannabis Use

Interactions between cannabinoid receptor pathways have been reported to exert anti-tumoral effects (see Chap. 4), while other research has demonstrated a possible tumor-promoting role in certain types of cancer particularly testicular germ cell tumors (TGCT) and HPV-related head and neck squamous cell carcinomas

Table 6.2 Likelihood of acute psychotic-like reactions/anxiety attacks with cannabis use

Risk factor	Likelihood of acute psychotic-like reaction/ anxiety attack
Initial **high** dose of THC Novice user No attention to set and setting Trauma-sensitive individual High risk or history of psychotic disorder	++++
Initial **high** dose of THC Novice user No attention to set and setting No history of trauma No history of psychotic disorder	+++
Initial **high** dose of THC Novice user Appropriate set and setting No history of trauma No history of psychotic disorder	++
Initial **moderate** dose of THC Novice user Appropriate set and setting No history of trauma No history of psychotic disorder	+/–
Initial **low** dose of THC Experienced user Appropriate set and setting No history of trauma No history of psychotic disorder	–

(HNSCC). A full discussion over the risks of cancer with cannabis use in healthy individuals is beyond the scope of this chapter and will only be briefly reviewed here. See Chaps. 1 and 2 for more details.

Epidemiological studies suggesting an association between cannabis use and nonseminomas or mixed testicular tumors have been known for some time [55, 64]. Low-strength evidence suggests that more than 10 years of cannabis use was associated with TGCT (OR, 1.36; 95% CI, 1.03–1.81; $P = 0.03$; I2 = 0%) and nonseminoma TGCT (OR, 1.85; 95% CI, 1.10–3.11; $P = 0.04$; I2 = 0%) [55]. Another study suggests the risk is higher with smoked cannabis compared with tobacco [102], suggesting the risk is linked with compounds found in cannabis rather than toxins produced from combustion of plant material. Cannabis use in young men should therefore be discouraged as it may increase the risk of testicular tumors.

Initial reports had not found an association between cannabis use and HNSCC [21]. However, 30% of HNSCC demonstrate human papillomavirus (HPV) infection, and the incidence is increasing [123]. A positive relationship between HPV-positive HNSCC and daily cannabis use, controlled for tobacco use, has been further demonstrated (OR 2.6, CI 1.1–6.6) with a strong dose-response relationship [48, 71, 121]. The possible molecular mechanisms for HNSCC may include CB1 and CB2 cannabinoid receptor activation via the p38 MAPK pathway [50]. Although an ongoing trial studying the efficacy of HPV vaccination against increased risks of oral HPV infection is still underway (ClinicalTrials.gov Identifier: NCT04199689), the FDA has nonetheless approved the use of an HPV vaccine for the prevention of oropharyngeal cancers. It is unclear whether vaccination will also confer protection after HPV exposure and concomitant cannabis use.

The increased risks of developing malignancies with cannabis use are of great concern, although there are other negative cancer-related consequences which need to be addressed. Cannabis use has been shown to reduce the response rate of nivolumab, a member of a growing family of checkpoint inhibitors [105]. This has raised many concerns, as this new class of drugs, as well as other immune modulators, are increasingly being recognized as highly effective treatments in oncology. Cannabis drug interactions, once thought to be mostly limited to the CYP450 enzyme family, are now entering a new and complex chapter, which is possibly related to CB1/CB2 receptor effects on multiple immune functions (see Chap. 1).

6.6 Contraindications and Precautions

Much has been written about the many contraindications to using cannabis. When added to the perceived risks of adverse events and lack of evidence for symptom management, this has led many to conclude that we should greatly limit medical cannabis use in general [7]. However, in the right patient, with a proper route of administration, judicious initial choice of product, and slow titration, the true contraindications to cannabis are few, and fewer still in the context of advanced cancer or end-of-life care (Table 6.3). Although pregnancy and lactation remain absolute

Table 6.3 Medical cannabis contraindications

Initial high THC dose[a] Smoke inhalation	Initial high THC dose[a] Oral route of administration	Initial low THC dose[a] Oral route of administration	Initial high CBD dose[b] Oral route of administration	Initial low CBD dose[b] Oral route of administration
Below age 25 Personal or family history of psychosis Current Cannabis Use Disorder (CUD) Active substance abuse disorder Unstable cardiovascular disease Pregnant or breastfeeding[c] Respiratory disease (if inhaled) Drug interaction issues (CYP1A2)	Below age 25 Personal or family history of psychosis Current CUD Active substance abuse disorder Unstable cardiovascular disease Pregnant or breastfeeding[c] Drug interaction issues	Below age 25 Personal or family history of psychosis Current CUD Active substance abuse disorder Pregnant or breastfeeding[c]	Pregnant or breastfeeding[c]	Pregnant or breastfeeding[c]

[a]No cutoff has been established in order to define a high dose or low starting dose of THC, although data suggests benefits with doses as low as 0.5 mg [8], while some authors consider a starting dose above 5 mg to be associated with significant adverse effects in cannabis-naive individuals [69]

[b]No cutoff has been established in order to define an initial high or low starting dose of CBD (see Chap. 7)

[c]Pregnancy/breastfeeding: Both CBD and THC metabolites are found in human milk [17, 78]. Data from animal studies support embryo-fetal development toxicity [20, 59, 75]

contraindications, the age limit for using cannabis in order to reduce effects on brain development, which has been established at approximately 25 years, may not be relevant for a patient with a limited life expectancy.

Pulmonary diseases have been a major concern since the reintroduction of medical cannabis in Western medicine, where inhaling combusted plant material was considered the preferred method for most patients, no doubt a cultural by-product of recreational use. However, this was not always the case. In the nineteenth century, medical cannabis was essentially dispensed in tinctures and other diluted extracts. Since most patients require long-acting formulations to manage chronic symptoms, the inhaled route should be used sparingly. Thus, the pulmonary contraindications can be avoided in most clinical situations. There are, of course, exceptions to the rule. See Chap. 7 for more details on choice of product and route of administration.

Psychiatric conditions are also a major concern. There is little doubt that the use of unopposed high-potency THC products in patients with an established psychotic disease or at clinical high risk of psychosis (CHR) is extremely imprudent. Trauma-sensitive patients, such as victims of child abuse, may encounter repressed memories in their field of awareness and experience panic attacks or dissociative states when using higher psychoactive doses of THC. Uncontrolled major depression or severe anxiety disorders may also worsen with cannabis, particularly with prolonged use of high-potency THC products. Incidently, cannabis is not considered a primary treatment regimen for these conditions, and patients should be encouraged to explore standard pharmacological approaches and counseling.

It is important to note that no study to date has demonstrated an increased risk of harm when high-dose CBD with small sub-psychoactive amounts of THC are used in any of these psychiatric conditions. See further section on medical history for advice on screening and counseling for patients presenting psychiatric disorders.

The cardiovascular effects of THC are well known, causing orthostatic hypotension, supine hypertension, and reflex tachycardia [87]. Doses of THC as low as 0.5 mg have been shown to reduce systolic blood pressure [8], although the effects are usually mild and of short duration. As a rule, patients with unstable cardiovascular disease (e.g., malignant hypertension, unstable angina, or arrhythmias that have not been investigated) should avoid cannabis products altogether, while individuals with stable cardiovascular disease should avoid high initial doses of THC to avoid significant hypotension and possible syncopal reactions. Table 6.4 lists other precautions that need to be considered before initiating cannabis.

6.7 Managing Physician Expectations

Though there are few comparative studies looking into the effectiveness and tolerability of cannabis versus standard pharmacological approaches, patient and physician acceptance is growing. A 1997 survey of oncologists highlighted that only 30% would consider prescribing cannabis to their patients [97]. This contrasts with a more recent survey done in 2018, where 46% of oncologists indicated that they now recommend cannabis clinically [28]. However, only 30% of those surveyed felt sufficiently informed to counsel patients on cannabis use in the 2018 study.

Table 6.4 Medical cannabis precautions

Initial high THC dose Smoke inhalation	Initial high THC dose Oral route of administration	Initial low THC dose Oral route of administration	Initial high CBD dose Oral route of administration	Initial low CBD dose Oral route of administration
Current active mood or anxiety disorder Risk factors for cardiovascular disease Heavy users of alcohol or taking high doses of benzodiazepines or other sedating medications Drug interaction issues	Current active mood or anxiety disorder Risk factors for cardiovascular disease Heavy users of alcohol or taking high doses of benzodiazepines or other sedating medications Drug interaction issues	Previous negative reaction to THC use	Drug interaction issues	unspecified

Introducing cannabis (or other cannabinoids) as a treatment modality can seem quite complex at first, since the use of "whole plant medicine" requires the modern clinician to step outside of the traditional one-molecule to one-receptor paradigm. Cannabinoids have multiple targets, and the clinical conditions that may eventually be treated with them covers a wide spectrum, with little available evidence to support its use at the present time.

One also needs to remember that cannabis is still not considered a first-line therapy for any clinical condition. However, results from preclinical research have now established that the endocannabinoid system plays a significant role in modulating many different physiological functions and may even have disease-modifying effects. These early studies have caused a surge in interest for the use of cannabis for many cancer-related issues, including symptom management, drug sparing, and disease-modifying effects (see Chaps. 4 and 5). The benefits of using cannabis for these purposes can vary widely, however, and many will find that mild psychoactivity can also be helpful (see Chap. 8). Thus, in a carefully evaluated and monitored cancer patient, cannabis should be regarded as a tool whose main purpose is to better cope with a life-threatening illness.

Cancer patients often face either scheduled or unforeseen hospitalizations. Dealing with hospitalized patients who are already using cannabis offers the opportunity to inquire on a patient's cannabis knowledge, evaluate current dosage, and screen for problematic use. Although the effects of cannabis withdrawal are usually mild in patients taking small doses of cannabinoids, it may become a significant issue with prolonged use at higher doses, which is why it may be prudent to continue ongoing treatment or offer a substitute approved cannabinoid (see Chap. 7 for more details).

6.8 Managing Patient Expectations

Patients with advanced cancer or in end-of-life settings who wish to explore the possible benefits of medical cannabis often have different expectations than with other pharmacological treatments. In circumstances where patients are unsure of what they wish to gain with cannabis, they should be encouraged to regard this option as a means to improve overall functioning or help them better cope with a multitude of mild symptoms, rather than as an incisive treatment for a single ailment. Cannabis may be helpful in the following circumstances:

- Cancer symptom management including pain, sleep disturbance, anxiety, and poor appetite. Endocannabinoid signaling participates in the modulation of many physiological functions in the CNS and peripheral organ systems. As a result, patients experiencing multiple symptoms originating from different brain areas or organ systems may respond more favorably to cannabis [2]. (see Chap. 5).
- Reducing the unwanted effects of cancer treatment including chemotherapy-induced nausea and vomiting and radiation- or chemotherapy-induced neuropathy (see Chap. 5).

- Drug-sparing effects [15, 82] (see Chap. 5).
- End-of-life distress (see Chap. 8).

Most patients wish to avoid any significant psychoactivity, at least initially, since these effects may interfere with their contact with others and reality. However, with experience, some may become accustomed to these effects and obtain unintended benefits. This is demonstrated by a recent review that has shown that approximately 80% of medical cannabis patients report using it "recreationally" on occasion [110]. See Chap. 8 for more information on the possible benefits of cannabis psychoactivity.

The use of cannabis in cancer and palliative care *cannot* presently be recommended for the following purposes:

- Cure for cancer.
  Even if preclinical studies have demonstrated anti-tumor effects, there is actually no clinical evidence that cannabinoids can alter the outcome for any type of cancer. It may in fact promote certain types of cancer. Some cannabis cancer advocates suggest using high-dose cannabinoid extracts (Phoenix Tears/Rick Simpson Oil). Patients should be cautioned that there is little evidence that these products are effective and are often produced with petroleum solvents. Furthermore, the doses suggested by these advocates may produce significant side effects (see Chap. 4).
- Substitute for primary treatment regimens.
  Studies suggest that cannabinoids are safe when used in conjunction with most chemotherapeutics, and preclinical evidence have shown that they may even provide synergistic effects in some situations [27]. Patients should be encouraged to see cannabinoids as an addition to their primary treatment and not a substitute. The recent discovery of significant interactions between cannabinoids and checkpoint inhibitors is an important reminder that "natural" compounds are not necessarily benign (see Chaps. 2 and 4).

6.9 Patient Evaluation

This section is intended to provide clinicians with a method for approaching and documenting the evaluation of a patient who is being considered for medical cannabis. A dual focus is taken in order to provide the appropriate tools from a medical-legal perspective, including recommendations for documentation, and also to provide an updated model for patient care based on an open and non-judgmental approach to medical cannabis counseling. The following section will review the key clinical questions intended for an effective interview. A further section will present additional information for a more detailed medical evaluation. A quick summary is also provided at the end of this chapter.

This will allow the reader to either obtain a quick overview of the subject, acquire the necessary talking points for a patient-centered interview, or take a deeper dive into a more detailed assessment of a patients' medical history.

Clinicians wishing to counsel patients and prescribe medical cannabis should first check with regulatory bodies about the legal status in their jurisdiction as well as rules and regulations that pertain to authorizing medical cannabis from both a medical, administrative, and legal perspective. Some resources to help you with this include the Society of Cannabis Clinicians in the USA or the Canadian Consortium for the Investigation of Cannabinoids in Canada. Many European advocacy groups such as PLEAcommunity (https://www.pleacommunity.org.uk/) in the UK offer an overview of the regulatory landscape.

6.10 The Initial Interview: Key Clinical Questions and Commentary

Owing to its complex composition, different administration methods, and range of effects, the use of cannabis may require more counseling than with most standard pharmaceuticals. In some cases, the evaluation may need two or more sessions, or it can also be managed by a multidisciplinary team composed of several professionals that assist the prescribing physician or nurse practitioner. These may include either a pharmacist or trained nurse. An experienced "budtender" can also be useful in guiding patients on product choice, quantity, vaporizer use, and advice on preventing accidental overdoses. This section will provide a series of suggested questions and topics intended to broach the subject of medical cannabis with patients. This is accompanied by a short commentary and references to further sections providing more detailed information.

- Assess social situation/context/beliefs
  - What do you know about medical cannabis?
  - What are your thoughts about medical cannabis?
  - Have you ever considered medical cannabis for your symptoms?
  - Have you ever discussed medical cannabis with your family?
  - How do you think your family would react if you were to start using medical cannabis?
    Commentary:
    Many patients and their caregivers are unaware that cannabis was widely used as medicine in the nineteenth and early twentieth centuries, long before prohibition. Lingering stigma surrounding its use may require education on the difference between medical and recreational cannabis.
- Religion and culture
  - In your religious or cultural community, is it accepted to use cannabis for medical purposes?
  - How is cannabis regarded in your community?
    Commentary:

In certain situations, it may be necessary to explore religious or cultural beliefs which may regard cannabis as an intoxicant and address potential barriers to use.

- Driving
  - Do you currently drive?
  - If so, is it daily or only on an occasional basis?
  - Do you depend on your ability to drive to maintain your household (childcare) and income (if still working)?
    Commentary:
    It is important to be aware of your patient's current driving status and reliance on this as this may be a limiting factor for some patients to use medical cannabis in some jurisdictions. It is equally important to be aware of the particular laws/regulations around the use of both medical and adult use cannabis and driving. It is also important to remember that many "high CBD" products can contain enough THC to produce detectable serum levels surpassing legal driving limits. For more information, see further section: Detailed medical evaluation/neurological effects.
- Occupation and safety-sensitive positions or tasks
  - Do you currently work?
  - What type of work do you do?
  - Is this a safety-sensitive job or industry? Is there a possibility of getting drug tested at work?
  - Can this have an impact on your employment status?
    Commentary:
    It is important to understand the current occupational status of your patient prior to authorizing medical cannabis. In general, the abilities required to drive an automobile are also prerequisites for other safety-sensitive tasks, such as operating machinery, precision work, data management, and childcare. Working memory plays an important role in following instructions. The psychoactive effects of THC on working memory and divided attention are thus particularly important factors to consider in these situations [44]. While the tendency to "hyperfocus" is a well-known and appreciated side effect of THC-induced impairment of divided attention, it comes at a price of not being able to "zoom out", see the bigger picture of what's happening in your immediate surroundings and reconsider the most important task to devote the bulk of your awareness to.
- Travel
  - Do you intend to travel outside the country?

    Commentary:

    International travel with any type of controlled substances can be risky. Most countries, including the USA, have a zero-tolerance policy with respect to illegal drugs. Travelling with a small quantity of cannabis, even with a doctor's authorization, can lead to denial of entry or severe penalties in many countries. Although Canada is the only G20 country that has legalized cannabis for medical and recreational use, this applies only to cannabis purchased in the regulated Canadian market. Importing cannabis while travelling to Canada, however, is not permitted. The legal status of approved cannabinoids such as nabiximols can also vary between countries. Hence, patients should always verify the legal status of their prescribed cannabinoids in the countries they aim to visit in the USA.

- Social considerations
  - Do you or does anyone in your house use supplemental oxygen?
  - Do you have young children in your house?
  - Do you have a safe space to store your medication including opioids, benzodiazepines, and other potential drugs of abuse?

    Commentary:

    Having cannabis in a home can have several unforeseen consequences. Aromatic terpenes found in dried cannabis flowers can produce a discernible odor which is why it should be kept in an airtight container. Smells from topical salves or creams can also be temporarily noticeable. Vaporization produces much less odor than with combustion but can be noticed in close vicinity. The absence of any odor is one of the advantages of ingestibles and oils. Storing cannabis safely is an important factor to consider when children are living in the house. Smoking is not compatible with home oxygen, and it may also be the case with vaporization. Vape pens and vaporizers contain heating elements which can reach high temperatures, and several injuries have been reported after nasal cannula ignited as a result of vape pen use [63]. For more information, see further section: Detailed medical evaluation/pulmonary effects.

- Financial
  - Are you aware of the financial costs of using medical cannabis?

    Commentary:

    Medical cannabis can be expensive. The average cost of medical cannabis according to the 2020 Canadian Cannabis Survey by Health Canada was estimated to be $93 CAD ($75 USD) per month. Some patients may prefer to produce their own cannabis. However, this requires a certain level of botanical knowledge. In Canada, patients may also choose to allow a third person to cultivate their cannabis medicine. Some private and public insurers have started reimbursing the cost of medical cannabis.

- Prior cannabis experience
  - Have you ever used cannabis previous to your diagnosis?
  - If so, remote or recent?
  - Why did you stop using cannabis?

- Was it for medical or recreational purposes?
- Did you previously have a negative experience using cannabis?
  Commentary:
  Approaching the subject of prior experience requires answers to the "what, where, how, when, and why."

Many cancer patients have prior cannabis experience or may have already begun self-medicating without clinical supervision. This is an important opportunity to determine proper vs improper cannabis use and whether they are using cannabis medicinally or recreationally or to treat cannabis withdrawal symptoms. For more information, see further section: Cannabis history.

6.11 Detailed Medical History

This section will examine, in greater detail, the possible clinical implications of the physiological effects of cannabinoids. It is intended to provide further clarifications on the subjects broached earlier in the chapter.

6.11.1 Neurological Effects and Driving Performance

Cannabis, and THC specifically, produces several neurophysiological effects which can impair balance, coordination, working memory, and divided attention, among others [44]. The most important risks associated with these effects are related to driving and safety-sensitive tasks. Some jurisdictions have "per se" limits that accept a certain level of THC and/or CBD in your system; others have a "zero tolerance" policy such as Australia. Driving while under the influence (DUI) of cannabis is a serious public safety issue. The critical issue of predicting the duration of impairment after a single dose of THC remains unresolved, however, since this will vary according to dose, the method of administration, gender, chronicity of use, and level of tolerance. As such, there is no clear answer to the question: "After how much time is it safe to drive after consuming cannabis?" since complex prediction models based on these variables may be necessary to accurately assess the required time to return to a safe level of driving performance. The College of Family Physician of Canada Preliminary Guidance document [36] suggests waiting 4 hours after inhalation (Level II), 6 hours after oral ingestion (Level II), and 8 hours after inhalation or oral ingestion if the patient experiences euphoria (Level II) [36].

Several recent publications have looked at pooling these factors into regression analysis which can provide us with some further guidance. For example, a 2021 review estimated that near-complete recovery of cognitive skills after taking a 20 mg dose of inhaled THC would require 7 hours but that safety-sensitive tasks could be safely undertaken after only 5 hours [73]. A 2014 review found that driving performance was reduced 5–6 hours after smoking cannabis. Although the maximum impairment occurred within the first 2 hours after smoking, the authors suggest abstaining from driving for at least 8 hours after experiencing a subjective "high" from inhaled cannabis [81]. These studies have taken into consideration the many variables which can influence the duration of impairment. However, of all these factors, the dose of THC is undoubtedly the single most important to consider in order to determine the duration of impairment. Unlike alcohol, however, the dose-dependent effect of THC on driving performance does not correlate with blood/plasma levels, making this a poor measurement of impairment [79]. The pharmacokinetics of the highly lipophilic THC molecule are more complex since it tends to accumulate in fatty tissue, and the brain in particular, thus reducing access to hepatic enzymes responsible for breaking down THC to inactive metabolites and producing plasma levels unrelated with actual brain tisue concentrations. This has been demonstrated in postmortem examinations of individuals involved in fatal motor vehicle accidents. Researchers found high levels of THC in brain areas involved in executive functioning, decision-making, vision, memory, and coordination, while blood or plasma levels were found to be nearly undetectable in many cases [79]. In addition, frequent cannabis users with higher baseline THC blood levels will exhibit higher blood levels after an acute inhaled dose while often demonstrating lower impairment than in infrequent users. Frequent cannabis users may also have a tendency to overestimate their driving ability. In one study, more than half of cannabis patients admitted to driving within 2 hours of consuming cannabis while feeling subjectively "high" [25]. Experienced cannabis users often claim to be aware of their level of intoxication and try to compensate by becoming "hyper-cautious." However, the evidence suggesting an increased ability to overcome THC-induced driving impairment remains inconsistent [10, 23, 62, 119]. While certain trials have indeed found that experienced cannabis users tend to exhibit less impairment than infrequent users after acute administration of THC, there is emerging evidence that chronic heavy users with a significant "body burden" and persistently higher levels of THC blood/plasma levels continue to show signs of impairment up to 7 days after last use [62]. The addition of CBD has been suggested as a counterweight to certain adverse effects caused by THC. However, evidence has shown that adding equal parts of CBD does not prevent THC-induced driving impairment [10]. The use of CBD-dominant cannabis, however, was not shown to impair driving (using 215 mg of vaporized dried cannabis from Bedrocan 9% CBD <1% THC:13.75 mg CBD and <2.15 mg THC) [11].

Until further studies can provide clearer guidelines, several rules of thumb can help guide clinicians in addressing their patients' concerns about driving and cannabis use, particularly for cannabis-naive patients who are especially sensitive to the psychoactive effects of THC. Inexperienced cannabis patients should probably avoid driving for a period of at least 8 hours after an inhaled dose, and probably longer after an oral dose, even if they do not feel subjectively intoxicated.

Guidelines for experienced or heavy cannabis users are more complex, however. Tolerance to THC is difficult to assess and can vary greatly from one individual to the next. In these situations, it is difficult to determine exactly how much time is required for their driving performance to return to a safe level. Therefore, frequent users need to be reminded that they may not be able to accurately evaluate their ability to drive and they can still pose risks even if they do not notice subtle signs of intoxication. Hence, cancer patients using daily high doses of THC-dominant cannabis products should consider avoiding driving altogether.

6.11.2 Cardiovascular Effects

THC has been shown to stimulate the sympathetic nervous system and inhibit the parasympathetic nervous system. It increases heart rate, myocardial oxygen demand, supine blood pressure, and platelet activation. It is also associated with endothelial dysfunction and oxidative stress. CBD, on the other hand, has been shown to reduce heart rate and blood pressure, improve vasodilation, and reduce inflammation and vascular hyperpermeability in preclinical diabetic models [87]. However, at very low doses (0.5 mg), THC has been shown to produce transient bradycardia [8]. A recent review of cardiovascular toxicity of cannabis has demonstrated that cannabis use is strongly associated with orthostatic hypotension and tachycardia. However, no serious cardiovascular events were noted [117]. Conversely, THC has also been associated with increased supine blood pressure immediately after use, possibly resulting from sympathetic nervous system stimulation and inhibition of the parasympathetic nervous system. Other potential cardiovascular effects include vascular inflammation, platelet activation, and carboxyhemoglobin generation that can result from inhaled smoke [87]. Risks of acute coronary syndromes and other serious cardiovascular events, including dysrhythmias, have been reported with inhaled cannabis [91, 92]. These risks seem particularly important with synthetic cannabinoids [90].

Some patients will experience peripheral vasodilation and symptomatic hypotension, even with small doses of THC. Patients need to be informed about this when initiating cannabis. Those with unstable cardiovascular disease should be counseled against the use of THC unless cleared by their cardiologist. CBD does not appear to have any positive or negative effects on cardiovascular function, however. The risks of cannabis use and serious cardiovascular outcomes are still being debated. Sudies trying to establish a link between recreational cannabis use and myocardial infarction, arrhythmias, or cerebrovascular events have yielded inconsistent results. In the prospective CARDIA (Coronary Artery Risk Development in Young Adults) study, which spanned over 25 years, cumulative lifetime use of cannabis was not associated with adverse cardiovascular outcomes. Studies with hospitalized patients which have suggested an increased risk have been plagued with a high probability of selection bias [87]. Most other studies were short term and retrospective in nature and examined the effects of smoked and unregulated cannabis of unknown potency. Concomitant tobacco use is also a known factor in up to 97% of subjects. In a similar fashion to tobacco, combustion of cannabis flowers produces polyaromatic compounds and carbon monoxide, which has been associated with a variety of negative cardiovascular outcomes, including cardiomyopathy, angina, myocardial infarction, arrhythmia, cardiac failure, pulmonary edema, and sudden death. However, it has been postulated that cannabis and tobacco may have a synergistic effect which may contribute to a type of peripheral arteriopathy [87]. Randomized clinical trials studying orally administered, regulated cannabis products have not demonstrated significant cardiovascular adverse events. However, recreational use of high-potency edibles leading to emergency department visits has been shown to produce cardiovascular symptoms (8%) compared with inhalation (3%). Synthetic cannabinoids such as Spice or K2 are often laced with fentanyl and other toxins, and the use of these compounds has also shown to produce serious cardiovascular adverse events. As a reminder, studies suggesting potential harms associated with cannabis use have examined the effects on recreational cannabis users with little or no knowledge of the actual dose of THC. The effects on blood pressure and heart rate vary according to dose. Small doses of 0.5 mg and 1 mg resulted in a mild transient decrease in diastolic blood pressure of approximately 5 mm Hg, which returned to baseline after 60 minutes and 150 minutes for the 0.5 mg and 1 mg doses, respectively [8]. THC has generally been considered to produce tachycardia. However, in this study, subjects also experienced a significant decrease in heart rate with the 0.5 mg dose, while the 1 mg dose resulted in an increase in heart rate, suggesting that THC may in fact have a biphasic effect. High-dose THC has been associated consistently with tachycardia and increased blood pressure immediately after use, possibly resulting from sympathetic nervous system stimulation and inhibition of the parasympathetic nervous system. While in other circumstances, postural hypotension has also been reported. Other potential cardiovascular effects include vascular inflammation, platelet activation, and carboxyhemoglobin generation that can result from inhaled smoke [92]. Risks of acute coronary syndromes and other serious cardiovascular events, including dysrhythmias, have been reported with inhaled cannabis, although concomitant tobacco use was often a cofounder [84, 90].

However, CBD has been shown to reduce heart rate and blood pressure and improve vasodilation in models of endothelial dysfunction. In diabetic models, it has also been shown to reduce inflammation and vascular hyperpermeability [87].

6.11.3 Pulmonary Effects

Smoking is never a recommended form of cannabis consumption, although inhalation of vaporized cannabis is not thought to cause the same side effects as inhalation of combusted smoke and is not known to worsen underlying COPD or other chronic lung conditions. Ideally, those with underlying respiratory illnesses should be counseled to use ingested forms of cannabis products and only use the vaporized inhaled route if necessary.

Although current tobacco use is not a contraindication to the use of medical cannabis, it may indicate that the patient has an underlying respiratory illness and may benefit from screening and counseling.

Inhaling cannabis via combustion may worsen COPD but has not been shown to contribute to the development of lung malignancies. It does however increase the risk of CYP 1A2 inhibition and poses a fire safety risk with the use of supplemental oxygen. For these reasons, we do not recommend inhalation via the combustion route but via inhalation of vaporized cannabis products if inhalation is needed and desired, although vape pens have also been associated with fires when using supplemental oxygen.

If the patient has difficulty generating sufficient negative pressure to use a conventional handheld portable vaporizer, a different type of device may be desired/indicated. For example, the Volcano™ vaporizer is one of the four approved devices for cannabis flower inhalation by Health Canada. It is a tabletop vaporizer that pushes vapor into a chamber bag which allows for easy inhalation, similar to other nebulized medicines. Vape pens have become very popular as they are practical and discrete. However, safety concerns with long-term use and contaminated products remain an issue and cannot be recommended until formal FDA approval. The use of high-potency cannabis distillates (shatter, rosin, etc.) is evidently discouraged. A recently marketed hand held device, the Syqe™ inhalor, containing precise individual doses of dried cannabis in cartridge form, has also been approved by Health Canada.

6.11.4 Gastrointestinal Effects

Patients who wish to avoid inhalation but who are unable to take cannabis products via the oral route because of dysphagia (i.e., esophageal cancer) or malabsorption syndromes may benefit from sublingually administered cannabis [61]. Patients with liver dysfunction or disease remain candidates for the use of medical cannabis, including both THC and CBD, although few clinical studies provide clues for dosage adjustment. In rats, cirrhosis increases CB1 expression in endothelial cells, and it has been suggested that this may increase the hypotensive action of THC in this patient population [3, 4]. Furthermore, active metabolites of CBD have been shown to accumulate in moderate to severe hepatic impairment and may require lower starting dose and slower titration [108]. Cannabis does not seem to have a negative impact in the progression of alcoholic or HCV-associated cirrhosis or fatty liver disease, however [3–5, 107].

Although some studies and guidelines caution about the use of cannabis in patients with liver fibrosis/cirrhosis, this may be more of a theoretical risk and may not be clinically significant especially within the cancer care/palliative care setting.

6.11.5 Immune System Modulatory Effects

Cannabinoid receptors have been identified in immune cells such as monocytes, macrophages, basophils, lymphocytes, and dendritic cells. THC has been known to modulate immune function and inflammation. Other phytocannabinoids such as cannabidiol (CBD) and cannabinol (CBN) have also been shown to alter the functional activities of the immune system [86]. However, the use of cannabinoids as immune modulators is complex and is not completely understood. Although legislation has passed in at least seven US states that forbids denial of transplantation listing based on patient cannabis use, most providers require a documented period of abstinence before surgery. In transplant patients, the use of CBD for the prevention of GVHD did not show any improvement or deterioration of their condition [122]. Significant drug-drug interactions with CBD and calcineurin inhibitors (cyclosporin, tacrolimus, pimecrolimus) may exist, leading to increased calcineurin inhibitor concentrations and toxicity, and careful monitoring in these patients using medical cannabis is required [31, 58, 89].

The risks of aspergillosis from inhaled cannabis have been reported in immunocompromised patients [46]. These patients should be encouraged to avoid inhaled cannabis products.

Although THC and CBD may have immunomodulatory effects, this is of uncertain clinical significance. In our experience, patients who are immunocompromised or with autoimmune disease are able to safely use non-inhaled forms of medical cannabis for symptom management, including both THC and CBD. However, patients undergoing immunotherapy for cancer management with checkpoint inhibitors should avoid using cannabis as it may increase the chance of treatment failure [105] (see Chap. 2).

6.12 Detailed Psychiatric History

Cancer and palliative care patients may be at risk for mental health issues, either from the grief which accompanies the diagnosis, as a result from the disease itself or treatment side effects. Cancer patients may also be at higher risk of developing delirium, and several precautions must be taken to avoid both acute and chronic psychiatric adverse events. However, depression, anxiety, and insomnia are all common syndromes in advanced cancer and palliative care for which low doses of cannabis may actually be safe and effective as an adjunctive treatment or if other approaches have failed to provide sufficient relief (see Chap. 5 for more information)

Despite the high prevalence of cannabis use in mental health patients, there is currently limited evidence regarding the safety and efficacy of THC or CBD for the treatment of psychiatric disorders. However, available trials report potential therapeutic effects of CBD in certain conditions, such as alcohol and drug use disorders, chronic psychosis, and certain anxiety disorders [19, 96]. A 2019 review concluded that high doses of CBD seem to be well tolerated and have not been shown to negatively affect outcomes in mental health disorders [41]. Caution is advised when interpreting these results, since many of these studies used high doses of purified CBD in the order of 300–600 mg or more during a single administration or for a period of less than 2 weeks [41]. Most products marketed as "high-CBD" "CBD-dominant" or "CBD oil" products often contain small amounts of THC that can vary according to the source material. Hemp-derived cannabis products cannot legally contain more than 0.3% THC by dry weight. However, products labeled as "high CBD" can also be derived from genetically dissimilar Cannabis Sativa (L.) species, and are not subject to these regulations in North America. As such, many "high-CBD"'products may contain much higher concentrations of THC (1% or more). In some cases, taking a larger dose of CBD in the hopes of experiencing CBD-related effects may in fact produce clinically significant THC-related effects. For example, a 300 mg dose of hemp derived CBD with a 0.3% THC potency actually provides approximately 1 mg of THC. This is a sufficient dose to produce therapeutic effects in many individuals.

Non-hemp derived "high-CBD" products are often described according to their CBD/THC (or THC/CBD) ratios. These vary widely and usually fall into the range of 20:1 or 25:1 but may sometimes be as low as 2:1. Thus, standard CBD doses of 20–50 mg in some of these products may expose patients to significant amounts of THC which may produce subjective effects. Patients attempting to replicate high-dosage CBD regimens (300 mg or more) with many standard cannabis-derived "high-CBD" products may inadvertently be taking large psychoactive doses of THC of 15 mg or more. Future regulations will undoubtedly improve labeling standards. Until such time, patients must remain cautious and carefully scrutinize product labels and calculate the precise dose of THC in milligrams they are actually taking.

6.12.1 *Screening for Clinical High Risk for Psychosis (CHR)*

Identifying patients who may be at higher risk of developing serious psychiatric adverse events is particularly important when considering the use of cannabis and THC in particular. Of these, the risk of psychosis is of special concern. Screening for patients at clinical high risk for developing psychosis (CHR) may therefore be required in some circumstances where it is suspected [94]. This is important, since studies have indicated that approximately 29–36% of CHR patients will eventually transition to an overt psychotic illness [45]. Using a few simple screening questions can help predict high-risk patients (see appendix: clinical high risk for psychosis checklist). If any doubt persists, patients should be referred for psychiatric evaluation.

Secondary causes of psychotic reactions can add further risks for patients who will be taking significant doses of THC. See Table 6.5.

6.12.2 *Possible Protective Effects of CBD in THC-Induced Psychotic-Like Symptoms*

THC and CBD have been shown to have opposite effects on regional brain activation across a variety of cognitive tasks in healthy individuals. Preclinical studies have shown that the addition of CBD in adolescent mice may protect against the long-term health effects of THC [80], and several human studies have demonstrated that the addition of CBD may reduce THC-induced psychotic-like symptoms when co-administered [77, 83, 116]. However, many questions remain unanswered. The "protective" dose of CBD needed to reduce the psychotic-like effects of THC has not been determined, particularly in individuals taking high doses of THC. A recent clinical study where subjects were given 8 mg of THC demonstrated that a lower 4 mg dose of CBD actually increased THC psychoactivity while much higher doses of CBD (400 mg) were required to obtain an opposite effect [101]. Another human experimental study has also confirmed that high doses of CBD (600 mg) seem to reduce the pro-psychotic properties of a 10 mg dose of THC [43]. Two other trials using smaller doses of THC (1.25 mg and 1.5 mg respectively) given intravenously demonstrated that pretreatment with CBD (2.5 mg and 600 mg respectively) was associated with a reduction of psychotic-like symptoms [56]. More studies are therefore needed to determine not only the protective dose of CBD but also whether CBD needs to be given simultaneously or as a pretreatment. Furthermore, there is no evidence that suggests CBD may be used as an effective "antidote" for treating THC-induced psychotic-like symptoms.

Table 6.5 Secondary causes of psychosis (adapted from Matskevich and Keshavan [72])

Substance induced	Iatrogenic	Illnesses
Cocaine THC Synthetic cannabinoids LSD MDMA Mescaline (PCP) Heavy metals (lead, mercury, arsenic) Withdrawal (alcohol, benzodiazepines)	Occurring with standard dosages: Amphetamines (ADHD) Glucocorticoids (usually within days of starting medication) More likely with toxic serum levels: Antidepressants Opioids Anticonvulsants Antipsychotics Antiparkinsonian agents Antihistamines Antibiotics Antimalarials Antiemetics Anticholinergic Rx and benzodiazepines (elderly)	Seizure disorders Brain tumors (particularly temporal and limbic) Genetic disorders (Prader-Willi, Huntington, Fahr's disease) Chronic subdural hematoma Traumatic brain injury Autoimmune disease (SLE, MS) Wilson's disease Endocrine (Cushing, thyroid) Nutritional (vitamin B and D deficiency) Sleep disorders (narcolepsy) Infectious (syphilis, HIV)

6.12.3 Anxiety and Depression

Prevalence of cannabis use is increased in patients with anxiety and depression. Recreational cannabis use has been associated with an increased risk of depression, anxiety, and suicidal ideation in those with social phobia. However, most publications used retrospective or observational data on recreational cannabis users who were consuming products of unknown potency. There are no randomized trials that have looked at the therapeutic potential of low-dose THC with or without CBD in any mental health disorder.

Patients should be counseled against using THC as a primary treatment for depression or anxiety and encouraged to consider first-line therapies. In advanced cancer and palliative care, an experienced cannabis user may consider THC as a therapeutic option for breakthrough or episodic symptoms, with oversight from a knowledgeable cannabis physician. Similarly, CBD may be considered as an adjunct in patients who have failed first-line therapies or who have only achieved a partial therapeutic response.

6.12.4 Bipolar Disease

Cannabis use is more frequent in individuals with bipolar disease and is associated with younger age at onset of the first manic episode. It may also worsen the occurrence of depressive or manic symptoms in those diagnosed with bipolar disorder [18, 49]. A prospective study found that individuals who consumed cannabis at baseline had a nearly threefold risk of developing mania during the 3-year follow-up (OR 2.86, 95% CI 1.34–6.09), with those consuming cannabis 3–4 times per week having the highest risk [100]. Other studies have also shown a dose-related effect of cannabis use on mental health outcomes, but precise knowledge of the amount of THC and/or CBD being used by these individuals is mostly unavailable. Future studies using standardized products may provide a clearer picture of the risks and/or benefits of THC, CBD, and other minor cannabinoids on the development and control of many mental health disorders. However, using high-CBD products with negligible amounts of THC may be considered under close supervision. In end-of-life settings, the risk vs benefits of administering higher doses of THC need to be evaluated on an individual basis.

6.12.5 Post-traumatic Stress Disorder

The use of cannabis has been very popular with patients suffering from post-traumatic stress disorder (PTSD) as well and has been reported to help with sleep and reduce nightmares. Although the available data does not seem to demonstrate a clear benefit [24, 53], this may in fact be due to unsupervised use of high-potency products. Further research is needed to clarify the role of cannabinoids for this condition. Patients should be advised to use the lowest effective dose of THC or synthetic cannabinoid for any condition.

Survivors of medical trauma, including myocardial infarction, have been known to develop symptoms of PTSD [99]. The many negative cognitive effects of THC on memory have been known for decades; however, they may play a positive role in preventing traumatic memory encoding (aversive memory extinction) for patients undergoing treatments which may be traumatic or difficult to endure. See Chap. 8 for more details.

6.12.6 Addiction Issues

Patients with a history of drug or alcohol abuse need to be warned that cannabis can also cause addiction, like any drug which produces euphoria via dopamine signaling and reward networks [68]. However, the risks of developing cannabis use disorder may be less relevant in advanced cancer and palliative care settings, unless long-term survival is expected. If high daily doses of THC are being used, or if a patient is presenting signs of a cannabis use disorder, screening tools such as the CAGE or CUDIT-R (provided in the appendix) may be useful. See Chap. 7 for more details.

6.12.7 Tolerance

Tolerance to the psychoactive effects of THC can occur quite rapidly over the course of several weeks. In most cases, however, tolerance to the benefits for symptom management (pain, anxiety, sleep) seem to remain consistent. Furthermore, a recent study suggests cannabinoids do not increase pain sensitivity, unlike opioids [103]. It is recommended to regularly assess the daily dose of THC in all medical cannabis patients. See Chap. 7 for more details.

6.12.8 Use of Cannabis in Mild Cognitive Impairment or Dementia

The safety of cannabis use in the elderly and dementia patients is of particular concern in oncology [66]. Few studies have looked at cannabis and THC tolerability in older dementia patients. Two small studies have investigated the safety and efficacy of synthetic THC (dronabinol) as treatment for the behavioral disturbances in dementia patients [115, 120]. Both studies found that doses of THC up to 5 mg were found to be effective and safe. In a 2015 RCT, ten dementia patients presenting clinically relevant neuropsychiatric symptoms, including agitation and/or aggression received either 0.75 mg or 1.5 mg THC twice daily. Low 0.75 mg dose decreased blood pressure, whereas the 1.5 mg dose increased systolic BP significantly (average 5.1 mmHg) [114]. In another similar randomized trial, THC doses of up to 4.5 mg daily were well tolerated in dementia patients; however, no benefit was shown in neuropsychiatric symptoms [6]. A recent review of cannabis use in older populations showed that short-term low-dose cannabis use was well tolerated in older adults without prior serious mental illness. However, longer-term cannabis use in this population may be detrimental to their mental health, although a direct causal link has not been established [2, 111]. In one study involving the elderly, 184 patients began cannabis treatment, of which 63.6% were female, and the mean age was 81.2 ± 7.5 years (median age: 82). There was a low dropout rate due to side effects, and after 6 months of treatment, 58.1% were still using cannabis. Of these patients, 33.6% reported adverse events, the most common of which were dizziness (12.1%), sleepiness and fatigue (11.2%). Of the respondents, 84.8% reported some degree of improvement in their general condition [1].

6.13 Dealing with Trauma-Sensitive Patients

Trauma sensitivity is an increasingly recognized premorbid condition which has been associated with an increased risk of negative psychological outcomes during meditative practices [109]. Sources of trauma include past sexual, physical and psychological abuse, traumatic death of a loved one, internet-assisted victimization, disasters, accidents, and animal attacks. The exact prevalence of past trauma can vary. One survey suggests that 20% of youth have experienced more than one type of trauma [95], while another survey has reported that two thirds of children reported at least one traumatic experience by age 18 and 13.4% developed symptoms of post-traumatic stress [38]. What is certain is that traumatic experiences are common and often underestimated.

Mindfulness-based cognitive therapy and other forms of psychotherapy which integrate mindfulness meditation have reported an increased risk of anxiety, panic attacks, and dissociative experiences in individuals who have experienced trauma, and certain authors have realized that precautions need to be taken when patients wish to practice mindfulness meditation strategies [109].

Neuroimaging studies have begun to shed light on the mechanics of meditative states, which share certain similarities with the effects of THC. Modulations in the default mode network (DMN) seem to play a central role in both the benefits and negative outcomes of meditation and psychedelic experiences, including psychoactive effects produced by THC-induced altered states of consciousness and psychosis [9, 30, 54]. Both meditative practices, psychedelics, and THC have been shown to reduce DMN connectivity [26, 47, 118], which may explain the similar effects on reduced ego identification and a "healthy" distancing from thought content (see Chap. 8 for more details). This shared neurocognitive effect may explain why some trauma-sensitive patients who consume cannabis may be at increased risk of comparable adverse events. This mechanism, which may be responsible for THC-induced psychotic-like reactions, seems to be partially reversed by the addition of CBD, according to one study [116].

Default mode activity has also been suggested to represent a neurobiological substrate for Freudian constructs such as *ego identification* [35, 93]. This would explain why a sudden deactivation of this important hub of self-awareness could result in the flooding of repressed traumatic memories. Hence, trauma-sensitive mindfulness strategies have been proposed in order to screen potential candidates who may be at higher risks of adverse events as a result of meditative practices [109]. It is reasonable to speculate that trauma-sensitive individuals may also be at risk when consuming THC.

Screening for trauma may be delicate, and some patients may not fully understand the meaning or relevance of past trauma and abuse. In addition, mild PTSD symptoms may go unnoticed, and it must be remembered that many trauma survivors minimize their own distress and might not mention it. A trauma-sensitive checklist has been provided in the appendix.

6.14 Medication History

Cannabis is not a first-line treatment for any condition at this time [57]. Patients should be reminded that primary treatment regimens must be optimized before considering Cannabis-Based Medicines, including non-pharmacological approaches such as physiotherapy, occupational therapy, acupuncture, and psychological counseling [36]. A careful review of past and current treatments should be undertaken in order to confirm adherence to established clinical guidelines.

Clinically relevant interactions between THC as a drug-drug interaction (DDI) "victim" of CYP 2C9 and 3A4 inhibitors are important to consider in a frail patient population, since several potent inhibitors such as clarithromycin and ketoconazole can increase THC plasma levels significantly [104]. CBD is metabolized mainly by 2C19 and 3A4 but is much less likely to be a "victim" of DDI interactions since few subjective effects occur as a result of increased bioavailability. Studies have indeed shown that strong 3A4 inhibitors nearly double CBD bioavailability [29], although this effect may not clinically relevant. CBD as a DDI "perpetrator" may be more significant, although doses required to inhibit CYP450 enzymes may be supratherapeutic [29, 74]. See Chap. 2 for more details.

Other clinically significant interactions include:

- Opioids and other CNS depressants [40] (increased sedation and risk of falls)
- Immunotherapy/checkpoint inhibitors. Cannabis consumption has considerable immunomodulatory effects with several studies suggesting that cannabis consumption correlated with a significant decrease in time to tumor progression and overall survival in patients using this class of medication [14, 106].

6.15 Cannabis History

If cannabis use is remote, inquire into the reason for use. If it was for social use in youth, then move on. If the patient was a prolonged daily user, this requires investigating if there were any signs of a cannabis use disorder (CUD) [12]. It is also important to ask if the patient has ever had any adverse effects with cannabis in the past (anxiety, paranoia). If this is the case, it is recommended to avoid initiating products containing significant amounts of THC.

If the patient is currently using cannabis, this requires a more detailed questionnaire. It is important to determine "what, where, how, when, and why."

What type of cannabis are they using?

Is it THC dominant, CBD dominant, or balanced ratio? And more importantly, what daily dose of THC are they taking? Estimating the daily dose of THC used by patients may not always be easy. Many medical cannabis patients are unaware of the daily dose in milligrams of THC they are actually taking, particularly when inhalation is the primary method of administration. When regulated edible products are being used, this is usually straightforward. For patients using inhalation, an approximate inhaled dose can be calculated based on the potency of the cannabis strain used by the patient. As an example, the total daily dose of THC for a patient smoking 3 grams of cannabis per day containing 15% THC is approximately 450 mg. As a reminder, the average doses of THC used in clinical trials rarely surpassed 30–40 mg per day [69]. In the case of illicit cannabis, THC potency is usually unknown and must be approximated based on available law enforcement data. In the USA, the average potency of cannabis has increased from approximately 4% in 1995 to approximately 14% in 2014 [42], while in Canada, the average potency of legal cannabis was estimated to be 18% in 2018 [34].

If the patient is indeed presently using large daily doses of THC, check for signs and symptoms of cannabis use disorder (CUD) and aberrant drug behavior. Further questioning may reveal if they have developed tolerance or dependence. Cannabis withdrawal symptoms may occur in almost 50% of regular cannabis users [16], and though they are usually mild, a subset of users may present with a clinically relevant syndrome [88]. The CAGE or CUDIT-R questionnaire can be useful (see appendix). Patients should be encouraged to try a "tolerance-break (T-break)" and discontinue cannabis for a few weeks. Nabilone and CBD have been studied for cannabis use disorder and may be used to reduce withdrawal symptoms [51, 98]. See Chap. 7 for patient monitoring.

Where is their cannabis coming from?

Are they using cannabis from the legal or black market? If purchasing from unregulated community sources, there is the possibility of contaminants or even additives in the product which is unlikely to be tested or properly labeled. Studies have repeatedly shown that unregulated cannabis products contain heavy metals, pesticide residues and other contaminants well above acceptable regulated levels [39, 70].

How are they using cannabis?
Inhalation of combusted plant material is still the most popular method, but others are gaining ground. It is important to ask about all methods of ingestion including:

- Vaporization of dried cannabis flower
- Vaporization of concentrated extracts (often referred to as "dabbing")
- Sublingual application
- Topical application
- Sublingually or oral-mucosally administered
- Suppositories

When do they use cannabis?
Understanding a patients' pattern of cannabis use is important and may reveal reasons for their underlying use as well as their risk of having already developed tolerance and/or dependency. Are they using cannabis daily, on a regular basis, or just episodically in response to well-defined symptoms? If they use it daily, determine if it is consumed in the early morning and regularly throughout the day or just in the evening or before bed. Do they use it before meals, prior to activity, or only in the evenings?

Why are they using cannabis?
This is an important question which certain chronic users may find difficult to answer. Some will claim it is purely for recreational purposes or else for wellness, relaxation, or unwinding. However, it may also be a form of self-treatment for a previously diagnosed medical condition or may be used to treat an undiagnosed physical or mental health issue. It is also important to determine if they are using cannabis purely habitually in order to avoid the unpleasant effects of cannabis withdrawal syndrome. Additionally, some may be using it for creative, spiritual, or religious reasons as well. See Chap. 8 for other possible benefits of cannabis psychoactivity. This line of questioning is an important opportunity for the patient to recognize the many possible reasons why they are in fact using cannabis and receive information on alternative treatments or counseling. It is also an opportunity for the physician to provide recommendations for safer use if they discern symptoms of CUD, aberrant drug behavior, or habitual use.

6.16 Conclusion

If you feel that your patient may benefit from a therapeutic trial of medical cannabis, then ensure that their expectations are well aligned with clinical intention. "SMART" goals are a practical method to evaluate a therapeutic trial. Patients hoping for a cannabis cancer cure need to be reminded of the known risks and unproven benefits. Always provide practical advice to patients on this subject, explaining why this is not an appropriate clinical option and why it may be dangerous. Rick Simpson Oil (AKA Phoenix Tears) provides massive doses of cannabinoids, is often produced through an extraction process using toxic solvents, and can be very costly. Drug-sparing effects of cannabinoids are an interesting avenue for patients wishing to reduce opioid side effects. Patients wishing for symptom management may receive more benefits if several mild symptoms are present. Thus, a multimodal symptom management strategy to improve quality of life may provide greater benefits. Psychoactive doses may not be necessary to obtain physiologic effects or benefits in most cases. Patients wishing to explore higher dose cannabis psychoactivity need to understand that this therapeutic window has its own risk and benefit profile. Several unexpected (or desired) effects of cannabis treatment may appear at higher doses, but this exploration requires close monitoring. Medical cannabis embraces the concept of whole plant medicine, which places it outside the traditional medical system. However, patients often feel empowered when they achieve a level of knowledge with cannabis, since it involves a wide range of products, uses, effects, and routes of administration. For many, it provides them with a feeling of at least some control over their treatment. It also helps give them a sense of identity as an individual, and not just a patient in the medical system.

If both clinician and patient are comfortable after a thorough history and expectations are aligned with a realistic therapeutic outcome, then one can proceed with a therapeutic trial.

Chapter Summary

- Medical cannabis often requires slow titration and a prolonged trial period.
- Early initiation of cannabis may be preferable in cancer patients in order to become habituated to the physical and psychoactive effects.
- Evaluation should begin with an inquiry into patient knowledge and beliefs about cannabis.
- Prior experience with cannabis can provide important clues on tolerability or abuse.
- Pregnant or lactating mothers should not use any cannabis products containing either THC or CBD.
- Patients who are currently being treated with checkpoint inhibitors should not use any cannabis products containing either THC or CBD pending further evidence.
- Patients with unstable cardiovascular disease should avoid taking THC.
- THC is contraindicated in patients with active and unmanaged psychiatric disorders such as schizophrenia and other psychotic illnesses.
- Cannabis is not a first-line treatment for depression, bipolar disorder, and generalized anxiety disorder.
- Chronic recreational use of THC has been associated with exacerbation of depression and anxiety as well as psychosis and worsened global functioning in bipolar disease.
- Small doses of THC may be beneficial for the management of anxiety, depression, and insomnia in carefully selected patients.
- CBD has some anxiolytic and antipsychotic properties, although at higher doses. Currently available high-CBD products may contain significant amounts of THC at these doses.

- Trauma-sensitive individuals and survivors of abuse may be at risk of adverse psychological effects when taking THC.
- Cannabis can be safely used in most other stable cancer patients.
- Low doses of cannabis are safe in the elderly.
- Cannabis for symptom management should be used as an adjunct to standard therapy.
- Preclinical evidence for the anti-tumor effects of cannabinoids have not yet been demonstrated conclusively in humans.
- Most of the long-term risks of using cannabis may not be relevant in advanced cancer and palliative care or for patients with a limited life expectancy.
- Driving impairment and impact on safety-sensitive tasks may diminish with prolonged use but may not return to baseline.
- International travel while carrying cannabis products is prohibited.
- Medical cannabis can be expensive, although some insurers allow partial or full reimbursement with certain medical conditions.
- Patients often find that exclusive use of orally administered cannabis products is sufficient to control their symptoms.
- Inhaled cannabis may provide benefits in limited situations.
- Smoking cannabis is discouraged, particularly in immunocompromised individuals (fungal contaminants).
- Smoking is hazardous while using supplemental home oxygen, and the use of vape pens is discouraged in this context as well.
- CBD is a potent CYP inhibitor and may either increase certain drug effects or lower prodrug metabolism.
- Patients already using high doses of THC should be screened for possible cannabis use disorder (CUD) and counseled accordingly.

References

1. Abuhasira R, Ron A, Sikorin I, Novack V. Medical cannabis for older patients—treatment protocol and initial results. J Clin Med. 2019;8 https://doi.org/10.3390/jcm8111819.
2. Abuhasira R, Schleider LB-L, Mechoulam R, Novack V. Epidemiological characteristics, safety and efficacy of medical cannabis in the elderly. Eur J Intern Med. 2018;49:44–50. https://doi.org/10.1016/j.ejim.2018.01.019.
3. Adejumo AC, Adegbala OM, Adejumo KL, Bukong TN. Reduced incidence and better liver disease outcomes among chronic HCV infected patients who consume cannabis. Can J Gastroenterol Hepatol. 2018a;2018:9430953. https://doi.org/10.1155/2018/9430953.
4. Adejumo AC, Ajayi TO, Adegbala OM, Adejumo KL, Alliu S, Akinjero AM, Onyeakusi NE, Ojelabi O, Bukong TN. Cannabis use is associated with reduced prevalence of progressive stages of alcoholic liver disease. Liver Int. 2018b;38:1475–86. https://doi.org/10.1111/liv.13696.
5. Adejumo AC, Alliu S, Ajayi TO, Adejumo KL, Adegbala OM, Onyeakusi NE, Akinjero AM, Durojaiye M, Bukong TN. Cannabis use is associated with reduced prevalence of non-alcoholic fatty liver disease: a cross-sectional study. PLoS One. 2017;12:e0176416. https://doi.org/10.1371/journal.pone.0176416.
6. Ahmed AIA, van den Elsen GAH, Colbers A, Kramers C, Burger DM, van der Marck MA, Olde Rikkert MGM. Safety, pharmacodynamics, and pharmacokinetics of multiple oral

doses of delta-9-tetrahydrocannabinol in older persons with dementia. Psychopharmacology. 2015;232:2587–95. https://doi.org/10.1007/s00213-015-3889-y.
7. Allan GM, Ramji J, Perry D, Ton J, Beahm NP, Crisp N, Dockrill B, Dubin RE, Findlay T, Kirkwood J, Fleming M, Makus K, Zhu X, Korownyk C, Kolber MR, McCormack J, Nickel S, Noël G, Lindblad AJ. Simplified guideline for prescribing medical cannabinoids in primary care. Can Fam Physician. 2018;64:111–20.
8. Almog S, Aharon-Peretz J, Vulfsons S, Ogintz M, Abalia H, Lupo T, Hayon Y, Eisenberg E. The pharmacokinetics, efficacy, and safety of a novel selective-dose cannabis inhaler in patients with chronic pain: a randomized, double-blinded, placebo-controlled trial. Eur J Pain. 2020;24:1505–16. https://doi.org/10.1002/ejp.1605.
9. Alves PN, Foulon C, Karolis V, Bzdok D, Margulies DS, Volle E, Thiebaut de Schotten M. An improved neuroanatomical model of the default-mode network reconciles previous neuroimaging and neuropathological findings. Commun Biol. 2019;2:1–14. https://doi.org/10.1038/s42003-019-0611-3.
10. Arkell TR, Lintzeris N, Kevin RC, Ramaekers JG, Vandrey R, Irwin C, Haber PS, McGregor IS. Cannabidiol (CBD) content in vaporized cannabis does not prevent tetrahydrocannabinol (THC)-induced impairment of driving and cognition. Psychopharmacology. 2019;236:2713–24. https://doi.org/10.1007/s00213-019-05246-8.
11. Arkell TR, Vinckenbosch F, Kevin RC, Theunissen EL, McGregor IS, Ramaekers JG. Effect of cannabidiol and Δ9-tetrahydrocannabinol on driving performance: a randomized clinical trial. JAMA. 2020;324:2177–86. https://doi.org/10.1001/jama.2020.21218.
12. Artigaud L, Fener C, Bisch M, Schwan R, Schwitzer T, De Ternay J, Adamson SJ, Rolland B, Laprévote V. Screening tools for cannabis use disorders and their adaptation to DSM-5: a literature review. Encéphale. 2020;46:382–9. https://doi.org/10.1016/j.encep.2020.02.010.
13. Azcarate PM, Zhang AJ, Keyhani S, Steigerwald S, Ishida JH, Cohen BE. Medical reasons for marijuana use, forms of use, and patient perception of physician attitudes among the US population. J Gen Intern Med. 2020;35:1979–86. https://doi.org/10.1007/s11606-020-05800-7.
14. Bar-Sela G, et al. Cannabis Consumption Used by Cancer Patients during Immunotherapy Correlates with Poor Clinical Outcome. Cancers (Basel). 2020;12.
15. Babalonis S, Lofwall MR, Sloan PA, Nuzzo PA, Fanucchi LC, Walsh SL. Cannabinoid modulation of opioid analgesia and subjective drug effects in healthy humans. Psychopharmacology. 2019;236:3341–52. https://doi.org/10.1007/s00213-019-05293-1.
16. Bahji A, Stephenson C, Tyo R, Hawken ER, Seitz DP. Prevalence of cannabis withdrawal symptoms among people with regular or dependent use of cannabinoids: a systematic review and meta-analysis. JAMA Netw Open. 2020;3:e202370. https://doi.org/10.1001/jamanetworkopen.2020.2370.
17. Baker T, Datta P, Rewers-Felkins K, Thompson H, Kallem RR, Hale TW. Transfer of inhaled cannabis into human breast milk. Obstet Gynecol. 2018; https://doi.org/10.1097/AOG.0000000000002575.
18. Bally N, Zullino D, Aubry J-M. Cannabis use and first manic episode. J Affect Disord. 2014;165:103–8. https://doi.org/10.1016/j.jad.2014.04.038.
19. Beale C, Broyd SJ, Chye Y, Suo C, Schira M, Galettis P, Martin JH, Yücel M, Solowij N. Prolonged cannabidiol treatment effects on hippocampal subfield volumes in current cannabis users. Cannabis Cannabinoid Res. 2018;3:94–107. https://doi.org/10.1089/can.2017.0047.
20. Benevenuto SG, Domenico MD, Martins MAG, Costa NS, de Souza ARL, Costa JL, Tavares MFM, Dolhnikoff M, Veras MM. Recreational use of marijuana during pregnancy and negative gestational and fetal outcomes: an experimental study in mice. Toxicology. 2017;376:94–101. https://doi.org/10.1016/j.tox.2016.05.020.
21. Berthiller J, et al. Marijuana smoking and the risk of head and neck cancer: pooled analysis in the INHANCE consortium. Cancer Epidemiol Biomarkers Prev. 2009;18:1544–51.
22. Bhattacharyya S, Morrison PD, Fusar-Poli P, Martin-Santos R, Borgwardt S, Winton-Brown T, Nosarti C, O'Carroll CM, Seal M, Allen P, Mehta MA, Stone JM, Tunstall N, Giampietro

V, Kapur S, Murray RM, Zuardi AW, Crippa JA, Atakan Z, McGuire PK. Opposite effects of delta-9-tetrahydrocannabinol and cannabidiol on human brain function and psychopathology. Neuropsychopharmacology. 2010;35:764–74. https://doi.org/10.1038/npp.2009.184.
23. Bonar EE, Cranford JA, Arterberry BJ, Walton MA, Bohnert KM, Ilgen MA. Driving under the influence of cannabis among medical cannabis patients with chronic pain. Drug Alcohol Depend. 2019;195:193–7. https://doi.org/10.1016/j.drugalcdep.2018.11.016.
24. Bonn-Miller MO, Brunstetter M, Simonian A, Loflin MJ, Vandrey R, Babson KA, Wortzel H. The long-term, prospective, therapeutic impact of cannabis on post-traumatic stress disorder. Cannabis Cannabinoid Res. 2020; https://doi.org/10.1089/can.2020.0056.
25. Borodovsky JT, Marsch LA, Scherer EA, Grucza RA, Hasin DS, Budney AJ. Perceived safety of cannabis intoxication predicts frequency of driving while intoxicated. Prev Med. 2020;131:105956. https://doi.org/10.1016/j.ypmed.2019.105956.
26. Bossong MG, Jansma JM, van Hell HH, Jager G, Kahn RS, Ramsey NF. Default mode network in the effects of Δ9-tetrahydrocannabinol (THC) on human executive function. PLoS One. 2013;8:e70074. https://doi.org/10.1371/journal.pone.0070074.
27. Bouquié R, Deslandes G, Mazaré H, Cogné M, Mahé J, Grégoire M, Jolliet P. Cannabis and anticancer drugs: societal usage and expected pharmacological interactions – a review. Fundam Clin Pharmacol. 2018;32:462–84. https://doi.org/10.1111/fcp.12373.
28. Braun IM, Wright A, Peteet J, Meyer FL, Yuppa DP, Bolcic-Jankovic D, LeBlanc J, Chang Y, Yu L, Nayak MM, Tulsky JA, Suzuki J, Nabati L, Campbell EG. Medical oncologists' beliefs, practices, and knowledge regarding marijuana used therapeutically: a nationally representative survey study. J Clin Oncol. 2018;36:1957–62. https://doi.org/10.1200/JCO.2017.76.1221.
29. Brown JD, Winterstein AG. Potential adverse drug events and drug–drug interactions with medical and consumer cannabidiol (CBD) use. J Clin Med. 2019;8:989. https://doi.org/10.3390/jcm8070989.
30. Buckner RL, DiNicola LM. The brain's default network: updated anatomy, physiology and evolving insights. Nat Rev Neurosci. 2019;20:593–608. https://doi.org/10.1038/s41583-019-0212-7.
31. Cabral GA, Rogers TJ, Lichtman AH. Turning over a new leaf: cannabinoid and endocannabinoid modulation of immune function. J Neuroimmune Pharmacol. 2015;10:193–203. https://doi.org/10.1007/s11481-015-9615-z.
32. CMA Policy. (Latest update approved by CMA Board in February 2020). Authorizing Cannabis for Medical Purposes, 2013.
33. Santé Canada. Information for health care professionals: Cannabis and cannabinoids. 2018. https://www.canada.ca/en/health-canada/services/drugs-medication/cannabis/information-medicalpractitioners/information-health-care-professionals-cannabis-cannabinoids.html.
34. Canada, H. Canadian Cannabis Survey 2020: Summary. (2020). https://www.canada.ca/en/healthcanada/services/drugs-medication/cannabis/research-data/canadian-cannabis-survey-2020-summary.html.
35. Carhart-Harris RL, Friston KJ. The default-mode, ego-functions and free-energy: a neurobiological account of Freudian ideas. Brain. 2010;133:1265–83. https://doi.org/10.1093/brain/awq010.
36. CFPC. Authorizing dried cannabis for chronic pain or anxiety. PRELIMINARY GUIDANCE. College of Family Physicians of Canada 28, 2014.
37. Cooper ZD, Bedi G, Ramesh D, Balter R, Comer SD, Haney M. Impact of co-administration of oxycodone and smoked cannabis on analgesia and abuse liability. Neuropsychopharmacology. 2018;43:2046–55. https://doi.org/10.1038/s41386-018-0011-2.
38. Copeland WE, Keeler G, Angold A, Costello EJ. Traumatic events and posttraumatic stress in childhood. Arch Gen Psychiatry. 2007;64:577–84. https://doi.org/10.1001/archpsyc.64.5.577.
39. Dryburgh LM, Bolan NS, Grof CPL, Galettis P, Schneider J, Lucas CJ, Martin JH. Cannabis contaminants: sources, distribution, human toxicity and pharmacologic effects. Br J Clin Pharmacol. 2018;84:2468–76. https://doi.org/10.1111/bcp.13695.

40. Dunn KE, Bergeria CL, Huhn AS, Speed TJ, Mun CJ, Vandrey R, Campbell CM. Within-subject, double-blinded, randomized, and placebo-controlled evaluation of the combined effects of the cannabinoid dronabinol and the opioid hydromorphone in a human laboratory pain model. Neuropsychopharmacology. 2021;46:1451–9. https://doi.org/10.1038/s41386-021-01007-4.
41. Elsaid S, Kloiber S, Le Foll B. Effects of cannabidiol (CBD) in neuropsychiatric disorders: a review of pre-clinical and clinical findings. Prog Mol Biol Transl Sci. 2019;167:25–75. https://doi.org/10.1016/bs.pmbts.2019.06.005.
42. ElSohly MA, Mehmedic Z, Foster S, Gon C, Chandra S, Church JC. Changes in cannabis potency over the last two decades (1995–2014) – analysis of current data in the United States. Biol Psychiatry. 2016;79:613–9. https://doi.org/10.1016/j.biopsych.2016.01.004.
43. Englund A, Morrison PD, Nottage J, Hague D, Kane F, Bonaccorso S, Stone JM, Reichenberg A, Brenneisen R, Holt D, Feilding A, Walker L, Murray RM, Kapur S. Cannabidiol inhibits THC-elicited paranoid symptoms and hippocampal-dependent memory impairment. J Psychopharmacol. 2013;27:19–27. https://doi.org/10.1177/0269881112460109.
44. Figueiredo PR, Tolomeo S, Steele JD, Baldacchino A. Neurocognitive consequences of chronic cannabis use: a systematic review and meta-analysis. Neurosci Biobehav Rev. 2019; https://doi.org/10.1016/j.neubiorev.2019.10.014.
45. Fusar-Poli P, et al. Predicting psychosis: meta-analysis of transition outcomes in individuals at high clinical risk. Arch Gen Psychiatry. 2012;69:220–9.
46. Gargani Y, Bishop P, Denning DW. Too many mouldy joints – marijuana and chronic pulmonary aspergillosis. Mediterr J Hematol Infect Dis. 2011;3:e2011005. https://doi.org/10.4084/MJHID.2011.005.
47. Garrison KA, Zeffiro TA, Scheinost D, Constable RT, Brewer JA. Meditation leads to reduced default mode network activity beyond an active task. Cogn Affect Behav Neurosci. 2015;15:712–20. https://doi.org/10.3758/s13415-015-0358-3.
48. Ghasemiesfe M, Barrow B, Leonard S, Keyhani S, Korenstein D. Association between marijuana use and risk of cancer: a systematic review and meta-analysis. JAMA Netw Open. 2019;2:e1916318. https://doi.org/10.1001/jamanetworkopen.2019.16318.
49. Gibbs M, Winsper C, Marwaha S, Gilbert E, Broome M, Singh SP. Cannabis use and mania symptoms: a systematic review and meta-analysis. J Affect Disord. 2015;171:39–47. https://doi.org/10.1016/j.jad.2014.09.016.
50. Gillison ML, Chaturvedi AK, Anderson WF, Fakhry C. Epidemiology of human papillomavirus-positive head and neck squamous cell carcinoma. J Clin Oncol. 2015;33:3235–42. https://doi.org/10.1200/JCO.2015.61.6995.
51. Haney M, Cooper ZD, Bedi G, Vosburg SK, Comer SD, Foltin RW. Nabilone decreases marijuana withdrawal and a laboratory measure of marijuana relapse. Neuropsychopharmacology. 2013;38:1557–65. https://doi.org/10.1038/npp.2013.54.
52. Hindley G, Beck K, Borgan F, Ginestet CE, McCutcheon R, Kleinloog D, Ganesh S, Radhakrishnan R, D'Souza DC, Howes OD. Psychiatric symptoms caused by cannabis constituents: a systematic review and meta-analysis. Lancet Psychiatry. 2020;7:344–53. https://doi.org/10.1016/S2215-0366(20)30074-2.
53. Hindocha C, Cousijn J, Rall M, Bloomfield M, et al. The effectiveness of cannabinoids in the treatment of posttraumatic stress disorder (PTSD): a systematic review. J Dual Diagn. 2020;16:120–39. https://doi.org/10.1080/15504263.2019.1652380.
54. Hua JPY, Karcher NR, Merrill AM, O'Brien KJ, Straub KT, Trull TJ, Kerns JG. Psychosis risk is associated with decreased resting-state functional connectivity between the striatum and the default mode network. Cogn Affect Behav Neurosci. 2019;19:998–1011. https://doi.org/10.3758/s13415-019-00698-z.
55. Huang Y-HJ, Zhang Z-F, Tashkin DP, Feng B, Straif K, Hashibe M. An epidemiologic review of marijuana and cancer: an update. Cancer Epidemiol Biomark Prev. 2015;24:15–31. https://doi.org/10.1158/1055-9965.EPI-14-1026.

56. Iffland K, Grotenhermen F. An update on safety and side effects of Cannabidiol: a review of clinical data and relevant animal studies. Cannabis Cannabinoid Res. 2017;2:139–54. https://doi.org/10.1089/can.2016.0034.
57. Institute of Medicine (US). Marijuana and medicine: assessing the science base. Washington, DC: National Academies Press (US); 1999.
58. Jaeger W, Benet LZ, Bornheim LM. Inhibition of cyclosporine and tetrahydrocannabinol metabolism by cannabidiol in mouse and human microsomes. Xenobiotica. 1996;26:275–84. https://doi.org/10.3109/00498259609046707.
59. Jutras-Aswad D, DiNieri JA, Harkany T, Hurd YL. Neurobiological consequences of maternal cannabis on human fetal development and its neuropsychiatric outcome. Eur Arch Psychiatry Clin Neurosci. 2009;259:395–412. https://doi.org/10.1007/s00406-009-0027-z.
60. Joy JE. Marijuana and Medicine: Assessing the Science Base. USA: National Academies Press; 1999.
61. Karschner EL, Darwin WD, Goodwin RS, Wright S, Huestis MA. Plasma cannabinoid pharmacokinetics following controlled oral Δ9-tetrahydrocannabinol and oromucosal cannabis extract administration. Clin Chem. 2011;57:66–75. https://doi.org/10.1373/clinchem.2010.152439.
62. Karschner EL, Swortwood MJ, Hirvonen J, Goodwin RS, Bosker WM, Ramaekers JG, Huestis MA. Extended plasma cannabinoid excretion in chronic frequent cannabis smokers during sustained abstinence and correlation with psychomotor performance. Drug Test Anal. 2016;8:682–9. https://doi.org/10.1002/dta.1825.
63. Lacasse Y, Légaré M, Maltais F. E-cigarette use in patients receiving home oxygen therapy. Can Respir J. 2015;22:83–5.
64. Lacson JCA, Carroll JD, Tuazon E, Castelao EJ, Bernstein L, Cortessis VK. Population-based case-control study of recreational drug use and testis cancer risk confirms an association between marijuana use and nonseminoma risk. Cancer. 2012;118:5374–83. https://doi.org/10.1002/cncr.27554.
65. Liu C, Sadat SH, Ebisumoto K, Sakai A, Panuganti BA, Ren S, Goto Y, Haft S, Fukusumi T, Ando M, Saito Y, Guo T, Tamayo P, Yeerna H, Kim W, Hubbard J, Sharabi AB, Gutkind JS, Califano JA. Cannabinoids promote progression of HPV-positive head and neck squamous cell carcinoma via p38 MAPK activation. Clin Cancer Res. 2020;26:2693–703. https://doi.org/10.1158/1078-0432.CCR-18-3301.
66. Lloyd SL, Striley CW. Marijuana use among adults 50 years or older in the 21st century. Gerontol Geriatr Med. 2018.
67. Lunney JR, Lynn J, Hogan C. Profiles of older medicare decedents. J Am Geriatr Soc. 2002;50:1108–12.
68. Lupica CR, Riegel AC, Hoffman AF. Marijuana and cannabinoid regulation of brain reward circuits. Br J Pharmacol. 2004;143:227–34. https://doi.org/10.1038/sj.bjp.0705931.
69. MacCallum CA, Russo EB. Practical considerations in medical cannabis administration and dosing. Eur J Intern Med. 2018;49:12–9. https://doi.org/10.1016/j.ejim.2018.01.004.
70. Maguire WJ, Call CW, Cerbu C, Jambor KL, Benavides-Montes VE. Comprehensive determination of unregulated pesticide residues in oregon cannabis flower by liquid chromatography paired with triple quadrupole mass spectrometry and gas chromatography paired with triple quadrupole mass spectrometry. J Agric Food Chem. 2019;67:12670–4. https://doi.org/10.1021/acs.jafc.9b01559.
71. Marks MA, Chaturvedi AK, Kelsey K, Straif K, Berthiller J, Schwartz SM, Smith E, Wyss A, Brennan P, Olshan AF, Wei Q, Sturgis EM, Zhang Z-F, Morgenstern H, Muscat J, Lazarus P, McClean M, Chen C, Vaughan TL, Wunsch-Filho V, Curado MP, Koifman S, Matos E, Menezes A, Daudt AW, Fernandez L, Posner M, Boffetta P, Lee Y-CA, Hashibe M, D'Souza G. Association of marijuana smoking with oropharyngeal and oral tongue cancers: pooled analysis from the INHANCE consortium. Cancer Epidemiol Biomark Prev. 2014;23:160–71. https://doi.org/10.1158/1055-9965.EPI-13-0181.

72. Matskevich AN, Keshavan MS. Medical Causes of Psychosis: Lessons for Individuals with Attenuated Psychosis Syndromes. In: Li H, Shapiro DI, Seidman LJ. editors, Handbook of Attenuated Psychosis Syndrome Across Cultures: International Perspectives on Early Identification and Intervention. Springer International Publishing. 2019, pp. 161–183. https://doi.org/10.1007/978-3-030-17336-4_8.
73. McCartney D, Arkell TR, Irwin C, McGregor IS. Determining the magnitude and duration of acute Δ9-tetrahydrocannabinol (Δ9-THC)-induced driving and cognitive impairment: a systematic and meta-analytic review. Neurosci Biobehav Rev. 2021;126:175–93. https://doi.org/10.1016/j.neubiorev.2021.01.003.
74. Millar SA, Stone NL, Yates AS, O'Sullivan SE. A systematic review on the pharmacokinetics of cannabidiol in humans. Front Pharmacol. 2018;9 https://doi.org/10.3389/fphar.2018.01365.
75. Mohiuddin M, Blyth FM, Degenhardt L, Di Forti M, Eccleston C, Haroutounian S, Moore A, Rice ASC, Wallace M, Park R, Gilron I. General risks of harm with cannabinoids, cannabis, and cannabis-based medicine possibly relevant to patients receiving these for pain management: an overview of systematic reviews. Pain. 2020; https://doi.org/10.1097/j.pain.0000000000002000.
76. Mongeau-Pérusse V, Jutras-Aswad D. Challenging CBD protective effect against THC-related outcomes: a call for robust clinical trials. Addiction. 2020; https://doi.org/10.1111/add.15254.
77. Morgan CJA, Gardener C, Schafer G, Swan S, Demarchi C, Freeman TP, Warrington P, Rupasinghe I, Ramoutar A, Tan N, Wingham G, Lewis S, Curran HV. Sub-chronic impact of cannabinoids in street cannabis on cognition, psychotic-like symptoms and psychological well-being. Psychol Med. 2012;42:391–400. https://doi.org/10.1017/S0033291711001322.
78. Moss MJ, Bushlin I, Kazmierczak S, Koop D, Hendrickson RG, Zuckerman KE, Grigsby TM. Cannabis use and measurement of cannabinoids in plasma and breast milk of breastfeeding mothers. Pediatr Res. 2021;1–8 https://doi.org/10.1038/s41390-020-01332-2.
79. Mura P, Kintz P, Dumestre V, Raul S, Hauet T. THC can be detected in brain while absent in blood. J Anal Toxicol. 2005;29:842–3. https://doi.org/10.1093/jat/29.8.842.
80. Murphy M, Mills S, Winstone J, Leishman E, Wager-Miller J, Bradshaw H, Mackie K. Chronic adolescent Δ9-tetrahydrocannabinol treatment of male mice leads to long-term cognitive and behavioral dysfunction, which are prevented by concurrent cannabidiol treatment. Cannabis Cannabinoid Res. 2017;2:235–46. https://doi.org/10.1089/can.2017.0034.
81. Neavyn MJ, Blohm E, Babu KM, Bird SB. Medical marijuana and driving: a review. J Med Toxicol. 2014;10:269–79. https://doi.org/10.1007/s13181-014-0393-4.
82. Nielsen S, Sabioni P, Trigo JM, Ware MA, Betz-Stablein BD, Murnion B, Lintzeris N, Khor KE, Farrell M, Smith A, Le Foll B. Opioid-sparing effect of cannabinoids: a systematic review and meta-analysis. Neuropsychopharmacology. 2017;42:1752–65. https://doi.org/10.1038/npp.2017.51.
83. Niesink RJM, van Laar MW. Does cannabidiol protect against adverse psychological effects of THC? Front Psych. 2013;4. https://doi.org/10.3389/fpsyt.2013.00130.
84. Rezkalla S, Kloner RA. Cardiovascular effects of marijuana. Trends Cardiovasc Med. 2019:29;403–7.
85. O'Shaughnessy WB. On the preparations of the Indian Hemp, or Gunjah. Prov Med J Retrosp Med Sci. 1843;5:363–9.
86. Pacifici R, Zuccaro P, Pichini S, Roset PN, Poudevida S, Farré M, Segura J, De la Torre R. Modulation of the immune system in cannabis users. JAMA. 2003;289:1929–31. https://doi.org/10.1001/jama.289.15.1929-b.
87. Page RL, Allen LA, Kloner RA, Carriker CR, Catherine M, Morris AA, Piano MR, Rana JS, Saucedo JF, et al. Medical marijuana, recreational cannabis, and cardiovascular health: a scientific statement from the American Heart Association. Circulation. 2020;142:e131–52. https://doi.org/10.1161/CIR.0000000000000883.
88. Preuss UW, Watzke AB, Zimmermann J, Wong JWM, Schmidt CO. Cannabis withdrawal severity and short-term course among cannabis-dependent adolescent and young adult inpatients. Drug Alcohol Depend. 2010;106:133–41. https://doi.org/10.1016/j.drugalcdep.2009.08.008.

89. Rein JL. The nephrologist's guide to cannabis and cannabinoids. Curr Opin Nephrol Hypertens. 2020;29:248–57. https://doi.org/10.1097/MNH.0000000000000590.
90. Richards JR. Mechanisms for the risk of acute coronary syndrome and arrhythmia associated with phytogenic and synthetic cannabinoid use. J Cardiovasc Pharmacol Ther. 2020;25:508–22. https://doi.org/10.1177/1074248420935743.
91. Richards JR, Bing ML, Moulin AK, Elder JW, Rominski RT, Summers PJ, Laurin EG. Cannabis use and acute coronary syndrome. Clin Toxicol (Phila). 2019;57:831–41. https://doi.org/10.1080/15563650.2019.1601735.
92. Richards JR, Blohm E, Toles KA, Jarman AF, Ely DF, Elder JW. The association of cannabis use and cardiac dysrhythmias: a systematic review. Clin Toxicol (Phila). 2020;58:861–9. https://doi.org/10.1080/15563650.2020.1743847.
93. Rizzolatti G, Semi AA, Fabbri-Destro M. Linking psychoanalysis with neuroscience: the concept of ego. Neuropsychologia. 2014;55:143–8. https://doi.org/10.1016/j.neuropsychologia.2013.10.003.
94. Salazar de Pablo G, Catalan A, Fusar-Poli P. Clinical validity of DSM-5 attenuated psychosis syndrome: advances in diagnosis, prognosis, and treatment. JAMA Psychiat. 2020;77:311–20. https://doi.org/10.1001/jamapsychiatry.2019.3561.
95. Saunders BE, Adams ZW. Epidemiology of traumatic experiences in childhood. Child Adolesc Psychiatr Clin N Am. 2014;23:167–84. https://doi.org/10.1016/j.chc.2013.12.003.
96. Scherma M, Masia P, Deidda M, Fratta W, Tanda G, Fadda P. New perspectives on the use of cannabis in the treatment of psychiatric disorders. Medicines (Basel). 2018;5 https://doi.org/10.3390/medicines5040107.
97. Schwartz RH, Voth EA, Sheridan MJ. Marijuana to prevent nausea and vomiting in cancer patients: a survey of clinical oncologists. South Med J. 1997;90:167–72. https://doi.org/10.1097/00007611-199702000-00001.
98. Shannon S, Opila-Lehman J. Cannabidiol oil for decreasing addictive use of marijuana: a case report. Integr Med (Encinitas). 2015;14:31–5.
99. Singh A, Agrawal S, Gargya S, Saluja S, Kumar A, Kumar A, Kalra K, Thind M, Saluja S, Stone LE, Ali F, Duarte-Chavez R, Marchionni C, Sholevar F, Shirani J, Nanda S. Posttraumatic stress disorder after myocardial infarction and coronary artery bypass grafting. Int J Crit Illn Inj Sci. 2017;7:84–90. https://doi.org/10.4103/IJCIIS.IJCIIS_27_17.
100. Skosnik PD. Cannabis use increases risk of developing symptoms of mania. Evid Based Ment Health. 2007;10:61. https://doi.org/10.1136/ebmh.10.2.61.
101. Solowij N, Broyd S, Greenwood L-M, van Hell H, Martelozzo D, Rueb K, Todd J, Liu Z, Galettis P, Martin J, Murray R, Jones A, Michie PT, Croft R. A randomised controlled trial of vaporised Δ9-tetrahydrocannabinol and cannabidiol alone and in combination in frequent and infrequent cannabis users: acute intoxication effects. Eur Arch Psychiatry Clin Neurosci. 2019;269:17–35. https://doi.org/10.1007/s00406-019-00978-2.
102. Song A, Myung NK, Bogumil D, Ihenacho U, Burg ML, Cortessis VK. Incident testicular cancer in relation to using marijuana and smoking tobacco: a systematic review and meta-analysis of epidemiologic studies. Urol Oncol. 2020;38:642.e1–9. https://doi.org/10.1016/j.urolonc.2020.03.013.
103. St. Pierre M, Russo EB, Walsh Z. No evidence of altered reactivity to experimentally induced pain among regular cannabis users. Clin J Pain. 2020;36:589–93. https://doi.org/10.1097/AJP.0000000000000844.
104. Stott C, White L, Wright S, Wilbraham D, Guy G. A Phase I, open-label, randomized, crossover study in three parallel groups to evaluate the effect of Rifampicin, Ketoconazole, and Omeprazole on the pharmacokinetics of THC/CBD oromucosal spray in healthy volunteers. Springerplus. 2013;2:236. https://doi.org/10.1186/2193-1801-2-236.
105. Taha T, Meiri D, Talhamy S, Wollner M, Peer A, Bar-Sela G. Cannabis impacts tumor response rate to nivolumab in patients with advanced malignancies. Oncologist. 2019. https://doi.org/10.1634/theoncologist.2018-0383.
106. Taha, T. et al. Cannabis Impacts Tumor Response Rate to Nivolumab in Patients with Advanced Malignancies. Oncologist (2019) https://doi.org/10.1634/theoncologist.2018-0383.

107. Tam J, Liu J, Mukhopadhyay B, Cinar R, Godlewski G, Kunos G. Endocannabinoids in liver disease. Hepatology. 2011;53:346–55. https://doi.org/10.1002/hep.24077.
108. Taylor L, Crockett J, Tayo B, Morrison G. A Phase 1, Open-Label, Parallel-Group, Single-Dose Trial of the Pharmacokinetics and Safety of Cannabidiol (CBD) in Subjects With Mild to Severe Hepatic Impairment. J Clin Pharmacol. 2019. https://doi.org/10.1002/jcph.1412.
109. Treleaven DA. Trauma-sensitive mindfulness: practices for safe and transformative healing, trauma-sensitive mindfulness: practices for safe and transformative healing. New York, NY: W W Norton & Co; 2018.
110. Turna J, Balodis I, Munn C, Van Ameringen M, Busse J, MacKillop J. Overlapping patterns of recreational and medical cannabis use in a large community sample of cannabis users. Compr Psychiatry. 2020;102:152188. https://doi.org/10.1016/j.comppsych.2020.152188.
111. Vacaflor BE, Beauchet O, Jarvis GE, Schavietto A, Rej S. Mental health and cognition in older cannabis users: a review. Can Geriatr J. 2020;23:242–9. https://doi.org/10.5770/cgj.23.399.
112. Vadhan NP, Corcoran CM, Bedi G, Keilp JG, Haney M. Acute effects of smoked marijuana in marijuana smokers at clinical high-risk for psychosis: a preliminary study. Psychiatry Res. 2017;257:372–4. https://doi.org/10.1016/j.psychres.2017.07.070.
113. van den Elsen GAH, Tobben L, Ahmed AI, Verkes RJ, Kramers C, Marijnissen RM, Olde Rikkert MG, van der Marck MA. Effects of tetrahydrocannabinol on balance and gait in patients with dementia: a randomised controlled crossover trial. J Psychopharmacol. 2017;31:184–91. https://doi.org/10.1177/0269881116665357.
114. van den Elsen GAH, Ahmed AIA, Verkes R-J, Kramers C, Feuth T, Rosenberg PB, van der Marck MA, Olde Rikkert MGM. Tetrahydrocannabinol for neuropsychiatric symptoms in dementia: a randomized controlled trial. Neurology. 2015;84:2338–46. https://doi.org/10.1212/WNL.0000000000001675.
115. Volicer L, Stelly M, Morris J, McLaughlin J, Volicer BJ. Effects of dronabinol on anorexia and disturbed behavior in patients with Alzheimer's disease. Int J Geriatr Psychiatry. 1997;12:913–9.
116. Wall MB, Pope R, Freeman TP, Kowalczyk OS, Demetriou L, Mokrysz C, Hindocha C, Lawn W, Bloomfield MA, Freeman AM, Feilding A, Nutt D, Curran HV. Dissociable effects of cannabis with and without cannabidiol on the human brain's resting-state functional connectivity. J Psychopharmacol (Oxford). 2019;33:822–30. https://doi.org/10.1177/0269881119841568.
117. Watanabe AH, Navaravong L, Sirilak T, Prasitwarachot R, Nathisuwan S, Page RL, Chaiyakunapruk N. A systematic review and meta-analysis of randomized controlled trials of cardiovascular toxicity of medical cannabinoids. J Am Pharm Assoc (2003). 2021; https://doi.org/10.1016/j.japh.2021.03.013.
118. Whitfield-Gabrieli S, Fischer AS, Henricks AM, Khokhar JY, Roth RM, Brunette MF, Green AI. Understanding marijuana's effects on functional connectivity of the default mode network in patients with schizophrenia and co-occurring cannabis use disorder: a pilot investigation. Schizophr Res. 2018;194:70–7. https://doi.org/10.1016/j.schres.2017.07.029.
119. Wickens CM, Watson TM, Mann RE, Brands B. Exploring perceptions among people who drive after cannabis use: collision risk, comparative optimism and normative influence. Drug Alcohol Rev. 2019;38:443–51. https://doi.org/10.1111/dar.12923.
120. Woodward MR, Harper DG, Stolyar A, Forester BP, Ellison JM. Dronabinol for the treatment of agitation and aggressive behavior in acutely hospitalized severely demented patients with noncognitive behavioral symptoms. Am J Geriat Psychiatry. 2014;22:415–9. https://doi.org/10.1016/j.jagp.2012.11.022.
121. Xie M, Gupta MK, Archibald SD, Stanley Jackson B, Young JEM, Zhang H. Marijuana and head and neck cancer: an epidemiological review. J Otolaryngol Head Neck Surg. 2018;47:73. https://doi.org/10.1186/s40463-018-0319-2.
122. Yeshurun M, et al. Cannabidiol for the Prevention of Graft-versus-Host-Disease after Allogeneic Hematopoietic Cell Transplantation: Results of a Phase II Study. Biology of Blood and Marrow Transplantation. 2015;21:1770–5.
123. Zhang ZF, Morgenstern H, Spitz MR, Tashkin DP, Yu GP, Marshall JR, Hsu TC, Schantz SP. Marijuana use and increased risk of squamous cell carcinoma of the head and neck. Cancer Epidemiol Biomark Prev. 1999;8:1071–8.

Chapter 7
Choosing a Product, Route of Administration, Initial Dosage, Titration, Monitoring and Management of Adverse Effects

Contents

7.1 Introduction 192
7.2 Terminology 193
7.3 General Considerations 194
7.4 Review of the Principal Active Ingredients of Cannabis 196
7.4.1 CBD 197
7.4.2 THC 197
7.4.3 THCA, CBDA, and Other Secondary Cannabinoids 198
7.5 Overview of the Main Routes of Administration of Cannabis Products 198
7.5.1 Oral Ingestion 199
7.5.2 Oromucosal Ingestion 201
7.5.3 Inhalation 201
7.5.4 Topical and Transdermal 204
7.5.5 Intra-rectal and Vaginal (Suppositories) 205
7.6 Considering the Initial Use of Approved Pharmaceutical Cannabinoids 205
7.7 Choosing a Cannabis Formulation 206
7.7.1 Word of Caution on Product Labeling 207
7.7.2 Regarding the Therapeutic Dose of THC 208
7.7.3 Regarding the Protective Effects of CBD on THC Psychoactivity 208
7.8 Cannabinoid Metabolism: Clinical Considerations Between Inhaled and Oral Routes of Administration 209
7.9 Treatment Selection According to Symptom or Clinical Setting 209
7.10 Precise Dosing Recommendations 217
7.10.1 Initial CBD Dosing 217
7.10.2 Initial THC Dosing 217
7.10.3 Considering Microgram THC Dosing 218
7.10.4 Proposed Dosing Protocols from Consensus Groups 218
7.10.5 Considering the Toxic Psychosis Threshold of THC 221
7.10.6 Considering the Use of High-Potency Extracts (Rick Simpson Oil, RSO, Phoenix Tears) 222
7.11 Dealing with Hospitalized Patients Already Taking Cannabinoid-Based Medicines 223
7.12 Estimating the Dose of THC in Unsupervised Patients 223
7.13 Patient Monitoring, Record Keeping, and Follow-Up Visits 224
7.13.1 Reporting Cannabis Side Effects 225

C. Cyr et al., *Cannabis and Cannabinoid-Based Medicines in Cancer Care*,
https://doi.org/10.1007/978-3-030-89918-9_7

7.14 Overview of Cannabis Use Disorder and Cannabis Withdrawal Syndrome........... 226
7.15 Conclusion........ 227
7.16 Chapter Summary........ 228
References........ 228

7.1 Introduction

Clinical trials studying the effects of cannabis have only begun to take into consideration the process of choosing a specific method of administration (oil, capsule, suppository, metered dosing device) and a specific formulation (THC rich, THC/CBD balanced, CBD rich). Furthermore, dosing regimens are not yet standardized, and studies with initial microgram dosing and slow titration of THC are still few in numbers. These crucial elements, considered the cornerstones for prescribing any type of medical treatment, have unfortunately been left to the exploration of individual patients who, for the most part, continue to self-medicate without any clinical supervision. Indeed, the most recent Health Canada Cannabis Survey in 2020 estimates that approximately 70% of self-identified medical cannabis patients still acquire their cannabis without a medical authorization. While more clinicians are developing a scientific curiosity about the role of cannabinoids in clinical practice, the bulk of the available knowledge for prescribing cannabis remains anecdotal or based on consensus recommendations from groups of experienced cannabis clinicians who mostly base their opinions on personal clinical experience and interpretation of the limited available data. Hence, much of the information contained in this chapter derives from such sources, pending the results from larger and better conducted RCTs.

Although many small clinical trials using medical cannabis have been carried out in the last 20 years, there are several reasons why this has not led to the publication of practical treatment guidelines. As mentioned above, product and formulation consistency varies widely from one study to the next, making reproducibility between trials extremely difficult to achieve (see Chap. 2 for more details). Furthermore, federal regulatory bodies continue to regard cannabis as an unapproved medication, placing researchers on an arduous bureaucratic journey in order to gain trial approval.

The third and possibly most important factor which prevents large-scale quality trials is strictly financial. The cannabis plant is still considered a non-patentable product, at least for the time being. Despite the fact that efforts have been undertaken to prevent “patent trolling” and the granting of a monopoly on specific cannabis cultivars, some do not regard cannabis genomics as something that should remain in the public domain [36]. Hence, several players in the cannabis industry are attempting an intellectual property land grab, with one recent request going as far as asking for a patent on all cannabis varieties containing the genetic sequences for the production of THCA and CBDA [30]. There is, however, an advantage to granting patents on certain genomic varieties of cannabis, as this would incentivize the industry to commit larger sums for large-scale trials and would theoretically provide much needed fuel for evidence-based medicine. This ethical debate remains open-ended for the time being.

No doubt future synthetically modified cannabinoids and endocannabinoid system modulators will provide adequate returns on investments to justify larger trials as well. However, as we've seen in Chaps. 1 and 2, it is possible that single compounds may encounter limited success if not combined with other cannabinoids to produce a desired effect. As such, the use of cannabis flowers or extracts will undoubtedly remain popular, even if synthetic derivatives provide evidence of efficacy.

Despite this hostile scientific environment, several clinical societies have acknowledged that the use of cannabis and cannabinoids may be beneficial in several settings, such as neuropathic pain (Canadian Pain Society, European Federation of Neurological Societies). Even without guidelines, physicians and patients often come to their own conclusions regarding the role of cannabis in clinical practice and dosing regimens, which are:

- Cannabis is most useful for improving overall functioning, treating multiple symptoms, and dealing with end-of-life distress.
- Most patients will use ingestible formulations as a baseline and a quick acting formulation for breakthrough or episodic symptoms without requiring increasing doses over time.

Results may vary from one individual to another, although observational trials with cancer patients have demonstrated a high level of tolerability and patient satisfaction with the use of medical cannabis.

This chapter will therefore deal with the practical aspects of prescribing Cannabinoid-Based Medicines: choosing a product type and formulation, route(s) of administration, initial dosage and titration, monitoring, and management of adverse events encountered at low and moderate dosage ranges. Specific adverse events with very high toxic dosage will be covered in Chap. 8. An overview of cannabis use disorder will also be provided, which might be more relevant for patients with chronic illness but could also be applicable in cancer care if long-term survival is expected.

7.2 Terminology

The term "endocannabinoidome" is still not widely used by clinicians and researchers, and in order to avoid confusion, its use to describe the *expanded* endocannabinoid system (ECS) will be restricted to the first chapter of this book. For the present chapter, the more commonly used term "endocannabinoid system (ECS)" will be used to describe most concepts relating to both the more specific canonical receptors and enzymes and the larger system of molecular targets and ligands. The "endocannabinoidome" will only be mentioned in order to point out a clinically relevant difference between these two related concepts.

"Cannabinoid-Based Medicines" will be used preferentially as a general umbrella term to describe all compounds containing either approved or non-approved cannabinoids derived from either natural or synthetically produced cannabis. The term "cannabis" and "medical cannabis" will only be used contextually when discussing the use of plant-based products specifically.

7.3 General Considerations

- Authorizing medical cannabis in jurisdictions where it has not yet been decriminalized may expose clinicians to negative medicolegal consequences. It is important to be familiar with regulations surrounding medical cannabis in your jurisdiction and to comply with all applicable rules and regulations. If you have questions about the process of authorizing the use of medical cannabis, it is recommended to reach out to your regulatory body or a reputable association, such as the Canadian Consortium for the Investigation of Cannabinoids (https://ccic.net/), the Association of Cannabis Clinicians (https://www.cannabisclinicians.org/) or Americans for Safe Access, which also also provides valuable information on regional state regulations (https://www.safeaccessnow.org/states).
- Diligent record keeping of the items discussed in this chapter is highly recommended. As medical cannabis remains outside the "mainstream" medical culture, it is important to clearly document reasons for authorizing medical cannabis and associated counseling.
- When traditional treatments have failed, a trial of Cannabinoid-Based Medicines or medical cannabis in cancer patients may be attempted to achieve certain legitimate goals, including:
  - Increasing overall functionality.
  - Helping to better cope with multiple cancer symptoms.
  - Dealing with end-of-life distress.
  - Patients may have other goals as well including regaining a sense of control or empowerment and reduction of other pharmaceuticals which may have had unintended or intolerable side effect profiles.
- If medical cannabis is authorized in legalized jurisdictions, the use of standardized regulated products reduces the risk of accidental overdosing and exposure to potential toxic contaminants. Patients should always be counseled against accessing cannabis from unregulated community sources (black market, gray market, cannabis clubs, unregulated dispensaries, friends, etc.).
- Legal cannabis producers have also been known to take a "static" approach to labeling THC and CBD values in order to save on costs, where a single potency label is pre-printed and applied across many batches which fall within a predetermined range.
- Approved Cannabinoid-Based Medicines include pharmaceutical cannabinoids (nabiximols, nabilone, dronabinol) which should always be considered if available. It is recommended to document that available pharmaceutical cannabinoids have been considered before proceeding with the use of medical cannabis instead.
- A trial of medical cannabis should only be undertaken in patients who have undergone an appropriate evaluation and for whom specific therapeutic goals have been set (See Chap. 6 for more information).
- The available data suggests that using cannabis as an anti-tumor agent or as a "Hail Mary pass" is not an appropriate therapeutic goal. (See Chap. 6 for more information.)

- Cannabis can be used for medical or recreational purposes. However, they differ in terms of products used, dosing, and intended effects. The role of the healthcare provider is to help the medical patient reach their intended goal. For the recreational user, the role of the healthcare provider is to provide information in order to limit any potential harm.
- Established cannabis users require a detailed review of their former and/or present use patterns. Current cannabis use does not preclude the authorization of medical cannabis, however. If current cannabis users are found to have cannabis user disorder or aberrant drug behavior, referral to the appropriate resource should be considered (See Chap. 6 for mor information).
- Cannabis dosing, choice of formulation, and frequency of use are highly individualized. Despite this, there are certain concepts that apply to all patients. A standardized approach and further recommendations will be reviewed in this chapter.
- For cannabis-naive individuals: start low, go slow, stay low (at least for THC).
- A dose of cannabis is defined by milligrams of THC and CBD, not grams of dried flower, number of puffs, drops of oil, or portions of edibles.
- Initial *microgram* dosing of THC (<1 mg) is a very safe starting point for most cannabis-naive individuals but requires specific products which permit this level of precise dosing (diluted oils, capsules, precise dosing inhaler devices).
- Oral or oral-mucosal ingestion of medical cannabis products is the mainstay of treatment for most chronic conditions.
- Inhaled cannabis is usually reserved for breakthrough or episodic symptoms. It may also be useful in exploring higher dose psychoactivity (see Chap. 8).
- Consistent administration procedures can reduce pharmacokinetic fluctuations and total cannabinoid exposure.
- Ingested cannabis products, especially CBD-dominant formulations, should be consumed with meals as this will increase absorption.
- Using precise metered formulations (capsules, sprays, metered dose inhalation devices) helps simplify cannabis administration and lowers the risk of involuntary intoxication.
- Combining different formulations and routes of administration is the rule rather than the exception.
- Patients often prefer higher CBD formulations for daytime use and higher THC for evening/nighttime use.
- Once patients identify their "lowest effective dose," this does not usually change over time. Tolerance to the euphoric effects of THC usually develops over a period of a few weeks, but this does not seem to extend to other therapeutic benefits including analgesia, anti-nausea, and sleep inducine effects.
- Patients should be warned that impairment can occur even with small doses of THC, not unlike with the use of benzodiazepines, opioids, etc. Healthcare providers and patients must be aware of legislation surrounding the use of medical cannabis and driving, working, or being involved in safety-sensitive situations.
- High-CBD preparations may contain sufficient amounts of THC that will lead to plasma levels surpassing legal driving limits.

- The terms "psychoactivity" and "euphoria" are not interchangeable:
  - Psychoactivity usually refers to any neurocognitive effect, which can be considered as either therapeutic (anxiolysis, sleep induction) or an adverse event (anxiety, paranoia, reduced memory) or even recreational in nature (euphoria, metacognition, insight catalysis). (See Chap. 8 for more information).
  - Euphoria, although commonly encountered at higher doses, is not the intended goal of treatment. It is not required to experience subjectively in order to achieve symptom control in most cases. Therapeutic effects may thus occur at doses below the threshold producing psychoactive or euphoric effects [1].
- Cannabinoid-Based Medicines may reduce the need for other medications (opioids, benzodiazepines, etc.), but results may vary. When initiating Cannabinoid-Based Medicines, other therapies should remain unchanged. Only after a patient has become stabilized on Cannabinoid-Based Medicines and the therapeutic effects have been identified should a taper of other pharmaceuticals be considered [63].
- The cost of approved Cannabinoid-Based Medicines are often covered by private and public insurers. However, the cost of unapproved medical cannabis products is only beginning to be eligible for reimbursement and may be prohibitive in many cases. Using the smallest effective dose is key to reducing costs.

7.4 Review of the Principal Active Ingredients of Cannabis

The cannabis plant contains an uncertified number of different compounds. Estimates vary between 400 and 500 different compounds which could be present in the cannabis plant, several of which might only be found in certain varieties such as the newly isolated tetrahydrocannabiphorol (Δ9-THCP) [14]. The chemistry of the cannabis plant is also quite unique. It contains several scientifically proven class of active compounds: terpenoids/terpenes, flavonoids, and cannabinoids. Terpenes are compounds which fall under the formula $(C_5H_8)_n$. The term is often used interchangeably with terpenoids, although strictly speaking, the latter are in fact modified terpenes that contain additional functional groups. Both have strong and often pleasant odors which often protect the host or attract pollinators. It is estimated that there are over 55,000 different chemical entities of terpenes and terpenoids, of which approximately 150 are found in the cannabis plant [8]. Many of these have shown to have therapeutic effects, at least preclinically, and several have exhibited anti-tumor properties. However, the estimated doses needed to block tumor formation in rodents were estimated to equal approximately 10% of their diet [8].

Presently, there is insufficient evidence to establish a link between terpenes, terpenoids, and any significant anticancer properties, at least with presently used dosages witnessed in clinical practice. This will require human trials in order to determine the dosage and timing required to establish its effectiveness when used in conjunction with standard chemotherapeutic and immunologic agents.

The class of compounds known collectively as cannabinoids, however, has been more closely studied. Of the 100 or so cannabinoids found in cannabis, only 2 have been studied clinically and at least enough to provide some preliminary guidance for their use. This book has focused primarily on two cannabinoids: cannabidiol (CBD) and tetrahydrocannabinol (THC), which are the two most abundant cannabinoids found in the majority of presently available cannabis varieties.

Over the course of the last 50 years or so, uninterrupted crossbreeding has led to plant hybridization which exhibits an ever increasing enzymatic activity directed towards the production of THC. However, recent interest in CBD has now driven the industry to create new hybrids which produce varying ratios of these two compounds. However, there are over one hundred other cannabinoids which have been isolated from the cannabis plant, such as cannabinol (CBN), cannabichromene (CBC), cannabigerol (CBG), and cannabivarin (CBV), all of which mostly exist in negligible amounts in presently available strains. Although hybrids geared towards their production are beginning to appear, further research will be required in order to validate the results from preclinical trials [37]. As such, this chapter will limit its scope to the management strategies of CBD and THC. Secondary cannabinoids will only be briefly discussed.

7.4.1 CBD

CBD is known for its antiepileptic and anxiolytic effects. While it is in this sense considered psychoactive, it does not impart the intoxicating effects that are known to occur with THC administration. CBD has also been shown to have anti-inflammatory and immunomodulatory effects in several studies [40, 57]. High dose CBD-rich formulations are most frequently prescribed for the treatment of refractory epilepsy, for control of anxiety, as an analgesic alternative, and to mitigate unwanted effects of THC. They are also known to have antipsychotic, antioxidant, and neuroprotective effects [40]. Approximately 65% of orally administered CBD is excreted unchanged in the feces, and 20% is excreted in the urine. Over 30 metabolites of CBD have been discovered [35].

7.4.2 THC

THC is still considered the primary psychotropic compound of cannabis and responsible for the euphoric effects (and the subjective "high" that recreational users seek). It interacts with the CB1 receptor as an agonist in the central nervous system and is known to influence many brain processes such as the modulation of pleasure, movement control, learning, memory, appetite, sleep regulation, and pain sensation [61]. THC-rich cannabis formulations are used for pain control, sleep disturbances, and appetite stimulation, as an antiemetic, and to help control spasticity in neurologic conditions like multiple sclerosis [40]. Approximately 65% of THC is excreted in the feces primarily as 11-hydroxy THC, the first of 18 major metabolites. These have been identified in the urine, which comprises another 20% of total THC excretion from the body [61].

7.4.3 *THCA, CBDA, and Other Secondary Cannabinoids*

There has been a growing interest in the use of non-decarboxylated cannabis compounds such as THCA, which are often obtained by extraction or "juicing" of fresh cannabis flowers. Until recently, THCA and CBDA were believed to be prodrugs and considered inert. THCA has not been known to exert agonistic activity at the CB1 receptor unless decarboxylated with heat to the active form Δ-9 THC. However, preclinical trials began to indicate that THCA may in fact bind to CB1 and possess anti-inflammatory, immunomodulatory, and neuroprotective as well as antineoplastic effects [50]. This has led to the promotion of THCA as a non-psychoactive and better tolerated alternative to the decarboxylated form Δ-9 THC. Although preclinical data may be promising, there remains some controversy as to the actual biological activity of THCA and its potential role in clinical practice. One confounding factor in anecdotal reports may be due to the observation that decarboxylation to Δ-9 THC can spontaneously occur at room temperature and small amounts of Δ-9 THC may in fact be producing modest CB1 receptor activity [68]. A 2017 study further backed this claim by showing that contamination by low levels of naturally occurring decarboxylation of THCA to Δ-9 THC may in fact explain CB1 activation [47]. Conversely, a more recent preclinical trial suggests that THCA may bind indirectly to CB1 and act as an allosteric CB1 receptor modulator [52]. For the time being, the therapeutic potential of THCA remains controversial.

7.5 Overview of the Main Routes of Administration of Cannabis Products

Medical cannabis products come in many forms. They are most commonly prescribed either in the form of unprocessed dried flowers for inhalation or for at-home processing to other formats, or as a decarboxylated cannabis extract diluted in food grade oil intended for oral ingestion. Cannabis oil can also be encapsulated in order to provide a familiar and more standardized product. Many other cannabis products can be made with decarboxylated extracts, such as edible food products, topical formulations, and rectal/vaginal suppositories.

Medical cannabis research is increasingly focused on developing alternative administration routes in order to increase bioavailability and reduce pharmacokinetic variability. Some recent initiatives have sought to identify new drug delivery mechanisms in order to avoid first-pass metabolism, such as intranasal gels and

Table 7.1 Characteristics of frequently used routes of administration for medical cannabis

Route and bioavailability	Forms	Method	Peak plasma concentration	Duration of effects
Oral ingestion Bioavailability 10–20%[a]	Bottled oil extract	Dosed using a syringe or dropper	1–3 hours	6–8 hours
	Cannabis oil capsules	Capsules filled with oil extracts	1–3 hours	6–8 hours
	Nabilone[b, c]	Capsules	60–90 minutes	8–12 hours
	Dronabinol[a]	Capsules	2 hours Range: 30 min to 4 hours	Up to 12 hours
Oromucosal/ sublingual	Nabiximols	Cannabinoids are absorbed from oral mucosa into systemic circulation	2–4 hours*	4–6 hours
	Oil extract	Patients are advised to leave cannabis oil under the tongue for 1–2 minutes for optimal absorption	1–3 hours	6–8 hours
Rectal	Suppository	Intra-rectal (lower 1/3)	2–8 hours	Undetermined[a]
Inhalation (smoke or vaporization) Bioavailability 5–56%, average 25–27%*	Dried cannabis	Vaporizer (ideal)	5–10 min	Half-life of 1.5–2 hours and the duration of effects is approximately 2–4 hours

[a][32]
[b][38]
[c][69]

formulations using nanotechnology [10]. However, the most frequently used methods remain the oral, oromucosal, and inhalation routes. They have their individual characteristics which will be reviewed below (see Table 7.1).

7.5.1 Oral Ingestion

Oral ingestion is the mainstay of treatment in most cases. It is the most common administration method recommended by physicians and used by medical cannabis patients. Edible cannabis products come in many forms. Some advocates suggest "juicing" fresh cannabis flowers, although no studies have demonstrated clinical benefits with using this method, particularly if the plant material has not been heated to produce decarboxylation of THC and CBD. Orally administered cannabis generally refers to products derived from the oily resin of the cannabis plant which is extracted either with solvents, supercritical CO_2, ice, heat, or mechanical compression. The extract which contains the active ingredients from the cannabis plant is then heated to produce decarboxylation. At this point, the activated extract can then be used in many ways: diluted into either food grade oil or glycerol compound (coconut, sunflower, medium chain triglyceride, etc.) for use in bottled cannabis oils, oromucosal sprays, edibles, capsules, and vape pens or mixed into a vehicle enhancer for skin absorption. The advantage of using this process is that the end product contains a precise amount of THC and/or CBD, which is usually measured in mg/ml. Concentrated undiluted extracts from the cannabis plant (butane hash oil, shatter, Phoenix Tears/Rick Simpson Oil, etc.) can contain over 90% cannabinoids by weight. Although popularity for these types of highly concentrated products is increasing for recreational and medical use, the increased risk of accidental overdose makes them improper alternatives for medical use in cannabis-naive or frail patients. The term "edibles" refers to food and beverage products that contain cannabis extracts. Their use is less common in jurisdictions where their sale is still prohibited. In which case, patients interested in using edibles have to procure cannabis oil or dried flowers in order to prepare their own edible products. Cannabis oil or extracts can be consumed in the following three ways:

- From a bottle, using a dosing syringe or dropper (oral or oromucosal)
- In fixed-dosage capsules
- In sublingual or oral-mucosal sprays, delivering a metered dose

In Canada the maximum concentration for THC-containing oil products is 30 mg/mL, while there is no upper limit set for CBD. Cannabis edibles are capped at 10 mg per portion. Diluted cannabis oil can be used to make capsules which is basically encapsulated oil, providing a consistent and standardized dose that can be easily incorporated into a patient's daily routine. In general, oils are provided to patients in a bottle. Patients are instructed to use a 1 mL syringe, draw up the appropriate amount, and place it in their mouth and swallow directly or mix it with a small amount of food. The overall bioavailability of orally administered THC varies from 5 to 20% and will vary according to food intake [35].

The presence of high-fat food has a dual effect on oral absorption: it increases the time to reach peak plasma concentration and also increases total cannabinoid absorption (area under the curve). In one study, the time to reach maximum plasma concentration was increased 3.5-fold with a high-fat meal and enhanced the overall level of a 5 mg dose of THC (fasting Tmax 1.9 +/− 1.1 h, fed Tmax 6.6 +/− 2.8 h). However, the peak plasma concentration was not significantly different in either fed or fasting state [43]. No differences were seen in cognitive or cardiovascular adverse effects in both groups. This study also demonstrated sex differences in absorption, where women given the same dose and meal presented significantly higher THC levels than men. Cannabis effects from oral administration parallel the Tmax curve and are experienced on average 1–3 hours post-consumption and can last 6–8 hours [44]. However, plasma concentrations fall much more quickly than subjective effects which makes this a poor measure of impairment in many cases [70].

Diluted cannabis oils are useful for initiating treatment and permit slow and precise titration. Once a maintenance dose is achieved, switching to capsules with standard dosages can be offered for convenience. The use of edibles depends on whether the portion contains an accurate and consistent dose of cannabinoids. Baked goods such as cookies and brownies are notoriously unpredictable in terms of potency. However, licensed medical cannabis producers have also produced gummies and mints with accurate dosages, and these may also be used instead of oils or capsules.

7.5.2 Oromucosal Ingestion

Very few truly oromucosal products are currently available on the market. This is due to the hydrophobic/lipophilic nature of cannabinoids. In order to properly act as an oral mucosal product it has to be modulated in order to allow for absorption. This is usually done by combining cannabinoids with other products such as alcohol or other compounds such as menthol which help in crossing the mucosal layers. Due to the lack of commercially available regulated products that are truly absorbed via the oral mucosa, it is not commonly used. Some healthcare providers encourage the patient to place the oil under the tongue and hold it there as long as possible (1–2 minutes), although patients are often tempted to swallow the oil or extract prematurely. Furthermore, studies have reported a wide-range bioavailability with this method. In one trial, Tmax for sublingual CBD was estimated to be between 1.64 and 4.2 hours [48], which suggests that the oromucosal route may not increase either speed to effect or bioavailability compared with the oral route. Thus, sublingual absorption with presently available products may not provide a clear pharmacokinetic advantage. Buccal strips and sprays are being developed and may provide more accurate pharmacokinetics.

7.5.3 Inhalation

Inhalation, when cannabis is drawn into the airway and lungs in smoke or vapor form, offers a more rapid rate of absorption and ease of titration. The onset of effects may begin within seconds after inhaling, and peak concentration is attained within 3–10 min [31, 61]. The half-life of inhaled cannabis is approximately 1.5–2 hours, and the duration of effects is approximately 2–4 hours [44, 61].

Vaporization of cannabis has been suggested as a safer alternative to smoking. These devices are designed to heat dried cannabis at a safe temperature which allows for the release of cannabinoids and other secondary compounds without the need for combustion. The potential advantages of using approved vaporizers include the formation of a smaller quantity of toxic by-products such as carbon monoxide, polycyclic aromatic hydrocarbons, and tar, as well as a more efficient extraction of Δ9-THC (and CBD) from the cannabis material [32]. Vaporization of high-potency cannabis extracts using "vape pens" is now widely available and becoming an increasingly popular delivery method. However, recent outbreaks of lung injury with the use of these and other vaping products have raised concerns over the use of harmful diluents and will require an ongoing effort to meet higher safety standards. Cannabis extracts diluted in food grade oils for oral administration are not formulated to be vaporized in any type of device.

Approved vaporizing devices using dried cannabis flower reduce the likelihood of producing harmful by-products caused by higher temperatures and minimize the risk of throat and lung irritation associated with smoking (i.e., from combustion) [44]. Unlike electronic cigarettes, the vaporization of dried cannabis flowers does not rely on vaporized liquids that contain nicotine, propylene glycol, or glycerin, all of which may be linked to lung toxicity [42]. Patients who cannot access a vaporizer and decide to smoke should avoid adding tobacco to their cannabis as it increases the risk of developing dependence to nicotine and may increase the risk of developing cannabis arteritis [42, 51]. Thankfully, smoking cannabis is rapidly losing its appeal. It is important to repeat that the use of edible products can bypass the lungs altogether, and this is generally becoming the preferred alternative for chronic symptoms. According to the 2020 Canadian Cannabis Survey by Health Canada, the use of inhalation continues to drop in popularity, and nearly 50% of medical cannabis patients now prefer orally administered products. Thus, the pulmonary contraindications can be avoided in many, if not most, cases. There are, of course, exceptions to the rule.

The pharmacokinetics of inhaled cannabis also vary widely, according to the depth of inhalation and breath hold. THC bioavailability has been estimated to be between 5% and 56% [35]. There are four methods for inhaling cannabis:

- Vaporization with dried flower (acceptable)
- Vaporization of diluted cannabis extracts (in MCT, PEG, etc.) with vape pens
- Vaporization of high-potency distillates (Shatter, wax, etc.) with "dabbing"
- Combustion of dried flower or cannabis extract

In Canada, there are four Health Canada-approved medical cannabis vaporizers: the Volcano Medic™, Mighty Medic™ and Volcano Medic 2™ by Storz & Bickel, and the Syqe™ medical inhaler (see Fig. 7.1). These devices are usually more expensive than many available commercial vaporizers used for recreational use.

7.5.3.1 Inhalation Techniques (Smoke or Vapor)

Trials looking into the possible benefits of inhaled medical cannabis have often used a cued-puff procedure, known as the "Foltin Puff Procedure," which requires a five-second breath inhalation followed by a ten-second breath hold [11, 73]. This standardized technique may not be amenable for all individuals, however. Patients should be advised to find a comfortable inhalation technique which works for them and keep the procedure as uniform as possible. After an initial puff, patients who do not experience effects after their first low-dose inhalation should inhale a second low-dose 15–30 minutes later. Waiting 15–30 minutes between each inhalation will help mitigate possible side effects since peak effects should occur in

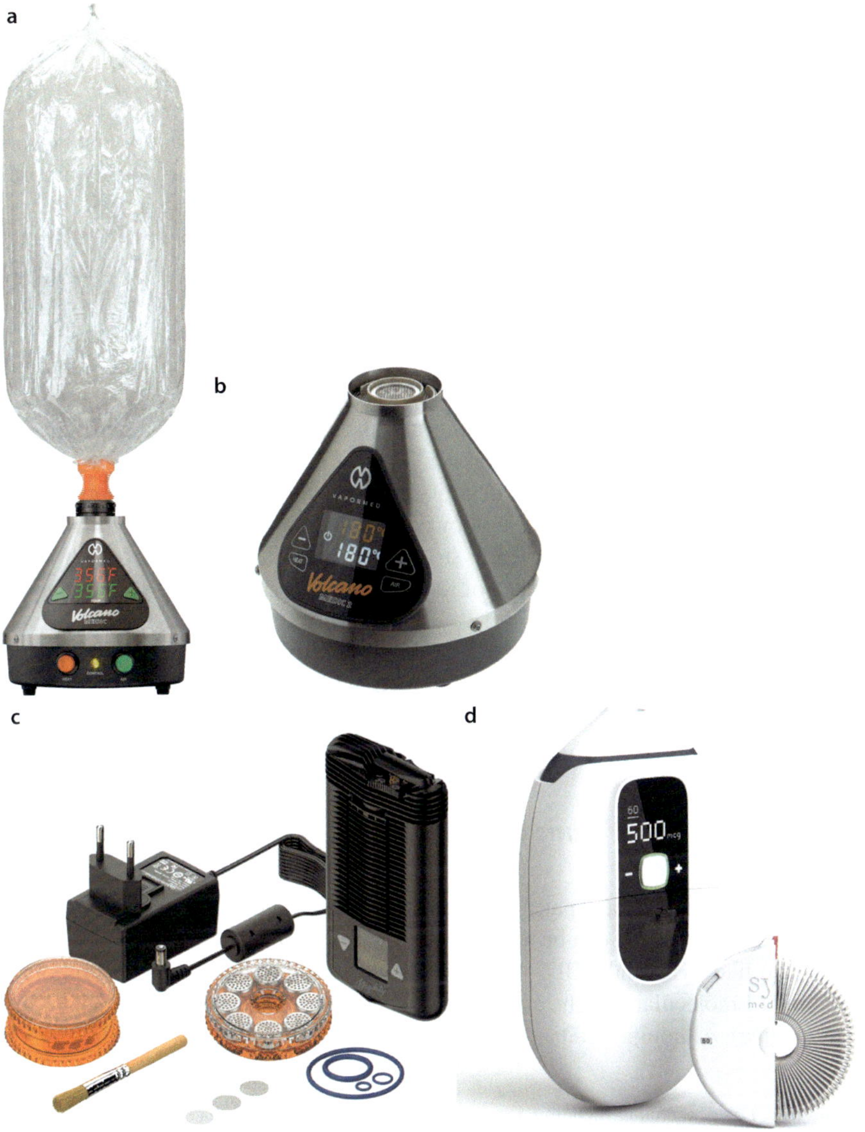

Fig. 7.1 Health Canada approved dried cannabis inhaler devices. (**a**) Volcano Medic™ shown with filling chamber and balloon, (**b**) Volcano Medic 2™, (**c**) Mighty Medic™ shown with filling chamber tool set, (**d**) Syqe™ medical cannabis inhaler device, shown with prefilled replacement cartridge containing dried cannabis

that time window. This approach will help patients safely determine the number of inhalations required to reach an effective dose. Cannabis-naive patients should also be advised to begin with a low-THC-potency product. See further for information on initial choice of product for inhalation. The Syqe™ inhaler device has addressed this issue by controlling breath duration and pressure.

7.5.3.2 Current Challenges for Calculating a Precise Dose of THC Using Dried Cannabis for Inhalation

Consuming dried cannabis by inhalation requires a prudent approach since risks of overdose are common when using high-potency products. The quantity of cannabis flower which contains a safe starting dose of 2.5 mg of THC can vary widely according to potency, humidity, and age of material. It has been known that THC breakdown occurs at room temperature and potency will reduce over time. Therefore, only approximate doses can reasonably be measured in many cases. For example, in order to quantify a 2.5 mg dose of THC with dried cannabis flower containing 25% THC, this would require only 10 mg of the plant material. Visually, this would resemble a small pea-sized amount which may be difficult to replicate from one dose to the next.

Larger and more approximate amounts can also be used, and this often simplifies the process. However, using much lower-potency products can allow for a wider margin of error. For example, the quantity of cannabis at 5% THC that provides a 2.5 mg dose equals 100 mg of dried flower which is much easier to manipulate. In some cases where low-potency THC strains are unavailable, blending with high-CBD strains can reduce the potency of the final product and provide a lower overall cannabinoid exposure (see Table 7.2).

The Syqe™ inhaler device uses cartridges prefilled with a precise amount of dried cannabis with a stop mechanism which activates once the preprogrammed dose is delivered.

7.5.4 *Topical and Transdermal*

Topical salves, creams, and patches are becoming more and more popular. However, deeper skin penetration can be a challenge for many drugs, particularly if they are lipophilic like THC and CBD. Another challenge to transcutaneous absorption is the limited molecular weight of the compound which cannot be greater than 500 daltons (Da). Although CBD and THC both have a molar mass of 314.2 Da, which

Table 7.2 Dried cannabis blending instructions for reducing THC concentration using high-potency strains and high-CBD strains (containing less than 1% THC)

THC % of initial product	Desired potency of final blend (%)	Mixing ratio of high-THC product and high-CBD (<1% THC) product
20	10	1:1
	5	1:2
	2.5	1:4
15	10	3:2
	7.5	1:1
	5	1:3
	2.5	1:6

falls under this threshold, no human studies have clearly demonstrated any significant systemic absorption of transdermal for both of these cannabinoids [35]. However, trials have shown possible benefits for localized dermatological conditions where the skin barrier is compromised, such as psoriasis and leg ulcers [10, 45]. Despite the fact that clinically relevant transdermal levels of cannabinoids have not yet been shown in vivo, promising in vitro studies have led many companies to develop a wide range of patents for topical CBD preparations. Enhancers are usually added to these compounds which may increase solubility and increase absorption by disrupting the skin's outer layer. Anecdotal reports have also found topical application useful either for joint pain/symptoms or for cutaneous symptoms such as shingles, eczema plaques, psoriatic plaques, etc. Small case series have also shown clinical benefits of using topical oils containing THC and CBD in malignant wounds and pyoderma gangrenosum [46].

7.5.5 Intra-rectal and Vaginal (Suppositories)

There are theoretical pharmacokinetic advantages with intra-rectal or vaginal delivery systems. The rectum has two venous drainage systems. The upper and middle thirds of the rectum drain primarily into the superior rectal veins and then borrow the portal circulation which empty into the liver. However, the lower third of the rectum drains into the middle and lower rectal veins which then drain directly into the inferior vena cava [5]. Vaginal venous drainage borrows the vaginal venous complex which drains into the internal iliac veins [66]. Thus, venous return in the lower third of the rectum and the vagina both bypass the portal circulation and therefore avoid first-pass metabolism. Plasma concentrations of Δ9-THC through rectal administration are also dose- and vehicle-dependent and vary according to the chemical structure of the THC ester [31]. While studies have shown that Δ9-THC itself is not well absorbed through the rectal mucosa, the prodrug Δ9-THC hemisuccinate seems to be well absorbed with a bioavailability ranging from 52% to 61% or twice that of the oral route [9]. Another small trial comparing 10 mg of oral vs rectal Δ9-THC hemisuccinate showed that total systemic exposure of THC (area under the curve) through the rectal route was 2.4 times higher compared with oral administration [23, 24].

7.6 Considering the Initial Use of Approved Pharmaceutical Cannabinoids

Many national regulatory authorities have approved several pharmaceutical cannabinoids. Presently, the available products include two synthetic THC analogues and a natural cannabis extract. Access to either product may vary depending on the jurisdiction. Clinicians should consult their local pharmacy in order to determine availability and insurance coverage.

Approved pharmaceutical cannabinoids should always be considered in clinical situations where they have been shown to be effective in clinical trials, since they are often covered by private or public insurance (see further Sect. 7.9). It is suspected, at least anecdotally, that dronabinol and nabilone are less well tolerated than natural cannabis compounds. Furthermore, it is not known if the addition of CBD would mitigate the side effects from the use of these synthetic THC analogues.

Dronabinol (Marinol®, Syndros®, Reduvo®, Adversa®) is a synthetic THC analogue in capsule form that is considered chemically similar to natural THC. It is approved by the FDA in the USA for HIV/AIDS-related anorexia and chemotherapy-induced nausea and vomiting. It is the enantiomer form (−) trans-Δ^9 THC and does not contain any other THC isomers or any CBD. It is considered to possess similar dose-related effects compared to THC. It does not contain any other secondary cannabinoids. The recommended adult starting dose of dronabinol is 2.5 mg orally twice daily one hour before lunch and dinner. Elderly patients may consider initiating dronabinol with 2.5 mg daily one hour before dinner or bedtime to reduce the risk of CNS effects.

Nabilone (Cesamet®) is a synthetic THC analogue in capsule form with an on-label indication for the treatment of nausea and vomiting associated with cancer chemotherapy for patients who have failed to respond adequately to conventional antiemetic treatments (Canada). Physicians have also prescribed nabilone (off-label use) for the treatment of AIDS-related anorexia, neuropathic pain, or pain in palliative care patients. Additional benefits observed in clinical practice include the improvement of sleep-related disturbances and spasms. Unlike dronabinol, nabilone does not possess an identical chemical structure as THC and has been shown to be a much more potent analogue. Like dronabinol, nabilone is an isolated active compound and does not contain either CBD or other secondary cannabinoids. It is available in 0.25, 0.5, and 1 mg capsules. The recommended starting dose for CINV is 1–2 mg twice a day, with the first dose given at bedtime.

Nabiximol (Sativex®) is a natural cannabis extract available in a buccal spray that contains 2.7 mg of THC and 2.5 mg of CBD per spray. Nabiximol is currently approved in Canada (not in the USA) as an adjunctive treatment for the symptomatic relief of neuropathic pain and spasms associated with multiple sclerosis in adults who have not responded to other therapies. Nabiximols may also be useful as an adjunctive analgesic treatment in adult patients with advanced cancer who experience moderate to severe pain during high-dose opioid therapy for persistent background pain. The recommended starting dose is one spray in the morning and one spray in the afternoon/evening.

7.7 Choosing a Cannabis Formulation

The term cannabis *formulation* relates to the composition of the different cannabinoids found in a specific product. While there is no accepted nomenclature for describing different cannabis formulations, clinicians and patients usually describe three main types, which are defined by the amount (or ratio) of the primary cannabinoids THC and CBD contained in the product (Table 7.3):

- CBD rich
- Balanced THC/CBD
- THC rich

7.7.1 Word of Caution on Product Labeling

Although many jurisdictions require that the amounts or ratios of THC and CBD be clearly indicated on the container, labeling requirements often do not specify in which order this ratio should be expressed. Labels may indicate content as either THC/CBD or inverted as CBD/THC and thus require careful examination in order to avoid confusion.

Furthermore, industry standards for testing are inconsistent, even in regulated markets, and caution must be exercised, particularly when purchasing "CBD-rich" or "CBD-dominant" products derived from plant species other than hemp. Cannabis (aka marijuana) and hemp are part of the same plant family, and both can produce significant amounts of CBD. However, hemp is legally defined as being the plant *Cannabis sativa L.* species which contains no more than 0.3%

Table 7.3 Cannabis formulations based on THC and CBD content

THC rich (THC dominant)	Contains primarily THC with more or less 1% relative CBD[a]
THC/CBD balanced (mixed ratio THC/CBD)	Contains varying ratios of both cannabinoids (1:2, 1:4, 2:1, etc.)[b]
CBD-rich products (high-CBD, CBD-dominant, full-spectrum CBD, broad-spectrum CBD)	May contain varying amounts of THC depending on the source material: *Cannabis sativa* (L.): usually contains more or less 1% THC including other secondary cannabinoids and terpenes[c] Hemp-derived CBD (aka full-/broad-spectrum CBD): legally required to contain no more than 0.3% THC by dry weight (USA and Canada) and contain other secondary cannabinoids and terpenes CBD isolates: heavily processed and purified products, usually in powder form and containing no other compound (not available in Canada)

[a]There is no accepted standard for the allowable amount of CBD in what is defined as a THC-rich product

[b]There is presently no clear evidence which indicates any clear benefit derived from using a specific THC/CBD ratio in any clinical setting. There is some data that suggests that the dose of CBD intended to mitigate THC adverse events may be much higher than previously thought [49]

[c]In Canada, the *Cannabis Act* and its regulations do not distinguish between CBD derived from industrial hemp and CBD derived from cannabis with greater than 0.3% THC. As such, there is no accepted lower limit of THC which defines a "CBD-rich" product. These may therefore contain higher amounts of THC which, in some cases, might produce impairment while using standard doses of CBD. See below for further explanations

THC on a dry weight basis, according to the Agriculture Improvement Act of 2018 (also known as the 2018 Farm Bill). Hemp has also been removed from the definition of marijuana in the Controlled Substance Act (CSA), and it is no longer considered a controlled substance under the CSA. This has provided the industry with a federal regulatory framework which guarantees accurate labeling of hemp-derived products in terms of maximum THC potency. Hemp is a not-too-distant cousin of *Cannabis sativa* and exhibits a clearly distinguishable profile at the genome-wide level [59], with a reduced level of activity of THCA synthase [13]. This limits the enzymatic activity of hemp species to produce THC's acid precursor THCA. However, regulations are still lacking concerning *Cannabis sativa* strains producing higher CBD-to-THC ratios. A 2017 study of US medical dispensary cannabis products reported that many high-CBD products were inaccurately labeled [7]. In this study, only 31% of products were accurately labeled, and 18 of the 84 samples of "CBD-rich" extracts contained THC concentrations up to 6.43 mg/ml. Hence, purchasing CBD-rich products in unregulated markets may put patients at risk of involuntary exposure to doses of THC at levels which may produce impairment or intoxication.

7.7.2 Regarding the Therapeutic Dose of THC

The pharmacokinetic-pharmacodynamic relationship between the dose of THC and therapeutic or subjective effects are complex and ill-defined. This is particularly the case with oral administration which significantly increases plasma levels of secondary active metabolites compared to the inhaled route. As such, the dose of THC required to produce either therapeutic or subjective effects can vary widely from one individual to another (See Sect. 7.8).

7.7.3 Regarding the Protective Effects of CBD on THC Psychoactivity

Studies have suggested that CBD may reduce some of the unwanted effects of THC. However, both the amount and timing of administration of CBD required to reduce psychoactivity remain unclear [49]. In one human trial, small doses of CBD were actually found to enhance THC effects. In the same study, a larger dose of 400 mg of CBD was required to reduce the subjective effects of a single 8 mg dose of THC [65]. Impairment can therefore still occur using "high-CBD" products if there is a significant amount of THC present.

Until formal regulatory frameworks address these issues, ensuring patient safety requires the use of properly tested products and a diligent reading of the label to determine potency. Patients need to be reminded that CBD and THC dosing is based on milligrams of active compounds and not ratios or percentages. It is then only a matter of calculating a safe starting dose.

7.8 Cannabinoid Metabolism: Clinical Considerations Between Inhaled and Oral Routes of Administration

THC first enters the body as Δ-9 THC, the decarboxylated and active form of the prodrug THCA. When inhaling cannabis, this occurs when THCA is heated by combustion or another heat source such as an electronic vaporizer device. Other formulations, including ingestible products, need to be preheated before packaging in order to activate THCA. Hence, cannabis oils, capsules, and edibles have all been decarboxylated prior to packaging in order for the end product to be effective.

Studies aimed at determining the plasma concentrations of Δ-9 THC required to produce subjective effects have provided wide-ranging results. Various pharmacodynamic models have suggested that plasma levels of Δ-9 THC between 7 and 29 mg/ml are required to produce a 50% subjective psychoactive "high" [16]. Other studies suggest that plasma levels of Δ-9 THC range between 2 and 250 ng/ml for the inhaled route and 1 and 8 ng/ml for the oral route in order to produce a 50% psychoactive "high" effect [33, 71]. The discrepancy between inhaled and oral Δ-9 THC levels required to produce psychoactive effects may depend on the presence of secondary active metabolites formed by first-pass hepatic metabolism. Of these, 11-hydroxy THC (11-OH THC) has been suggested as a prime suspect. It has been suggested that 11-OH THC may be more psychoactive than Δ-9 THC and may also cross the blood-brain barrier more easily. This compound is formed by the actions of cytochrome P450 enzymes CYP3A4, 2C9, and 2C19. However, genetic polymorphisms of 2C9 are relatively frequent, affecting up to 40% of the population in some areas [58]. These widespread mutations result in a reduced transformation of Δ-9 THC into 11-OH THC, which further complicates the search for a precise threshold dose of oral THC.

An oral dose of 2.5 mg of THC was long considered the psychoactive threshold for subjective effects [44]; more recent studies have suggested that some individuals may perceive subjective effects with doses as low as 0.5 mg, however [1]. Thus, the lowest possible threshold dose of THC remains elusive, which explains why a low starting dose is considered a more prudent approach when initiating cannabis products containing THC.

7.9 Treatment Selection According to Symptom or Clinical Setting

Choosing a specific cannabis formulation and dosing regimen may seem like a daunting task. Cannabis is a complex amalgamation of many active compounds with a wide range of interindividual differences in regard to bioavailability, metabolism, effect, and tolerability. Prior exposure also plays a significant role in initial product choice. Hence, cannabis does not fit well within the typical medical model for drug prescribing.

Initial choice of a cannabis formulation relies in great part on clinical trials primarily using THC. For this reason, conditions that have shown to respond well to this cannabinoid should be treated initially with synthetic THC analogues such as dronabinol or nabilone (see prior Sect. 7.7). In cases where these medications are considered ineffective or not well tolerated, a trial of medical cannabis can then be attempted. Nabiximols, if it is available, can be an interesting next step for patients, since it contains an equal ratio of CBD and THC extracted from the plant material. Although no comparative studies have been carried out between nabiximols and dronabinol or nabilone, some authors suggest that it offers a better tolerability profile than its synthetic counterparts [44]. Accordingly, certain symptoms such as neuropathic pain or chemotherapy-induced nausea and vomiting may respond better to THC-rich products rather than CBD. However, in some situations where THC is not well tolerated, anecdotal observations suggest that CBD may provide some benefits in these settings as well.

For these reasons, it is important to remember that medical cannabis is a highly individualized treatment option that often requires several trials of different formulations and routes of administration before finding optimal benefits. It is also worth noting that many patients often use more than one cannabis formulation in their treatment regimen. Some may use medical cannabis on a prn basis as well. As an individualized treatment, the age-old mantra of "Start Low and Go Slow" rings true here. The goal of establishing a "lowest therapeutic dose" can mitigate the risk of side effects and the development of tolerance. This goal can be achieved by following the initiation and dose titration protocols which have been proposed as preliminary guidance and adjusted according to patient overall health status and prior experience (see Table 7.1).

Disclaimer Most of the following suggestions concerning the initial choice of cannabis formulation is based mostly on shared clinical experience among patients and cannabis clinicians and is not currently based on comparative clinical trials.

- *Chronic pain (cancer and noncancer related)*
  - *Therapeutic goals:*

    Reduce pain
    Improve functionality
    Reduce the use of opioids and other medications for pain control if not tolerated
    Improve overall health-related quality of life
  - *Related conditions:*

    Cancer-related pain
    Somatic, nociceptive, and visceral pain
    Neuropathic pain (central and/or peripheral neuropathic pain)
  - *Recommended treatment and route of administration:*

    Initial treatment with approved pharmaceuticals

    - Consider nabiximols for moderate/severe pain related to advanced cancer.
    - Consider nabilone for chronic pain.

Secondary trial of cannabis extracts for oral administration

- Start with CBD-rich products if side effects were reported with previous THC or nabilone use.
- Consider THC/CBD balanced in other cases.
- For more experienced prescribers, consider recommending patients to purchase one THC-rich bottle and one CBD-rich bottle and try mixing products with varying ratios of THC to CBD until the desired effect is achieved.

Introduction of inhaled cannabis formulations

- Consider THC/CBD balanced and/or THC-rich PRN for breakthrough pain.

- *Neuropathic pain*
  - *Therapeutic goals:*

    Reduce pain
    Improve functionality
    Improve activities of daily life
    Reduce the use of opioids and other medications for pain control if not tolerated
    Improve overall health-related quality of life

  - *Related conditions:*

    Diabetic neuropathy
    Multiple sclerosis pain

  - *Recommended treatment and route of administration:*

    Initial treatment with approved pharmaceuticals
    Consider nabiximols for neuropathic pain related to multiple sclerosis (on-label indication approved by Health Canada).
    Secondary trial of cannabis extracts for oral administration

    - Start with CBD-rich products if side effects were reported with previous THC or nabilone use.
    - Consider THC/CBD balanced (see special considerations).
    - More experienced prescribers can recommend patients to order two different types of bottled cannabis oil, one THC-rich product and one CBD-rich product. This will allow patients to trial different THC/CBD ratios until they find the most beneficial combination. For patients who are new or sensitive to THC, consider first initiating treatments with CBD before introducing THC.

    Introduction of inhaled cannabis formulations
    Consider THC/CBD balanced or THC-rich PRN (for breakthrough pain).
    Special considerations

THC is generally preferred by patients with fibromyalgia and neuropathic pain. • Consider an increase in THC dose if little relief and no adverse reactions were reported. This can be achieved by ordering two different types of bottled cannabis oil and by using a higher ratio of THC to CBD (e.g., 2:1).

- *Chemotherapy-induced nausea and vomiting (CINV)*
  - *Therapeutic goals:*

    Reduce nausea
    Reduce vomiting
    Decrease anxiety and associated anticipatory nausea
    Improve health-related quality of life

  - *Related conditions:*

    Nausea and vomiting caused by cancer treatments
    Symptoms related to chronic inflammatory bowel disease
    Side effects from other medications

  - *Recommended treatment and route of administration:*

    Initial treatment with approved pharmaceuticals
    Consider nabilone for nausea and vomiting induced by chemotherapy.
    Secondary trial of cannabis extracts for oral administration
    For delayed emesis, consider THC-rich formulations.
    Introduction of inhaled cannabis formulations
    For acute emesis, consider vaporizing THC/CBD balanced 1–2 hours before chemotherapy. For anticipatory nausea, consider vaporizing CBD-rich 1–2 hours before appointment.
    Special considerations
    Nabilone (Cesamet®) is an FDA-approved on-label treatment for CINV. It is important to note that heavy use of THC-rich products has also been associated with the inducement of nausea and vomiting (hyperemesis syndrome).

- *Appetite stimulation*
  - *Therapeutic goals:*

    Stimulate appetite
    Increase weight
    Cessation of rapid weight loss

  - *Related conditions:*

    Cancer-related anorexia-cachexia syndrome
    Significant weight loss
    HIV/AIDS
    Loss of appetite as a side effect of medication
    Anorexia nervosa

– *Recommended treatment and route of administration:*

Initial treatment with approved pharmaceuticals
A trial of nabilone or dronabinol can be considered in this setting.
Secondary trial of cannabis extracts for oral administration

- Start with CBD-rich products if side effects were reported with previous THC or nabilone use.
- Consider THC-rich 1 hour before meals.

Introduction of inhaled cannabis formulations
Consider THC-rich 30 min before meals.
Special considerations
Consider a therapy of THC/CBD balanced oil combined with vaporization of THC/CBD balanced PRN if a THC-rich therapeutic regimen is not well tolerated.

- *Anxiety*
- There is little evidence to support the use of cannabis for the treatment of anxiety. However, a 2018 review suggests that cannabis may be effective to relieve anxiety when it is associated with other conditions such as chronic pain or MS-related spasms [6].

– *Therapeutic goals:*

Reduce anxiety
Improve mood
Reduce reactivity to stress
Improve sleep
Reduce panic attacks

– *Related conditions:*

Generalized anxiety disorder
Obsessive-compulsive disorder
Attention deficit disorder (ADD)
Attention deficit hyperactivity disorder (ADHD)
Anorexia nervosa
Panic attacks

– *Recommended treatment and route of administration:*

Initial treatment with approved pharmaceuticals
Neither nabilone nor dronabinol is approved for the treatment of anxiety. However, nabilone has shown some efficacy in the treatment of anxiety [25, 67], and low doses can be considered if well tolerated.
Secondary trial of cannabis extracts for oral administration

- Start with CBD-rich products if side effects were reported with previous THC or nabilone use.
- Low doses of THC have been found to decrease anxiety levels [12].

  - Consider adding THC if needed.

  Introduction of inhaled cannabis formulations
  Consider THC-rich 30 min before meals.
  Special considerations
  Consider a therapy of THC/CBD balanced oil combined with vaporization of THC/CBD balanced PRN if a THC-rich therapeutic regimen is not well tolerated.

- *Depression*
- Although some authors suggest that cannabis may one day play a role in the treatment of psychiatric illnesses [60], there is little evidence to support the use of cannabis for depression at this time. In fact, chronic recreational cannabis use has been associated with worsened symptoms of depression [6, 39]. Although THC may produce varying degrees of euphoria which can be experienced as a welcome reprieve for depressed patients, it is unclear if tolerance to this effect will occur with prolonged use [22]. Close monitoring of depressed patients who are increasing their dosage may help detect the early onset of tolerance. In which case, patients should be asked directly which of the desired effects of cannabis they may be "chasing." If tolerance is suspected, a THC or "T" break may be in order. (See Sect. 7.14).

  – *Therapeutic goals:*

    Reduce anxiety
    Improve mood
    Reduce reactivity to stress
    Improve sleep
    Reduce panic attacks

  – *Recommended treatment and route of administration:*

    Initial treatment with approved pharmaceuticals
    Neither nabilone nor dronabinol are approved for the treatment of depression. However, a trial was started to assess the efficacy of dronabinol for the treatment of depression and/or anxiety in older adults but was halted due to the prohibitive cost of the drug [28].
    Secondary trial of cannabis extracts for oral administration
    Consider CBD-rich products.
    Introduction of inhaled cannabis formulations
    Consider CBD-rich PRN.
    Special considerations

    - If needed, consider slowly adding THC once an appropriate dosage of CBD has been determined. While lower doses of THC may alleviate symptoms of depression, higher doses may worsen them. Tolerance to euphoric effects should be monitored closely.

- Consider the addition of THC by ordering two different types of bottled cannabis oil, one THC-rich and one CBD-rich, or select a THC/CBD product with a higher ratio of CBD to THC (2:1 or 4:1 ratio).

- *Post-traumatic stress disorder (PTSD)*
- Cancer patients often need to endure difficult and sometimes traumatizing investigations and treatments, and commonly meet unexpected and distressing events during the course of their illness. These may produce clinical states ressembling PTSD. Although it is still unclear if cannabis is effective for this medical condition [6], several observational studies have shown that cannabis may provide benefits for those suffering from PTSD [34]. Furthermore, cannabis may help prevent traumatic memory formation by way of aversive memory extinction (see Chap. 8 for more information).

  – *Therapeutic goals:*

    Reduce nightmares/flashbacks
    Reduce depression and anxiety related to PTSD
    Reduce triggers sensitivity
    Improve social functioning

  – *Related conditions:*

    Flashbacks
    Insomnia
    Nightmares
    Panic attacks
    Paranoia
    Difficulty concentrating

  – *Recommended treatment and route of administration:*

    Initial treatment with approved pharmaceuticals:
    A recent review on the use of nabilone for the treatment of PTSD found that the two available RCTs have demonstrated that nabilone may be effective for the treatment of several PTSD-associated symptoms, including a reduction in nightmares and an improvement in sleep time and quality. However, the current level of evidence is insufficient to draw any conclusions, and no guidelines were identified [17]. At least one trial is underway in order to determine the effectiveness of dronabinol in PTSD [55]. In this context, it may be advisable to begin with nabilone for nightmares or insomnia in PTSD patients.
    Secondary trial of cannabis extracts for oral administration:
    Consider THC/CBD balanced products.
    Introduction of inhaled cannabis formulations:
    Consider THC/CBD balanced or THC-rich PRN.
    Special considerations:

    - THC products are commonly preferred by patients with PTSD.

- Inhaled THC-rich products may alleviate difficulty falling asleep (sleep induction), while ingested THC-rich products may help with interrupted sleep (for sleep maintenance).
- Consider ordering two different types of bottled cannabis oil, one THC-rich product and one CBD-rich product, and mix them to obtain a THC/CBD ratio of 2:1. More experienced prescribers can help patients trial different THC/CBD ratios until they find the most beneficial combination. Also consider THC-rich dried cannabis to inhale PRN.
- Consider starting with CBD-rich products in case of anxiety and panic attacks.

- *Sleep disturbances*
  - *Therapeutic goals:*

    Improve sleep in quality and duration
  - *Related conditions:*

    Chronic pain
    PTSD
    Nightmares
    Flashbacks
    Anxiety
    Spasticity
    Restless leg syndrome
  - *Recommended treatment and route of administration:*

    Initial treatment with approved pharmaceuticals
    Consider nabilone at bedtime. Consider prescribing 0.5 mg doses and starting treatments with a half dose.
    Secondary trial of cannabis extracts for oral administration
    Consider THC-rich at bedtime (longer duration of action may provide better sleep maintenance).
    Introduction of inhaled cannabis formulations
    Consider THC-rich at bedtime (shorter onset of action may provide better sleep induction).
    Special considerations

    - Inhaled THC-rich products may alleviate difficulty falling asleep (sleep induction), while ingested THC-rich products may help with interrupted sleep (for sleep maintenance).
    - CBD has been shown to impact the circadian rhythm, and patients often report difficulty sleeping after taking CBD products before bed. Low-dose CBD may impair sleep quality over the long term, with evidence indicating it can have a stimulating effect, whereas high-dose CBD can have a sedative effect [2].
    - Consider THC/CBD balanced product only if THC is not tolerated.

7.10 Precise Dosing Recommendations

To date, no official guidelines have been published for the use of cannabis for any medical condition. Furthermore, there is no consensus on what constitutes a standard dose of either CBD or THC.

7.10.1 Initial CBD Dosing

Preclinical data suggests that the effective dose of CBD may lie between 0.1 and 1 mg/kg for pain conditions [19] and up to 20 mg/kg for seizure control [64]. For this reason, it is difficult to determine a standard CBD dose at the present moment, and patients must be guided by either subjective benefits, maximum tolerability, significant drug interactions, or affordability. Again, it is important to be reminded that most non-hemp derived "high CBD" products may contain appreciable amounts of THC. Careful product selection and label inspection of active ingredients are essential elements of harm reduction.

7.10.2 Initial THC Dosing

The Canadian Cannabis Act, which, in 2018, established the framework for recreational cannabis legalization in Canada, has determined that the maximum amount of THC per individual package would be set at 10 mg. This decision was considered a compromise between health officials who recommended a maximum dose of 2.5 mg, while industry advocates recommended a higher limit. Hence, the psychoactive threshold found between 2 and 3 mg of THC is considered a safe introductory dose for recreational use.

However, this may not be the case for the medical use of THC. The starting dose of nabilone, a potent THC analogue, has been established at 0.25 mg. However, no head-to-head comparisons between nabilone and other THC analogues or natural compounds have been attempted. Early trials undertaken with standard THC, such as nabiximols and dronabinol (another synthetic analogue but with a biologically similar level of CB1 receptor agonism as THC), have estimated that an initial 2.5 mg dose of THC represents the psychoactive threshold for most individuals. It was thus surmised from early trial subjects that the dosage range producing subjective effects must represent the lowest effective dose for symptom management. However, more recent trials and consensus statements are in fact challenging this assumption. A 2020 study has shown that a dose of THC as small as 0.5 mg may provide therapeutic benefits [1].

7.10.3 Considering Microgram THC Dosing

The starting dose and therapeutic window of THC for most medical applications is still being debated. Furthermore, as explained above, it is likely that pharmaceutical industry standards have overestimated the lowest effective dose threshold, due in part on the assumption that subjective psychoactivity was considered a prerequisite to achieve therapeutic benefit.

Recent trials using more precise inhaler devices have reported clinical benefits in patients using *microgram* doses of THC, even as low as 0.5 mg, while reducing exposure to unwanted side effects [1]. Use of standardized formulations and novel delivery methods which exhibit a more narrow pharmacokinetic range and provide a more predictable total cannabinoid exposure are thus beginning to demonstrate that patients can achieve significant therapeutic benefits with much lower initial doses of THC than previously thought [1]. It is not known if oral microgram doses of THC carry the same therapeutic potential as for the inhaled route, however.

Oral cannabis products come in many forms. Diluted oils sold in Canada are required to contain a maximum concentration of no more than 30 mg of THC per ml. At this maximum concentration, however, a single drop (20–30 drops per ml) contains at least 1 mg of THC. In some jurisdictions, such as in Thailand, recommended methods for obtaining even smaller volumes include using a toothpick dipped in THC-rich oils. Using less concentrated products (e.g., 10–20 mg of THC/ml) is another, and more pragmatic way of securely providing microgram THC dosing (<1mg). Standardized softgels or capsules are now available and contain a minimum starting dose between 2 and 3 mg of THC. Low-dose gummies and edibles containing 2–3 mg per portion can be halved or quartered, which make these products another interesting choice for initial microgram dosing of THC.

7.10.4 Proposed Dosing Protocols from Consensus Groups

A recent publication by a group of 20 cannabis clinicians from 9 countries has provided a consensus-based series of recommendations using a modified Delphi process (Table 7.4) [4]. Based on their collective experience, the initial use of CBD followed by low-dose THC was considered the primary strategy for initiating cannabis in most clinical settings involving chronic pain. Different dosing protocols were also proposed in regard to THC initiation, depending on patient frailty, experience, and need for timely symptom control. After initiation of treatment with CBD, a standard protocol is proposed using a THC starting dose of 2.5 mg, while a conservative protocol for frail patients starts with 1 mg or less of THC. A third more rapid protocol was also proposed for patients with cannabis experience or particularly severe symptoms who require a more rapid titration.

Another consensus-based series of recommendations for titrating cannabinoids and tapering opioids in chronic pain was also recently published (see Table 7.5) [63]. This protocol was designed for patients wishing primarily to introduce

Table 7.4 Disclaimer: The initial introduction of CBD has not yet been demonstrated clinically for these purposes. The following recommendations are based on preclinical evidence, observational data, and clinical experience

Slow protocol: (cannabis naive, frail, or polypharmacy patients, severe hepatic or renal failure)	Consider starting with a CBD-rich product at 5 mg bid Increase by 5 mg/dose every 2–3 days up to a maximum of 20 mg bid If benefits encountered, consider increasing CBD dose to 40 mg bid If little or no benefits encountered, maintain CBD dose of 20 mg bid before adding THC Consider adding nighttime THC at a starting dose of $\leq$1 mg HS Increase THC dose by 1 mg every 7 days until desired efficacy or tolerability (max 15–20 mg) Consider adding daytime THC at a starting dose of $\leq$1 mg am or pm Increase THC dose by 1 mg every 7 days until desired efficacy or tolerability (max 15–20 mg bid) THC doses above 30–40 mg per day have not shown to be beneficial and may increase adverse events [44] Consider taking cannabis oil with meals to increase absorption [48]
Standard protocol: (patients with prior cannabis experience, or with a low ECOG grade)	Consider starting with a CBD-rich product at 5–10 mg bid Increase by 5 mg/dose every 2–3 days up to a maximum of 20 mg bid If benefits encountered, consider increasing CBD dose to 40 mg bid If little or no benefits encountered, maintain CBD dose of 20 mg bid before adding THC Consider adding nighttime THC at a starting dose of 2–3 mg HS Increase THC dose by 2–3 mg every 7 days until desired efficacy or tolerability (max 15–20 mg/dose) Consider adding daytime THC at a starting dose of 2–3 mg am or pm Increase THC dose by 2–3 mg every 7 days until desired efficacy or tolerability (max 15–20 mg bid) THC doses above 30–40 mg per day have not shown to be beneficial and may increase adverse events [44] Consider taking cannabis oil with meals to increase absorption [48]
To mitigate side effects, *START LOW AND GO SLOW:* Extend the days in between dose increases, slow down titration, or go back to the previous dose if patients experience side effects	

Adapted from: Bhaskar et al., "Consensus recommendations on dosing and administration of medical cannabis to treat chronic pain: results of a modified Delphi process", 2021

Table 7.5 Adapted from: Sihota et al., "Consensus-Based Recommendations for Titrating Cannabinoids and Tapering Opioids for Chronic Pain Control", 2020. Disclaimer: The initial introduction of CBD has not yet been demonstrated clinically for these purposes. These recommendations are based on preclinical evidence, observational data, and clinical experience

Patient selection: When should cannabis be considered in a chronic pain patient?	If the patient has not achieve an acceptable level of pain control, despite optimal pharmacological, physical, and psychological therapy If the patient has experienced significant side effects to opioid medication If the patient has significant risk factors associated with increased adverse effects of opioid use
Treatment initiation: *Beginning with a CBD-rich product* Disclaimer: The consensus group acknowledges that the use of CBD has not been demonstrated clinically for these purposes. Recommendations are based on preclinical evidence, relative safety of CBD, and the possibility that the small amounts of THC present in these formulations may provide certain benefits	Consider starting with a CBD-rich product at 5 mg bid Increase the dose by 5 mg once or twice weekly No consensus was achieved on the maximum dose of CBD to be attained
Adding THC:	Consider adding THC if no benefits are encountered with CBD alone Initial THC dosing should begin with 0.5–3 mg HS Increase by 1–2 mg/dose once or twice weekly up to 40 mg per day divided bid or tid
Opioid reduction protocol Consider a reduction of opioids if the following conditions have been met:	Cannabis dosing has been optimized The patient demonstrates a significant improvement in functional capacity The patient wishes to reduce his/her opioid use In which case, reduce morphine equivalent dose by 5–10% every 1–4 weeks It is not recommended to begin tapering opioids during initial titration of cannabinoids or at any given dose of cannabinoids
Recommended follow-up	Follow-up is recommended once or twice a month until symptoms have reached a steady state After which, follow-up every 3 months is recommended
To mitigate side effects, *START LOW AND GO SLOW:* Extend the days in between dose increases, slow down titration, or go back to the previous dose if patients experience side effects	

cannabis in order to reduce their overall opioid use. Both protocols share many similarities in terms of initial product choice and THC dosing according to individual patient characteristics.

7.10.5 Considering the Toxic Psychosis Threshold of THC

Of all the acute side effects of THC, the one that is often considered most problematic is the risk of an acute psychotic-like reaction. Increasing trends in involuntary intoxications and ER visits are indeed alarming [62]. Until the turn of the millennium, cannabis was consumed mostly in the form of inhaled low-potency dried herb. The recent arrival of ultrahigh potency extracts and powerful synthetic CB1 receptor agonists has caught most of the population off guard and is in great part responsible for the rise of acute psychotic episodes [21, 29]. Accordingly, many public health authorities have begun to implement awareness campaigns and other safeguards [26, 27, 56].

Psychotic-like reactions caused by common non-psychotropic medications are actually quite common. According to the DSM-V, it has been estimated that in 7–25% of individuals presenting with a first episode of psychosis, the cause may be due to substance or medication. The most commonly implicated drugs include antiparkinsonian agents, cardiac medications, and corticosteroids [74]. However, the risk of psychosis with approved medications may develop using standard therapeutic doses and not necessarily related to overdosing. There is reason to believe that this may not the case with cannabis, at least in majority of individuals. Although psychotic reactions with recreational use are indeed common, randomized clinical trials looking into the effects of medical cannabis have not suggested that doses of THC below 2.5 mg are associated with an increased risk of psychosis. Although anecdotal reports of unexpected psychotic symptoms in patients using very small doses of THC do exist, it appears that an oral dose of 10–20 mg of THC is sufficient to achieve psychotropic effects, while a dose of 30–40 mg of THC in a cannabis-naive individual carries a high risk of marked intoxication [51]. The interindividual risk of experiencing psychosis with cannabis varies widely and is possibly linked to certain predisposing genetic factors and possible drug interactions which increase THC bioavailability [3, 20, 54]. Studies using low doses of THC have consistently demonstrated a high degree of tolerability in the majority of subjects, and again, these adverse effects are unlikely to occur with starting doses of 2.5 mg or lower [44]. In frail, advanced cancer or palliative care patients, we recommend even lower starting doses of less than 1 mg which should further mitigate this risk substantially (Table 7.1).

The role of CBD modulation on CB1 receptors has also been studied and shown to reduce psychotic-like symptoms in neuroimaging studies [18, 72]. Early studies using nabiximols had suggested that an equal amount of CBD and THC increased the toxic psychosis threshold, when comparing data with other approved cannabinoids such as dronabinol [44]. However, recent data suggests that a much higher dose of CBD may be necessary to provide significant antipsychotic effects [65]. For the time being, there is still no consensus on the protective effects of CBD on

THC-induced psychotic-like symptoms, and more research is necessary in order to establish precise dosing protocols of both THC and CBD that will insure more predictable outcomes [49].

7.10.6 Considering the Use of High-Potency Extracts (Rick Simpson Oil, RSO, Phoenix Tears)

As previously discussed in Chap. 4, the use of high-potency cannabis extracts, also known as Rick Simpson Oil (RSO) or Phoenix Tears, has been proposed by certain cannabis advocates as a cancer treatment alternative. However, in the opinion of the authors of this textbook, the use of high-potency extracts which often contain varying levels of cannabinoids cannot be regarded as a judicious adjunct or replacement for traditional treatments, particularly if the ongoing use of the latter is still offering a reasonable chance of remission. Concommitant use of cannabinoids with checkpoint inhibitors is also of concern as this has been shown to reduce treatment response. In situations where patients have exhausted every traditional treatment modality, the use of this alternative as a last resort option must be approached with extreme caution. Patients may wish to explore this course of action based on expectations from preliminary evidence suggesting that cannabinoids may hold disease-modifying effects in cancer. However, patients should be reminded that preclinical data also strongly suggests that certain cannabinoid combinations and/or concentrations may produce paradoxical effects and actually increase tumor growth and spread. Until further evidence emerges, the use of RSO must be considered a throw of the dice with several unpredictable outcomes: disease remission, disease progression, nul disease-modifying effect, and either adverse events or possible benefits from high-dose psychoactivity. See Chap. 4 for more information on patient counseling.

Disclaimer *The following information is intended to serve as a general reference for clinicians who wish to inform patients of the basic steps involved in producing and administering these products, and the further health risks involved. It must be made clear that no clinical trials have been carried out and that these proposed dosage protocols have been elaborated by non-medically trained individuals.*

Producing RSO usually entails the same steps as for most cannabis extracts: cannabis flowers usually containing varying amounts of THC, CBD, and minor cannabinoids are first washed using a solvent. Suggested compounds used to dissolve the resin from the plant material include naphtha, ether, butane, acetone, or alcohol. The solvent in the filtered liquid is then "purged" by evaporation through boiling, leaving behind the oil.

Warning Producing high-potency cannabis extract can be dangerous in untrained hands. Solvents such as naphtha can be toxic and *highly explosive*, and insufficient purging of the extract can leave behind toxic levels of residues.

Initial suggested treatment calls for a gradual increase in total daily cannabinoid doses up to a range of one thousand milligrams or more. This regimen is then usually continued for weeks or months at these high doses followed by lower-maintenance dosing.

Warning Rapid titration of THC in unprepared or cannabis-naive individuals may lead to marked intoxication causing anxiety, panic attacks, psychosis, and psychedelic experiences, accompanied by several acute cardiovascular complications such as hypotension and syncope.

7.11 Dealing with Hospitalized Patients Already Taking Cannabinoid-Based Medicines

The use of approved Cannabinoid-Based Medicines is seldom an issue when patients are hospitalized. Bridging personal or medical cannabis use to an institutional setting may be problematic in certain cases. However, this can usually be safely achieved, particularly if patients already have acquired sufficient cannabis experience and if they are using orally administered and regulated products. In certain jurisdictions where medical cannabis is legalized, protocols have been established in order to deal with these situations. Options include:

- Continued use of the patient's own products (smoked, vaporized, or other route of administration). This may often be the patient's preference. However, if unregulated or homegrown products are being used, it is important to ensure consistent potency and dosage. Smoked or vaporized products may not be permitted in certain institutions or only in designated areas.
- Switching to a non-inhaled route of administration. If the institution permits the use of non-inhaled medical cannabis products and the patient accepts to switch to an oral or oromucosal route, measures should be taken to ensure access to standardized cannabis products certified by either federal regulatory bodies or an independent third party, such as the Patient Focused Certification compliance program (https://patientfocusedcertification.org/) offered by Americans for Safe Access. When switching from the inhaled to oral route, it is suggested to start with a lower equivalent dose of THC in order to reduce the risks of adverse effects.
- Switching to an FDA-approved cannabinoid medicine. If the use of medical cannabis products is not permitted or available in an institution, a trial of an approved cannabinoid may be an option. There are three approved compounds, though they may not be available in all jurisdictions: dronabinol, nabilone, and nabiximols (see earlier Sect. 7.6).

7.12 Estimating the Dose of THC in Unsupervised Patients

Calculating the dose of cannabinoids, and THC in particular, may be challenging for patients using unregulated, inappropriately labeled, or homegrown cannabis products, since many are still using archaic methods for calculating a cannabis "dose," such as drops of oil, number of inhalations, or portions of edibles. Many patients are thus unaware of the actual dose in milligrams of THC or CBD they are *actually* taking.

In recent decades, the average THC potency has increased. In the Canadian market, the average THC potency of cannabis products was approximately 18% in 2018. In this situation, using this average can be a useful rule of thumb when guesswork is unavoidable.

An approximate dose of THC in milligrams can be surmised by a mathematical rule of three ($a \times b = x$), where:

- a is the product potency expressed in mg of THC by weight of product (mg or g) or volume (ml) (e.g., tincture containing 10 mg/ml of THC). If only the percentage of THC is known, this can be translated to mg (ex. 20% THC = 200 mg THC per gram of dried flower).
- b is the weight (mg or g) or volume (ml) of the portion or *dose* used by the patient (e.g., 0.5 ml).
- x is the estimated dose of THC in mg (e.g., 10 mg/ml × 0.5 ml = 5 mg per dose).

Regulated markets have in part addressed this issue, but many hurdles remain as testing requirements vary widely from one jurisdiction to the next. Unreliable labeling even in regulated markets continues to plague patients and healthcare providers who wish to maintain a stable dosage range with more predictable results. In one study, 26% of "CBD" products tested contained less than the amount indicated, while the THC content in some samples were judged to be sufficient to produce intoxication or impairment [7].

7.13 Patient Monitoring, Record Keeping, and Follow-Up Visits

Required monitoring and follow-up visits for medical cannabis patients vary according to jurisdiction. Most suggest a minimum initial follow-up visit after 1–3 months and then every 3 months until treatment stabilization. After which, yearly visits are required for stable patients. The exploration of cannabis formulations and administration methods may require some time. Advanced cancer and palliative patients may benefit from closer monitoring in order to reduce the time required to achieve a steady state in regard to tolerability and efficacy.

Record keeping is also important and should include the patient's choice of cannabis formulation, methods of administration, increase or decrease in dosage, frequency of doses, reported side effects, and any decrease in doses of other prescribed medications (if applicable). Consider the use of validated questionnaires for symptom burden (i.e., Edmonton Symptom Assessment System (ESAS), Brief Pain Inventory (BPI)) and/or quality-of-life assessments such as the EQ-5D-5L to facilitate monitoring of patient's symptoms.

7.13.1 *Reporting Cannabis Side Effects*

Cannabis is not a benign substance. Increasing doses of THC can produce a powerful disruption in neural connectivity which can affect cognitive and physiological functions (see Table 7.5). With the exception of seizure disorders, CBD doses used in most clinical situations have not been shown to produce significant side effects, but several have nonetheless been reported. Health Canada provides an online portal where patients, hospitals, healthcare providers, and industry can report cannabis side effects (Table 7.6):

https://www.canada.ca/en/health-canada/services/drugs-health-products/medeffect-canada/adverse-reaction-reporting/cannabis.html

The FDA Safety Information and Adverse Event Reporting Program provides the FDA 3500 form which can be used by healthcare professionals, consumers, and patients for voluntary reporting of adverse events, but these are only for products which fall under FDA regulations. Hence, much needed pharmacovigilance data is not being reported for cannabis products.

The best way to mitigate THC-induced side effects is to initiate treatment with low doses and titrate up slowly (please refer to Tables 7.1 and 7.4). Common side effects such as hypotension, palpitations, and dizziness can be managed by temporarily lying down. Anxiety and paranoid reactions are common in unprepared cannabis-naive individuals who take a large dose of THC. Medical treatment is rarely required in these situations. Relaxation techniques, retreating to a quiet environment free of external stimuli, or finding a gentle distraction such as music will usually suffice while waiting for these side effects to subside (see Chap. 8 for more information).

Table 7.6 Cannabis dose-related side effects

Most common	Common	Rare
Drowsiness Fatigue Dizziness Dry mouth Irritation of breathing passages (cough, phlegm – associated with smoking cannabis) Nausea Anxiety	Altered judgment or decreased attention Impaired motor coordination and motor performance Headaches Hypertension Euphoria Blurred vision Change in appetite Tachycardia Diarrhea Orthostatic hypotension Depression	Ataxia/discoordination Impaired short-term memory Impaired information processing Paranoia, hallucinations Panic attack Toxic psychosis

Adapted from [44]

7.14 Overview of Cannabis Use Disorder and Cannabis Withdrawal Syndrome

Cannabis use disorder (CUD) is a serious negative outcome related to chronic cannabis use and is associated with cognitive impairment, poor school or work performance, and psychiatric comorbidity such as mood disorders and psychosis. The DSM-V manual has amalgamated the diagnostic criteria of dependence and abuse into a single clinical entity "use disorder," which may be more sensitive in detecting problem use than the former diagnostic method [15, 53].

Cannabis use has been gradually increasing in the USA between 2002 and 2017, going from 10.4% to 15.3%. The overall prevalence in the general population of mild DSM-V CUD increased from 1.5% to 1.9% during the same period. However, the prevalence of moderate or severe DSM-V CUD has remained stable. For regular cannabis users, the risk of developing CUD increases significantly, but the prevalence of moderate (4–5 criteria) or severe (6+ criteria) DSM-V CUD has reduced slightly from 4.3% to 3.1% and from 2.4% to 1.3%, respectively, in this population [15].

If long-term survival is to be expected in cancer patients, this outcome needs to be discussed with the patient, and early signs of CUD should be monitored closely. See Table 7.7 for diagnostic criteria of CUD. Clinicians should keep a look out for telltale signs such as:

- Daily or near-daily use in the absence of clinically significant symptom burden or benefits
- Euphoria as the primary sought-after effect
- Increasing tolerance and use of high doses of THC-rich products
- Symptoms of withdrawal
- Social isolation and signs of anxiety or depression

Cannabis withdrawal syndrome (CWS) was newly added in the latest edition of the *Diagnostic and Statistical Manual of Mental Disorders*, the DSM-V. Although cannabis withdrawal symptoms have been generally regarded as mild or benign, recent evidence suggests that frequent users may experience more distressing symptoms and significant disability. The prevalence of CWS was estimated at 12.1% for chronic users [41]. The risk of developing CWS has also been shown to be increased in patients with prior mood or anxiety disorders, personality disorders, or a family history of depression. However, personal or family history of other substance use disorders did not increase the risk of CWS. The most commonly reported symptoms include:

Nervousness/anxiety
Hostility
Sleep difficulty
Depressed mood

Table 7.7 Cannabis use disorder (DSM-V)

Definition	A problematic pattern of cannabis use leading to clinically significant impairment or distress, as manifested by at least two of the following, occurring within a 12-month period:
Diagnostic criteria	1. Cannabis is often taken in larger amounts or over a longer period than was intended 2. There is a persistent desire or unsuccessful efforts to cut down or control cannabis use 3. A great deal of time is spent in activities necessary to obtain cannabis, use cannabis, or recover from its effects 4. Craving or a strong desire or urge to use cannabis 5. Recurrent cannabis use results in failure to fulfill role obligations at work, school, or home 6. Continued cannabis use despite having persistent or recurrent social or interpersonal problems caused or exacerbated by the effects of cannabis 7. Important social, occupational, or recreational activities are given up or reduced because of cannabis use 8. Recurrent cannabis use in situations in which it is physically hazardous 9. Cannabis use continues despite knowledge of having a persistent or recurrent physical or psychological problem that is likely to have been caused or exacerbated by cannabis 10. Tolerance, as defined by either: (1) a need for markedly increased cannabis to achieve intoxication or desired effect or (2) a markedly diminished effect with continued use of the same amount of the substance 11. Withdrawal, as manifested by either (1) the characteristic withdrawal syndrome for cannabis or (2) cannabis is taken to relieve or avoid withdrawal symptoms
Severity score	Severity is graded as either Mild, Moderate, or Severe depending if 2–3, 4–5, or 6+ of the above criteria are present

7.15 Conclusion

Cancer and palliative care patients are especially vulnerable to side effects which may explain, at least in part, the hesitation clinicians face when considering cannabis or other cannabinoid based medicines for these patients. Cannabis treatments have traditionally required extensive and time-consuming counseling which is necessary in order to avoid involuntary intoxications and monitor appropriate use. For many self-medicating patients, this "hit and miss" approach remains a challenge. However, the legal cannabis market has provided patients and clinicians with a variety of more precise cannabis formulations, which has greatly reduced the complexity of integrating this class of compounds in all areas of medicine. Pending further evidence, consensus groups have gathered the limited available clinical data in order to provide preliminary guidance on choosing a product formulation and dosing strategies. By doing so, it is hoped that clinicians will feel more comfortable to safely guide their patients in exploring the potential benefits of cannabis while reducing potentially undesirable outcomes.

7.16 Chapter Summary

- Dosing recommendations remain nascent.
- Suggested starting doses of CBD vary between 5 and 10 mg.
- Suggested maintenance doses for CBD vary between 40 and 100 mg/day and used in divided doses.
- Initial nighttime THC dosing is recommended to reduce exposure to adverse effects. Suggested starting for THC in most patients varies between 2 and 3 mg.
- In frail patients, starting doses of THC of less than 1 mg are recommended.
- Initial THC doses of 0.5 mg may also provide clinical benefits.
- Tolerance to adverse effects tends to occur rapidly.
- Tolerance to the therapeutic effects does not seem to develop when low doses of THC and CBD are used and remain stable over time.
- Most patients usually self-titrate to a sub-psychoactive threshold.
- Patients tend to vary their dosing ranges and occasionally take psychoactive doses. This is not necessarily a sign of misuse or abuse, but warrants closer monitoring.
- Rapid dose escalation or daily high-dose THC use may be a sign of tolerance to certain psychoactive effects such as euphoria, and this should entail a review of the patient's therapeutic objective.

Acknowledgments This chapter was inspired in great part by The Prescriber Guidebook (© Santé Cannabis), which was developed by the team of healthcare professionals and research personnel at Santé Cannabis, Quebec's premier medical cannabis clinic and research organization. The Prescriber Guidebook is one part of a comprehensive training and support program offered by Santé Cannabis. If you are interested in more in-depth medical cannabis training, please register to the Santé Cannabis Prescriber Training Portal: formation.santecannabis.ca.

References

1. Almog S, Aharon-Peretz J, Vulfsons S, Ogintz M, Abalia H, Lupo T, Hayon Y, Eisenberg E. The pharmacokinetics, efficacy, and safety of a novel selective-dose cannabis inhaler in patients with chronic pain: a randomized, double-blinded, placebo-controlled trial. Eur J Pain. 2020; https://doi.org/10.1002/ejp.1605.
2. Babson KA, Sottile J, Morabito D. Cannabis, cannabinoids, and sleep: a review of the literature. Curr Psychiatry Rep. 2017;19:23. https://doi.org/10.1007/s11920-017-0775-9.
3. Benyamina A, Karila L, Lafaye G, Blecha L. Genetic influences in cannabis use disorder and psychosis: dopamine and beyond. Curr Pharm Des. 2016;22:6392–6. https://doi.org/10.2174/1381612822666160831095707.
4. Bhaskar A, Bell A, Boivin M, Briques W, Brown M, Clarke H, Cyr C, Eisenberg E, de Oliveira Silva RF, Frohlich E, Georgius P, Hogg M, Horsted TI, MacCallum CA, Müller-Vahl KR, O'Connell C, Sealey R, Seibolt M, Sihota A, Smith BK, Sulak D, Vigano A, Moulin DE. Consensus recommendations on dosing and administration of medical cannabis to treat chronic pain: results of a modified Delphi process. J Cannabis Res. 2021;3:22. https://doi.org/10.1186/s42238-021-00073-1.

5. Birnbaum E. Surgical anatomy of the colon, rectum, and anus. In: Ratto C, Parello A, Donisi L, Litta F, editors. Colon, rectum and anus: anatomic, physiologic and diagnostic bases for disease management, Coloproctology. Cham: Springer; 2017. p. 9–19. https://doi.org/10.1007/978-3-319-09807-4_4.
6. Black N, Stockings E, Campbell G, Tran LT, Zagic D, Hall WD, Farrell M, Degenhardt L. Cannabinoids for the treatment of mental disorders and symptoms of mental disorders: a systematic review and meta-analysis. Lancet Psychiatry. 2019; https://doi.org/10.1016/S2215-0366(19)30401-8.
7. Bonn-Miller MO, Loflin MJE, Thomas BF, Marcu JP, Hyke T, Vandrey R. Labeling accuracy of cannabidiol extracts sold online. JAMA. 2017;318:1708–9. https://doi.org/10.1001/jama.2017.11909.
8. Booth JK, Bohlmann J. Terpenes in Cannabis sativa – from plant genome to humans. Plant Sci. 2019;284:67–72. https://doi.org/10.1016/j.plantsci.2019.03.022.
9. Brenneisen R, Egli A, Elsohly MA, Henn V, Spiess Y. The effect of orally and rectally administered delta 9-tetrahydrocannabinol on spasticity: a pilot study with 2 patients. Int J Clin Pharmacol Ther. 1996;34:446–52.
10. Bruni N, Della Pepa C, Oliaro-Bosso S, Pessione E, Gastaldi D, Dosio F. Cannabinoid delivery systems for pain and inflammation treatment. Molecules. 2018;23:2478. https://doi.org/10.3390/molecules23102478.
11. Chait LD, Corwin RL, Johanson CE. A cumulative dosing procedure for administering marijuana smoke to humans. Pharmacol Biochem Behav. 1988;29:553–7. https://doi.org/10.1016/0091-3057(88)90019-6.
12. Childs E, Lutz JA, de Wit H. Dose-related effects of delta-9-THC on emotional responses to acute psychosocial stress. Drug Alcohol Depend. 2017;177:136–44. https://doi.org/10.1016/j.drugalcdep.2017.03.030.
13. Cirovic N, Kecmanovic M, Keckarevic D, Keckarevic Markovic M. Differentiation of Cannabis subspecies by THCA synthase gene analysis using RFLP. J Forensic Legal Med. 2017;51:81–4. https://doi.org/10.1016/j.jflm.2017.07.015.
14. Citti C, Linciano P, Russo F, Luongo L, Iannotta M, Maione S, Laganà A, Capriotti AL, Forni F, Vandelli MA, Gigli G, Cannazza G. A novel phytocannabinoid isolated from Cannabis sativa L. with an in vivo cannabimimetic activity higher than Δ9-tetrahydrocannabinol: Δ9-Tetrahydrocannabiphorol. Sci Rep. 2019;9:20335. https://doi.org/10.1038/s41598-019-56785-1.
15. Compton WM, Han B, Jones CM, Blanco C. Cannabis use disorders among adults in the United States during a time of increasing use of cannabis. Drug Alcohol Depend. 2019;204:107468. https://doi.org/10.1016/j.drugalcdep.2019.05.008.
16. Cone EJ, Huestis MA. Relating blood concentrations of tetrahydrocannabinol and metabolites to pharmacologic effects and time of marijuana usage. Ther Drug Monit. 1993;15:527–32. https://doi.org/10.1097/00007691-199312000-00013.
17. Cowling T, MacDougall D. Nabilone for the treatment of post-traumatic stress disorder: a review of clinical effectiveness and guidelines, CADTH rapid response reports. Ottawa: Canadian Agency for Drugs and Technologies in Health; 2019.
18. Davies C, Bhattacharyya S. Cannabidiol as a potential treatment for psychosis. Ther Adv Psychopharmacol. 2019;9.
19. De Gregorio D, McLaughlin RJ, Posa L, Ochoa-Sanchez R, Enns J, Lopez-Canul M, Aboud M, Maione S, Comai S, Gobbi G. Cannabidiol modulates serotonergic transmission and reverses both allodynia and anxiety-like behavior in a model of neuropathic pain. Pain. 2018; https://doi.org/10.1097/j.pain.0000000000001386.
20. Decoster J, van Os J, Myin-Germeys I, De Hert M, van Winkel R. Genetic variation underlying psychosis-inducing effects of cannabis: critical review and future directions. Curr Pharm Des. 2012;18:5015–23. https://doi.org/10.2174/138161212802884591.
21. Di Forti M, Morgan C, Dazzan P, Pariante C, Mondelli V, Marques TR, Handley R, Luzi S, Russo M, Paparelli A, Butt A, Stilo SA, Wiffen B, Powell J, Murray RM. High-potency can-

nabis and the risk of psychosis. Br J Psychiatry. 2009;195:488–91. https://doi.org/10.1192/bjp.bp.109.064220.

22. D'Souza DC, Ranganathan M, Braley G, Gueorguieva R, Zimolo Z, Cooper T, Perry E, Krystal J. Blunted psychotomimetic and amnestic effects of Δ-9-tetrahydrocannabinol in frequent users of cannabis. Neuropsychopharmacology. 2008;33:2505–16. https://doi.org/10.1038/sj.npp.1301643.
23. ElSohly MA, Gul W, Walker LA. Pharmacokinetics and tolerability of Δ9-THC-Hemisuccinate in a suppository formulation as an alternative to capsules for the systemic delivery of Δ9-THC. MCA. 2018;1:44–53. https://doi.org/10.1159/000489037.
24. ElSohly MA, Stanford DF, Harland EC, Hikal AH, Walker LA, Little TL, Rider JN, Jones AB. Rectal bioavailability of delta-9-tetrahydrocannabinol from the hemisuccinate ester in monkeys. J Pharm Sci. 1991;80:942–5. https://doi.org/10.1002/jps.2600801008.
25. Fabre LF, McLendon D. The efficacy and safety of nabilone (a synthetic cannabinoid) in the treatment of anxiety. J Clin Pharmacol. 1981;21:377S–82S. https://doi.org/10.1002/j.1552-4604.1981.tb02617.x.
26. Fischer B, Malta M, Messas G, Ribeiro M. Introducing the evidence-based population health tool of the lower-risk cannabis use guidelines to Brazil. Braz J Psychiatry. 2019;41:550–5. https://doi.org/10.1590/1516-4446-2018-0239.
27. Fischer B, Russell C, Sabioni P, van den Brink W, Le Foll B, Hall W, Rehm J, Room R. Lower-risk cannabis use guidelines: a comprehensive update of evidence and recommendations. Am J Public Health. 2017;107:e1–e12. https://doi.org/10.2105/AJPH.2017.303818.
28. Forester B. Observational study of Dronabinol treatment for depression and/or anxiety in older patients (Clinical trial registration No. NCT03369639). clinicaltrials.gov, 2019.
29. Forti MD, Quattrone D, Freeman TP, Tripoli G, Gayer-Anderson C, Quigley H, Rodriguez V, Jongsma HE, Ferraro L, Cascia CL, Barbera DL, Tarricone I, Berardi D, Szöke A, Arango C, Tortelli A, Velthorst E, Bernardo M, Del-Ben CM, Menezes PR, Selten J-P, Jones PB, Kirkbride JB, Rutten BP, de Haan L, Sham PC, van Os J, Lewis CM, Lynskey M, Morgan C, Murray RM, Amoretti S, Arrojo M, Baudin G, Beards S, Bernardo M, Bobes J, Bonetto C, Cabrera B, Carracedo A, Charpeaud T, Costas J, Cristofalo D, Cuadrado P, Díaz-Caneja CM, Ferchiou A, Franke N, Frijda F, Bernardo EG, Garcia-Portilla P, González E, Hubbard K, Jamain S, Jiménez-López E, Leboyer M, Montoya GL, Lorente-Rovira E, Loureiro CM, Marrazzo G, Martínez C, Matteis M, Messchaart E, Moltó MD, Nacher J, Olmeda MS, Parellada M, Peñas JG, Pignon B, Rapado M, Richard J-R, Solano JJR, Díaz LR, Ruggeri M, Sáiz PA, Sánchez E, Sanjuán J, Sartorio C, Schürhoff F, Seminerio F, Shuhama R, Sideli L, Stilo SA, Termorshuizen F, Tosato S, Tronche A-M, van Dam D, van der Ven E. The contribution of cannabis use to variation in the incidence of psychotic disorder across Europe (EU-GEI): a multicentre case-control study. Lancet Psychiatry. 2019;6:427–36. https://doi.org/10.1016/S2215-0366(19)30048-3.
30. Grimm N, Scott B, Lyons G. Biotech Institute's Growing Patent Portfolio -- U.S. Patent No. 9,095,554 and the path forward [WWW Document]. Patent Docs. 2017. https://www.patentdocs.org/2017/11/biotech-institutes-growing-patent-portfolio-us-patent-no-9095554-and-the-path-forward.html. Accessed 8.2.21.
31. Grotenhermen F. Pharmacokinetics and pharmacodynamics of cannabinoids. Clin Pharmacokinet. 2003;42:327–60. https://doi.org/10.2165/00003088-200342040-00003.
32. Health Canada. Information for health care professionals: Cannabis and cannabinoids [WWW Document]. 2018. https://www.canada.ca/en/health-canada/services/drugs-medication/cannabis/information-medical-practitioners/information-health-care-professionals-cannabis-cannabinoids.html. Accessed 7.19.21.
33. Hollister LE, Gillespie HK, Ohlsson A, Lindgren JE, Wahlen A, Agurell S. Do plasma concentrations of delta 9-tetrahydrocannabinol reflect the degree of intoxication? J Clin Pharmacol. 1981;21:171S–7S. https://doi.org/10.1002/j.1552-4604.1981.tb02593.x.
34. Hindocha C, Cousijn J, Rall M, Bloomfield MAP. The Effectiveness of Cannabinoids in the Treatment of Posttraumatic Stress Disorder (PTSD): A Systematic Review. J Dual Diagn. 2020;16:120–39.

35. Huestis MA. Human cannabinoid pharmacokinetics. Chem Biodivers. 2007;4:1770–804. https://doi.org/10.1002/cbdv.200790152.
36. Hymes T. PHYLOS FALLOUT: open Cannabis project to shutter this month. Future Cannabis Project. 2019. https://futurecannabisproject.org/2019/05/phylos-fallout-open-cannabis-project-to-shut-down-ocp/. Accessed 8.2.21.
37. LaVigne JE, Hecksel R, Keresztes A, Streicher JM. Cannabis sativa terpenes are cannabimimetic and selectively enhance cannabinoid activity. Sci Rep. 2021;11:8232. https://doi.org/10.1038/s41598-021-87740-8.
38. Lemberger L, Rowe H. Clinical pharmacology of nabilone, a cannabinol derivative. Clin Pharmacol Ther. 1975;18:720–6. https://doi.org/10.1002/cpt1975186720.
39. Lev-Ran S, Roerecke M, Le Foll B, George TP, McKenzie K, Rehm J. The association between cannabis use and depression: a systematic review and meta-analysis of longitudinal studies. Psychol Med. 2014;44:797–810. https://doi.org/10.1017/S0033291713001438.
40. Ligresti A, De Petrocellis L, Di Marzo V. From phytocannabinoids to cannabinoid receptors and endocannabinoids: pleiotropic physiological and pathological roles through complex pharmacology. Physiol Rev. 2016;96:1593–659. https://doi.org/10.1152/physrev.00002.2016.
41. Livne O, Shmulewitz D, Lev-Ran S, Hasin DS. DSM-5 cannabis withdrawal syndrome: demographic and clinical correlates in U.S. adults. Drug Alcohol Depend. 2018;0 https://doi.org/10.1016/j.drugalcdep.2018.09.005.
42. Lopez-Quintero C, Pérez de los Cobos, J, Hasin DS, Okuda M, Wang S, Grant BF, Blanco C. Probability and predictors of transition from first use to dependence on nicotine, alcohol, cannabis, and cocaine: results of the National Epidemiologic Survey on Alcohol and Related Conditions (NESARC). Drug Alcohol Depend. 2011;115:120–30. https://doi.org/10.1016/j.drugalcdep.2010.11.004.
43. Lunn S, Diaz P, O'Hearn S, Cahill SP, Blake A, Narine K, Dyck JRB. Human pharmacokinetic parameters of orally administered Δ9-tetrahydrocannabinol capsules are altered by fed versus fasted conditions and sex differences. Cannabis Cannabinoid Res. 2019;4:255–64. https://doi.org/10.1089/can.2019.0037.
44. MacCallum CA, Russo EB. Practical considerations in medical cannabis administration and dosing. Eur J Intern Med. 2018;49:12–9. https://doi.org/10.1016/j.ejim.2018.01.004.
45. Maida V, Shi RB, Fazzari FGT, Zomparelli L. Topical cannabis-based medicines - a novel adjuvant treatment for venous leg ulcers: an open-label trial. Exp Dermatol. 2021; https://doi.org/10.1111/exd.14395.
46. Maida V, Shi RB, Fazzari FGT, Zomparelli L. Topical cannabis-based medicines – a novel paradigm and treatment for non-uremic calciphylaxis leg ulcers: an open label trial. Int Wound J. 2020;17:1508–16. https://doi.org/10.1111/iwj.13484.
47. McPartland JM, MacDonald C, Young M, Grant PS, Furkert DP, Glass M. Affinity and efficacy studies of Tetrahydrocannabinolic acid a at cannabinoid receptor types one and two. Cannabis Cannabinoid Res. 2017;2:87–95. https://doi.org/10.1089/can.2016.0032.
48. Millar SA, Stone NL, Yates AS, O'Sullivan SE. A systematic review on the pharmacokinetics of cannabidiol in humans. Front Pharmacol. 2018;9 https://doi.org/10.3389/fphar.2018.01365.
49. Mongeau-Pérusse V, Jutras-Aswad D. Challenging CBD protective effect against THC-related outcomes: a call for robust clinical trials. Addiction. 2021;116:207–8. https://doi.org/10.1111/add.15254.
50. Moreno-Sanz G. Can you pass the acid test? Critical review and novel therapeutic perspectives of Δ9-Tetrahydrocannabinolic acid A. Cannabis Cannabinoid Res. 2016;1:124–30. https://doi.org/10.1089/can.2016.0008.
51. Page RL, Allen LA, Kloner RA, Carriker CR, Catherine M, Morris AA, Piano MR, Rana JS, Saucedo JF, null null. Medical Marijuana, recreational cannabis, and cardiovascular health: a scientific statement from the American Heart Association. Circulation. 2020;142:e131–52. https://doi.org/10.1161/CIR.0000000000000883.
52. Palomares B, Garrido-Rodriguez M, Gonzalo-Consuegra C, Gómez-Cañas M, Saen-Oon S, Soliva R, Collado JA, Fernández-Ruiz J, Morello G, Calzado MA, Appendino G, Muñoz E.

Δ9-Tetrahydrocannabinolic acid alleviates collagen-induced arthritis: role of PPARγ and CB1 receptors. Br J Pharmacol. 2020;177:4034–54. https://doi.org/10.1111/bph.15155.
53. Patel J, Marwaha R. Cannabis Use Disorder. In: StatPearls. Treasure Island: StatPearls Publishing; 2021.
54. Pelayo-Terán JM, Suárez-Pinilla P, Chadi N, Crespo-Facorro B. Gene-environment interactions underlying the effect of cannabis in first episode psychosis. Curr Pharm Des. 2012;18:5024–35. https://doi.org/10.2174/138161212802884609.
55. Roepke S. Treating nightmares in posttraumatic stress disorder with Dronabinol: a randomized controlled study (THC PTSD-trial) (Clinical trial registration No. NCT04448808). clinicaltrials.gov, 2021.
56. Russell C, Rueda S, Room R, Tyndall M, Fischer B. Routes of administration for cannabis use - basic prevalence and related health outcomes: a scoping review and synthesis. Int J Drug Policy. 2017;52:87–96. https://doi.org/10.1016/j.drugpo.2017.11.008.
57. Russo Ethan B. Taming THC: potential cannabis synergy and phytocannabinoid-terpenoid entourage effects. Br J Pharmacol. 2011;163:1344–64. https://doi.org/10.1111/j.1476-5381.2011.01238.x.
58. Sánchez-Diz P, Estany-Gestal A, Aguirre C, Blanco A, Carracedo A, Ibáñez L, Passiu M, Provezza L, Ramos-Ruiz R, Ruiz B, Salado-Valdivieso I, Velasco EA, Figueiras A. Prevalence of CYP2C9 polymorphisms in the south of Europe. Pharmacogenomics J. 2009;9:306–10. https://doi.org/10.1038/tpj.2009.16.
59. Sawler J, Stout JM, Gardner KM, Hudson D, Vidmar J, Butler L, Page JE, Myles S. The genetic structure of Marijuana and Hemp. PLoS One. 2015;10:e0133292. https://doi.org/10.1371/journal.pone.0133292.
60. Scherma M, Masia P, Deidda M, Fratta W, Tanda G, Fadda P. New perspectives on the use of cannabis in the treatment of psychiatric disorders. Medicines (Basel). 2018;5 https://doi.org/10.3390/medicines5040107.
61. Sharma P, Murthy P, Bharath MMS. Chemistry, metabolism, and toxicology of cannabis: clinical implications. Iran J Psychiatry. 2012;7:149–56.
62. Shen JJ, Shan G, Kim PC, Yoo JW, Dodge-Francis C, Lee Y-J. Trends and related factors of cannabis-associated emergency department visits in the United States: 2006-2014. J Addict Med. 2019;13:193–200. https://doi.org/10.1097/ADM.0000000000000479.
63. Sihota A, Smith BK, Ahmed S-A, Bell A, Blain A, Clarke H, Cooper ZD, Cyr C, Daeninck P, Deshpande A, Ethans K, Flusk D, Le Foll B, Milloy M-J, Moulin DE, Naidoo V, Ong M, Perez J, Rod K, Sealey R, Sulak D, Walsh Z, O'Connell C. Consensus-based recommendations for titrating cannabinoids and tapering opioids for chronic pain control. Int J Clin Pract. 2020:e13871. https://doi.org/10.1111/ijcp.13871.
64. Silvestro S, Mammana S, Cavalli E, Bramanti P, Mazzon E. Use of Cannabidiol in the treatment of epilepsy: efficacy and security in clinical trials. Molecules. 2019;24:1459. https://doi.org/10.3390/molecules24081459.
65. Solowij N, Broyd S, Greenwood L, van Hell H, Martelozzo D, Rueb K, Todd J, Liu Z, Galettis P, Martin J, Murray R, Jones A, Michie PT, Croft R. A randomised controlled trial of vaporised Δ9-tetrahydrocannabinol and cannabidiol alone and in combination in frequent and infrequent cannabis users: acute intoxication effects. Eur Arch Psychiatry Clin Neurosci. 2019;269:17–35. https://doi.org/10.1007/s00406-019-00978-2.
66. Standring S, Gray H, editors. Gray's anatomy: the anatomical basis of clinical practice. 40 reprinted ed. Edinburgh: Churchill Livingstone Elsevier; 2009.
67. Tambaro S, Bortolato M. Cannabinoid-related agents in the treatment of anxiety disorders: current knowledge and future perspectives. Recent Pat CNS Drug Discov. 2012;7:25–40.
68. Taschwer M, Schmid MG. Determination of the relative percentage distribution of THCA and Δ(9)-THC in herbal cannabis seized in Austria - impact of different storage temperatures on stability. Forensic Sci Int. 2015;254:167–71. https://doi.org/10.1016/j.forsciint.2015.07.019.
69. Valeant Canada Limited. Cesamet® (Nabilone) product monograph, 2009.

70. Vandrey R, Herrmann ES, Mitchell JM, Bigelow GE, Flegel R, LoDico C, Cone EJ. Pharmacokinetic profile of oral cannabis in humans: blood and oral fluid disposition and relation to pharmacodynamic outcomes. J Anal Toxicol. 2017;41:83–99. https://doi.org/10.1093/jat/bkx012.
71. Wachtel SR, ElSohly MA, Ross SA, Ambre J, de Wit H. Comparison of the subjective effects of Delta(9)-tetrahydrocannabinol and marijuana in humans. Psychopharmacology. 2002;161:331–9. https://doi.org/10.1007/s00213-002-1033-2.
72. Wall MB, et al. Dissociable effects of cannabis with and without cannabidiol on the human brain's resting-state functional connectivity. J Psychopharmacol. 2019;33:822–30.
73. Wilsey B, Marcotte TD, Deutsch R, Gouaux B, Sakai S, Donaghe H. Low dose vaporized cannabis significantly improves neuropathic pain. J Pain. 2013;14:136–48. https://doi.org/10.1016/j.jpain.2012.10.009.
74. York EMA., PharmD, MPH, CGP Associate Clinical Professor St John's University, College of Pharmacy &. Health Sciences Queens, New York Clinical Specialist Rite Aid Pharmacy Whitestone, New, 2014. Nonpsychotropic Medication-Induced Psychosis. U.S. Pharmacist.

Chapter 8
Psychoactive Effects of Cannabinoid-Based Medicines: Exploration and Inquiry

Contents

8.1 Introduction.......... 236
8.2 Terminology.......... 240
8.3 Cannabis Psychoactivity: Current Challenges.......... 241
8.3.1 The Complicated Social, Cultural, and Spiritual History of Cannabis Psychoactivity.......... 241
8.3.2 The Evidence Remains Mostly Anecdotal.......... 243
8.3.3 Our Understanding of the Neurocognitive Effects of THC Has Only Just Begun.......... 243
8.3.4 Management Guidelines for Cannabis Psychoactivity Are Not Available.......... 244
8.3.5 Cannabis Psychoactivity Is Common in Medical Cannabis Patients.......... 244
8.3.6 Avoiding Psychoactivity Is Possible, but Difficult...for Now.......... 245
8.3.7 Precise Dosing Guidelines Are Only Beginning to Emerge.......... 245
8.3.8 Prior Experience with Cannabis May Influence Tolerance to Psychoactivity and Even Psychotic-Like Reactions.......... 246
8.4 Basic Precautions.......... 247
8.4.1 Introducing Cannabis Early in the Course of Life-Limiting Illnesses.......... 247
8.4.2 Preventing Involuntary Intoxications.......... 248
8.4.3 Low Initial THC Dosing: The Cornerstone of Harm Reduction.......... 249
8.4.4 Route of Administration: Oral Versus Inhaled.......... 249
8.5 Preparing Patients for Cannabis Psychoactivity.......... 250
8.5.1 Set and Setting.......... 251
8.5.2 Integration.......... 252
8.5.3 Trauma Sensitivity.......... 252
8.6 Dealing with an Involuntary Intoxication (Bad Trip).......... 253
8.7 Overview of the Specific Neurocognitive Effects Associated with Cannabis Psychoactivity.......... 255
8.7.1 Slowed Down Perception of Time.......... 255
8.7.2 Metacognition: Thinking About Thinking.......... 257
8.7.3 Metacognition Versus Mind Wandering.......... 258
8.7.4 Metacognition Versus Insight.......... 259
8.7.5 Introspective and Mystical/Spiritual Reflections.......... 260
8.7.6 Reduced Working Memory and Divided Attention.......... 261

C. Cyr et al., *Cannabis and Cannabinoid-Based Medicines in Cancer Care*,
https://doi.org/10.1007/978-3-030-89918-9_8

8.7.7 Heightened Sense of Awareness and Nonspecific Amplification: The Effects of THC on the Triad Network – Default Mode, Salience, and Central Executive 263
8.7.8 Aversive Memory Extinction 270
8.8 Other Benefits of Cannabis Use in End of Life Situations 271
8.8.1 Cannabis and Creativity 271
8.8.2 Higher-Order Problem-Solving 271
8.8.3 Delaying Palliative Sedation 272
8.8.4 Coping with Forced Confinement 273
8.9 Conclusion 274
References 274

8.1 Introduction

> "The ceremonial and religious use of psychedelics are much older than the recreational uses and abuses. For most of their history, they have been mysterious, dangerous substances and must be treated respectfully." – Humphrey Osmond

Americans, in general, are not dying "good deaths." Rather, they often face the dying process marked by needless suffering and disregard for their wishes or values [22]. While the complex social, political, and cultural hurdles which continue to prevent many patients from obtaining quality end-of-life care are beyond the scope of this textbook, one could argue that improving access to potentially beneficial treatments which address emotional, existential, and spiritual suffering would certainly be a step in the right direction. Hence, it is not surprising to witness the growing interest in integrating cannabis and psychedelics in cancer and palliative care [3, 35].

It has been said that psychedelic experiences are like "going into the basement of your life with a bright searchlight." Consequently, this inward journey requires adequate preparation and a series of grounding strategies which can be provided by a qualified psychedelic-assisted psychotherapy (PAP) specialist. Compared to cannabis, the use of traditional psychedelics like psilocybin may in fact be better tolerated for these purposes since they do not produce significant cardiovascular effects via CB1 receptor activation. For these reasons, this chapter will address the necessary precautions for exploring the psychedelic effects associated with higher doses of THC. However, lower dose cannabis psychoactivity may provide other interesting benefits which may be clinically useful in advanced cancer and palliative care.

The idea of inducing psychedelic experiences during the dying process probably predates the experiments carried out by Aldous Huxley with LSD in the 1960s and may even go back thousands of years. Huxley was first introduced to mescaline by Canadian psychiatrist Humphrey Osmond. While taking care of his wife Maria during her final days battling cancer, he became convinced of the benefits of using psychedelics as a means to better understand and cope with death. In a touching account where she was given LSD in her last hours, he later argued that psychedelic experiences in the dying may help create a deeply meaningful setting which enables closer human contact [35]. Huxley himself was later diagnosed with cancer and also used LSD during his final hours. In the following decade, further research aimed at exploring the effects of LSD on death anxiety were briefly carried out before psychedelic research was halted in the early 1970s [66, 67].

Although Huxley's experimentations offers a compelling argument for the use of psychedelics to address end-of-life anxiety, the information provided in this chapter should not be interpreted as a sanction for the precipitous use of psychedelic doses of THC to advanced cancer or palliative care patients. Rather, the aim is to impart healthcare providers, patients, and their caregivers with the ability to take the necessary precautions which may permit a safe and gradual introduction to the psycholytic and psychedelic effects of cannabis in certain carefully chosen individuals while preventing negative outcomes resulting from these unique experiences.

With increasing public awareness of the relative safety of psycholytic and psychedelic experiences associated with using moderate to higher-dose THC, clinicians may have no choice but to get acquainted with these peculiar effects. Surveys have indeed shown that 80% of medical cannabis patients regularly take psychoactive doses of cannabis and most do so without medical supervision [56, 124]. Although these effects seem to be generally well tolerated, the acute and long-term risks need to be taken into consideration before patients begin to explore higher-dose psychoactivity, particularly if long-term survival is expected.

Cannabis is like any medicine. Clinicians who choose to add it to their armamentarium must understand how to better predict and manage effects at all dosage ranges. While no official guidelines exist regarding the therapeutic windows of either THC or CBD, recent consensus statements from experienced cannabis clinicians have suggested that total daily THC doses beyond 30–40 mg are usually not required to obtain clinical benefits, at least for situations regarding symptom management, and are in fact associated with more adverse outcomes [13]. These recommendations place the standard "therapeutic" use of THC at a much lower dosage range than that encountered with recreational use. The use of much higher doses is associated with more pronounced psychoactivity and may cross the "toxic psychosis threshold" in inexperienced individuals. Hence, they are not advisable, at least if the intended goal is symptom control [79].

The subjective reactions encountered at higher THC doses have a curious paradoxical nature. They are reported to be aversive in some circumstances and meaningful in others [36]. Similar paradoxical reactions also occur with other psychedelics such as LSD or psilocybin when crossing their respective "toxic" threshold dose. Likewise, high doses of traditional psychedelics will produce either unpleasant psychotic-like reactions or, in more appropriate or controlled settings, may give rise to powerful meaningful experiences.

Every psychedelic compound is considered to have a threshold dose (THC, LSD, psilocybin, or other) which produces a complete dissolution of the ego (psycholytic effect). When this occurs, psychological boundaries and egoic defense mechanisms diminish or completely dissolve, and the subjective effects are accompanied by a state often described as one of heightened psychological vulnerability and suggestibility. It is important to remember that transient psychotic experiences, whether drug induced or not, do not necessarily equate with a negative outcomes. In fact, some authors suggest that occasional psychotic-like reactions that do not cause significant impairment or distress usually do not lead to a clinical diagnosis [38]. Hence, the distressing psychotic reactions witnessed in emergency rooms following intoxications with cannabis are most likely the result of mismanaged psychedelic experiences. While these effects are usually short lived in most individuals, the risks involved with repeated unsupervised experiences of this nature, particularly over a long period of time, have been clearly linked with developing chronic and persistent mental health problems [128].

Written accounts of higher-dose cannabis use conducted in a more controlled and secure environment have also been shown to exhibit diametrically different effects. When experienced as being positive, some authors have described them as states of "oceanic boundlessness," producing long-lasting meaningful insights [36]. As such, inexperienced individuals who are exposing themselves to repeated psychedelic experiences require close clinical monitoring and appropriate counseling in order to help with proper integration of their experiences.

The therapeutic effects of THC on the CB1 receptors found in the central nervous system are complex and do not readily produce psycholitic or psychedelic effects at small doses. In fact, THC may exhibit multiple therapeutic windows [49], with clinical benefits beginning even at very low "microgram" doses [5]. This first "low-dose" therapeutic window may occur as a result of gently supplementing the endocannabinoid system (ECS), which some authors have suggested can become deficient or disrupted in its ability to respond adequately to stress. In which case, a small nudge may gear neurotransmitter release downwards to a more homeostatic level [107]. This gentle agonistic activity at the CB1 receptor and slightly reduced neurotransmitter release in certain key regions of the CNS may in fact be reestablishing a more appropriate *endocannabinoid tone*. This would explain many of the reported clinical effects of THC on brain regions regulating physiological functions such as pain, sleep, mood, and appetite. Conversely, when patients do not respond at this dosage range, this may be an indication of a minimally impaired endocannabinoid system (ECS) or one which is not greatly involved in the disease process. The low dosage range of THC which has been found to aid in common symptom management may start as low as 0.5 mg with benefits rarely encountered beyond a total daily dose of 40 mg, as mentioned earlier [5, 79].

However, THC is most often used at a second, intermediary therapeutic window. Patients are more likely to skip the microgram dosage range unwittingly, since available formulations are often too potent to make this feasible. On the other hand, many others simply do not respond to low doses of THC and may be tempted to increase the dosage in order to obtain symptom relief. There is little data to support the use of higher doses of THC for symptom management. In fact, a higher "intermediate" dosage range may shift the homeostatic equilibrium of neurotransmitter release into a zone of increased altered brain connectivity and more pronounced subjective effects. In this dosage range, euphoria may be prominent while maintaining the sense of self and the ego's defense mechanisms below the psychedelic range. This is often considered a state of increased introspection and awareness of ego defenses such as projection, denial, and displacement. This may also be accompanied by a sense that one understands these reactions and the unconscious mechanisms and impacts of the choices which result from their activation [51]. The therapeutic benefits encountered at this dosage range remain controversial. Although many patients claim that euphoria and insight catalysis are subjectively beneficial, the long-term mental health risks need to be taken into consideration in otherwise young or healthy patients [11, 54]. The complex relationship between cannabis psychoactivity and negative cognitive and mental health outcomes is not yet fully understood and will not be dealt with in this chapter. Those who wish to explore this subject in more detail, however, must be reminded that studies looking into the negative impacts of prolonged cannabis use are mostly based on the observation of chronic heavy users and conclusions cannot yet be generalized to include medically supervised patients using standardized dosing regimens [89, 132]. In fact, observational studies of medical cannabis patients seem to indicate overall improvements in functionality and distinct neural activation patterns compared with "self-medicating" heavy users [89].

A third possible therapeutic window for THC may also exist and would be encountered at very high doses that produces the most pronounced effects on neural networks, possibly by dimerization of CB1 and 5HT2A receptors [59]. For the time being, the effects encountered at this dosage range have left many clinicians perplexed as to their potential clinical value and are relegated to the category of adverse effects or intoxication in clinical trials, as mentioned earlier. The integration of psychedelic effects encountered at these much higher doses of THC requires a deeper understanding of the impact of CB1 receptor agonists in neuropsychiatry, which will be covered in this chapter.

Many available cannabis products remain notoriously mislabeled and place patients at risk of involuntary overdoses. Until standardized formulations with more predictable pharmacokinetics replace presently available products, most patients using cannabis will experience some form of psychoactivity at one point or another, and this should always be considered as a possible outcome in cannabis-naive patients. While cannabis psychoactivity and psychedelic effects are often well tolerated in experienced cannabis users, these can be very traumatizing experiences in unprepared or cannabis-naive individuals. Unlike psilocybin or LSD, the dosage ranges of THC necessary to produce psychedelic effects vary widely and are often accompanied by other significant psychological symptoms such as paranoia, anxiety, dissociative states, and cardiovascular side effects such as hypotension and reflex tachycardia. Hence, cannabis may be a less desirable compound for inexperienced cancer patients who wish to explore the benefits of psychedelic experiences, particularly when introduced late in the course of the illness. However, in patients who are well accustomed to the psycholitic and dissociative effects of cannabis, this may provide a further option when nearing the threshold for palliative sedation.

Patients who wish to explore the psychoactive effects mentioned earlier must also be cautioned that tolerance to many effects such as euphoria can occur quite rapidly. Limiting the frequency of this dosage regimen, at least early in the course of the disease, will permit them to continue obtaining benefits and avoid significant drug tolerance. For patients with a history of well-tolerated psychoactive experiences using cannabis, the occasional use of moderate to high doses may, in many cases, gradually unlock constrained neural pathways and lead to a more favorable environment for introspection, creative problem-solving, and improved interpersonal connection. This chapter will therefore aim to demonstrate that cannabis may not only serve as an adjunct for symptom management but also provide an opportunity for deeper healing and increased acceptance of the dying process through insight catalysis.

8.2 Terminology

The term "endocannabinoidome" is still not widely used by clinicians and researchers, and in order to avoid confusion, its use to describe the *expanded* endocannabinoid system (ECS) will be restricted to the first chapter of this book. For the present chapter, the more commonly used term "endocannabinoid system (ECS)" will be used to describe most concepts relating to both the more specific canonical receptors and enzymes and the larger system of molecular targets and ligands. The "endocannabinoidome" will only be mentioned in order to point out a clinically relevant difference between these two related concepts.

"Cannabinoid-Based Medicines" will be used preferentially as a general umbrella term to describe all compounds containing either approved or non-approved cannabinoids derived from either natural or synthetically produced cannabis. The term "cannabis" and "medical cannabis" will only be used contextually when discussing the use of plant-based products specifically, and "THC" will be used when pertaining to psychoactivity.

The term "cannabis psychoactivity" has generated much debate. Many authors tend to use the term as a reference to the higher-dose "recreational" or "intoxicating" effects of cannabis, while others have proposed that the term should include the effects on all cognitive functions relating to mood, thoughts, and behaviors, including clinically relevant symptoms such as anxiety or insomnia and even the antipsychotic/anxiolytic properties associated with CBD. For the purposes of this chapter, the psychoactive effects of cannabis will refer specifically to THC-*induced* effects and not those related to symptom management. The exact dosage ranges of THC which produces specific psychoactive effects vary according to many individual factors. *Low*-dose anxiolytic and hypnotic effects, which are often reported with little or no subjective or objective signs of intoxication, are reviewed in Chap. 5. This chapter will focus on the potential benefits of further *moderate-to-high* psycholytic "recreational" doses and *very high* psychedelic dosing ranges.

Non-ordinary states of consciousness which lead to mystical or spiritual experiences are described in many ways. American psychologist Abraham Maslow described them as *peak experiences*: "rare, exciting, oceanic, deeply moving, exhilarating, elevating experiences that generate an advanced form of perceiving reality, and are even mystic and magical in their effect upon the experimenter." These types of experiences have also been associated with other activities, such as sensory deprivation, yogic practices, and even in high-level sporting events. Other authors and researchers have used similar scientific terminology such as "Mystical-Type Experiences" or "Non-dual Experiences." R.M. Bucke called it the "Cosmic Consciousness," Aldous Huxley refers to it as the Source of the "Perennial Philosophy," and William Miller calls it the trigger of "Quantum Change." Related philosophical terms also include Epiphany, Enlightenment, Transcendental Awareness, the Numinous, the Ground of Being, the One, the Ground Luminosity of Pure Awareness, the Void that Contains all Reality, oceanic boundlessness and the Nameless. At first glance, many of these expressions may seem better suited for shamanic rituals rather than for modern Western medicine. Thus, the accepted medical terminology describing these therapeutically induced states of consciousness remains to be determined.

Other terms used to describe the subjective features of cannabis psychoactivity which are not necessarily psychedelic in nature include: increased sense of connection with oneself or others, sensory enhancement, a heightened sense of awareness or dishabituation (a tendency to notice things which one is normally unaware), free play of the imagination, increased sensitivity to sound and greater appreciation of the subtleties of music, insight catalysis, increased tendency for self-exploration and enhanced creativity, to name a few [36]. However, recent neuroimaging studies have provided us with a better understanding of the mechanisms behind the unique subjective effects of cannabis psychoactivity, and a more neurobiologically driven terminology is slowly emerging. These include such terms as: activated reward pathways, emotional and attentional processing, activation of the default mode, salience and central executive networks, aversive memory modulation, metacognition, and other brain region-specific disruptions in connectivity.

Although a full comprehension of the effects of cannabis on the central nervous system is far from complete, and beyond the scope of this chapter, an attempt will be made to bridge the traditional vernacular with the current understanding of pronounced CB1 receptor activation on the neural networks involved in cannabis psychoactivity.

8.3 Cannabis Psychoactivity: Current Challenges

8.3.1 The Complicated Social, Cultural, and Spiritual History of Cannabis Psychoactivity

When William O'Shaughnessy returned from India in 1843, he published *On the Preparations of the Indian Hemp, or Gunjah*, which formally introduced cannabis to Western medicine. It became the first widely available compound to possess psychotomimetic properties and grew in popularity despite its reputation for causing serious and unpredictable adverse reactions. In France, where cannabis entered circulation following colonial excursions in Egypt at the end of the eighteenth century, its use also quickly spread, particularly as an object of curiosity among various intellectual circles. Cannabis social clubs sprung up where early experimenters began to investigate whether certain factors could reduce the unpredictability of the curious effects, long known as the *fantasia* [81]. The active compound responsible for cannabis psychoactivity was not to be discovered for another century, but many inferred that the varying potency of available products was clearly an important factor to consider, and every new arrival required a careful approach and re-titration. However, this troublesome variable did not deter their inquisitiveness, and further explorations helped to delineate several other external or "non-drug" factors that seemed to play a significant role in determining the outcome of cannabis psychoactivity. Psychiatrist Jacques Joseph Moreau, founding member of the famous Parisian *Club des Hashischins,* extensively documented the experiences of his guests who would ingest *heroic* doses of cannabis and found striking similarities with *mental alienation* (schizophrenia). He promptly noticed that these effects varied from one individual to the next but also observed that the same individual could present drastically different effects even when taking a similar dose. His book, *Du Haschich et de l'Aliénation Mentale: études psychologiques,* published in 1845, is considered one of the pioneering works of psychopharmacology and provided precious insights on the biological origins of psychotic illnesses and on the importance of *set* and *setting* when dealing with psychedelic experiences.

Consequently, the use of cannabis for purposes other than symptom management remains worrisome for many modern clinicians. There are clear risks involved with these dramatic experiences, particularly with frequent usage. Daily use often serves as a red flag in detecting cannabis use disorder in an otherwise young or healthy individual and has been implicated in the development of many chronic mental illnesses. This pattern of use may not carry the same long-term risks in an advanced cancer or palliative care patient, however.

Habitual cannabis users come in many forms. Many will eventually spiral into a lonely foray of nihilistic self-exploration, disconnecting from their community and friends. Others will fall prey to the clutches of paranoia, misinterpreting reality cues and eventually crystallizing a belief system which leads them into a chronic psychotic illness. However, others manage to become successful artists and business people, wearing tailored suits and who chose to live in the moment with a certain neurochemical assistance.

And then there are a few habitual cannabis users who choose a path outside of prevailing social norms, as decluttered and unhindered souls, living off the land, seeking connection with others and nature. This simple lifestyle does not necessarily equate with a low level of social functioning, as the Rastafari can attest. This religious community, whose faith has survived in a hostile environment for nearly a century, was finally given its right to exist without threat of violence when cannabis was legalized in Jamaica in 2015. Rastafarianism has long adopted cannabis as part of its sacraments and regards the plant not as a product for human consumption, but rather as nature's attempt to communicate with mankind. They have since learned to harness the empathogenic nature of cannabis and channel the experience towards increased relatedness and the development of a more compassionate view of the world.

Thus, the spiritual nature of the cannabis experience is fundamental to understanding its therapeutic possibilities. Presently, this intangible potential is seldom taken into consideration when discussing the uses of cannabis in medicine. This is regrettable, since death and grieving are areas of great concern for all physicians. The primary focus of cannabis as a means to reduce specific symptom burden and our reliance on standard scientific litmus tests may need to be challenged in order to fully integrate and appreciate this class of compounds.

8.3.2 The Evidence Remains Mostly Anecdotal

The benefits of cannabis psychoactivity are still being debated, even at lower or moderate dosage ranges [91]. These are often assessed in clinical trials, particularly the anxiolytic and hypnotic effects. However, they are still considered as having little therapeutic value when targeting mental health conditions primarily, and few comparative studies with standard treatments have been carried out. In one systematic review, however, small improvements in anxiety were noted in individuals with other coexisting conditions, such as chronic noncancer pain or multiple sclerosis [15].

Cannabis produces a wide range of other dose-dependent psychoactive effects. In addition to reduced anxiety and mild euphoria, which are often encountered at low-to-moderate doses [79], increased CB1 receptor activation in certain key brain networks eventually leads to a progressive unlocking of conscious control over several higher cognitive functions and loosening of the ego. At very high doses, a cascade of unique cognitive effects can eventually lead to complete *ego dissolution* or *ego death*, which are popular terms still used to describe the effects encountered with high-dose cannabis and traditional psychedelics such as LSD or psilocybin. While the pharmacological effects of these compounds may differ somewhat, recent preclinical and neuroimaging studies examining the effects of THC on the 5HT2A receptor are suggesting that the downstream effect on the neural networks and corresponding brain regions responsible for *dissolving* the ego may in fact be similar and are helping to further our understanding of consciousness beyond psychoanalytic concepts.

8.3.3 Our Understanding of the Neurocognitive Effects of THC Has Only Just Begun

Over the last 20 years, functional magnetic resonance imaging (fMRI) and other powerful technologies made it possible to examine living brains in increasingly sophisticated ways. Neuroscientists started searching for the mechanisms which explain our mental faculties and have made great strides in understanding the neural foundations of perception, attention, learning, memory, decision-making, motor control, and other classic categories of mental activity. For example, the prefrontal cortex, situated just behind the forehead, has long been seen as the seat of judgment. Behind it lies the motor cortex, responsible for planning and coordinating movement; to the sides, the temporal lobes, crucial for memory and the processing of emotion; above them, the somatosensory cortex; and behind them, the visual cortex. The amygdala is considered the seat of emotional processing, while the hippocampus is the brain region mostly involved in memory.

However, things may not be as clear-cut as it seems. For example, memory also requires brain networks other than the hippocampus, and the hippocampus is turning out to be key to a growing number of cognitive processes other than memory. The cerebellum was thought to be dedicated almost exclusively to motor control, but recent studies have found that it's also instrumental in attentional processes, emotional regulation, language processing, and decision-making [98]. The basal ganglia, another ancient part of the brain usually associated with motor control, has been similarly implicated in several high-level cognitive processes as well.

As we will see in a further section, recent functional neuroimaging studies are providing interesting clues that may help to explain the complex neurocognitive effects of THC on these neural networks, many of which are densely populated with CB1 receptors. And as a result, the endocannabinoid system is beginning to take on a greater role in our understanding of mental diseases, emotions, personality traits, dreams, and of consciousness itself [88].

8.3.4 Management Guidelines for Cannabis Psychoactivity Are Not Available

Managing cannabis psychoactivity may seem challenging for inexperienced clinicians. Most of us have not been trained in psychedelic medicine, and many are still unfamiliar with the unusual but necessary precautions aimed at avoiding serious adverse events [80, 125]. Mitigating acute adverse effects and long-term health risks requires careful monitoring, particularly in older or frail patients [4, 119], and detailed instructions on this subject can be found in Chaps. 6 and 7. This chapter will review basic precautions and focus on examining the characteristic features of cannabis psychoactivity, their underlying neurological mechanisms, and the possible clinical benefits for advanced cancer and palliative care patients.

Other cannabis-related issues lack clear guidance, such as managing involuntary intoxications, which will be dealt with in a later section. Cannabis use disorder is another possible outcome for any patient exploring the psychoactive effects of cannabis. However, unless long-term survival is expected, escaping the torments of a terminal illness and finding a space of deeper introspection and creative problem-solving by way of higher-dose cannabis psychoactivity may outweigh the need for sustained high levels of functionality in this patient population.

8.3.5 Cannabis Psychoactivity Is Common in Medical Cannabis Patients

Psychoactive effects related to the use of medical cannabis are common and usually well tolerated. Surveys have shown that approximately 80% of medical cannabis patients report voluntarily taking higher psychoactive doses, with the majority self-medicating without clinical supervision [116, 124]. Psychoactivity is also difficult to avoid with the use of presently available cannabis products containing any significant amount of THC, even in a regulated market. However, most patients who have access to standardized products eventually learn to self-titrate and after a period of experimentation can usually reduce the risks of experiencing levels of psychoactivity that will impair their relationship with the outside world.

Since most patients will experience these effects, broaching the subject, particularly with cannabis-naive individuals, is an important harm reduction intervention. Patients may be curious and wish to know "what it's like" to experience these unique effects. One way to begin describing the vast consciousness-altering world of cannabis psychoactivity is to describe one of the most consistently reported features of the experience: change in time perception [49, 119]. This effect has been shown to be unrelated to dose [7] and may vary subjectively from one experience to the other. This concept may assist in better understanding and further explaining the resulting impact of altered connectivity in other neural networks and their ensuing subjective effects. This will be dealt with in more detail in a further section.

8.3.6 Avoiding Psychoactivity Is Possible, but Difficult...for Now

Cannabis plant-based medicines have a bioavailability problem. Dried flowers and extracts often exhibit wide-ranging potency and pharmacokinetics, and *prescribing* medical cannabis with a reasonable level of accuracy remains an unresolved issue, even in structured regulatory frameworks. In Canada, cannabis for medical use is still authorized to patients solely in grams per day of dried flowers, without any further requirements pertaining to dosing of individual cannabinoids [71]. This practice is potentially hazardous since patients are free to choose the potency and the route of administration of any product. As seen in Chap. 6, unreliable testing and labeling persist in many jurisdictions, and, compounded with the inherently erratic pharmacokinetics of presently available cannabis products, maintaining plasma levels within a sub-psychoactive therapeutic window remains challenging [56, 71]. Fortunately, several of these pharmacological hurdles are now being addressed. Newer formulations including oil capsules with precise doses and natural cannabis-based compounds using nanoparticle technology are providing more predictable total drug exposure. Novel synthetic cannabinoids, including peripherally acting compounds, are also under development and will provide robust cannabinoid receptor activity without the risks of CNS cognitive impairment. When these new products reach the market, simplified prescribing regimens for cannabinoid based medicines will become more easily accessible and eventually resemble traditional pharmaceuticals. However, it is likely that many patients will prefer turning to "traditional" cannabis products, which will remain more affordable for many.

8.3.7 Precise Dosing Guidelines Are Only Beginning to Emerge

The definition of a standard "dose" of cannabis is still undetermined [55, 133]. This issue is particularly important since the risks of hypotension, syncope, psychosis, dissociative states, and anxiety attacks have been widely reported in inexperienced recreational cannabis users who often accidentally consume an unspecified or toxic dose. However, these dramatic events are extremely rare when medical cannabis patients are closely monitored and informed on the basic "start low, go slow, stay low" titration principle [79]. In fact, serious dose related adverse reactions should theoretically *never* occur with proper guidance and with the use of products that have been accurately tested for potency. The subject of initial dosage and titration is studied in more detail in Chap. 7.

8.3.8 Prior Experience with Cannabis May Influence Tolerance to Psychoactivity and Even Psychotic-Like Reactions

Few studies have looked at the overall tolerability of cannabis in infrequent versus frequent users. Earlier publications mentioned that "experienced" users would report having some control over the degree to which they are involved in the subjective effects of cannabis [119]. This was initially thought to be a consequence of behavioral compensation. However, recent data suggests that regular use of cannabis induces tolerance to certain effects, possibly via CB1 receptor downregulation. PET scan studies have also demonstrated that this desensitization may be more pronounced in cortical brain regions, while subcortical brain regions remain mostly unaffected [25]. This may explain why heavy users display reduced impairments in some neurocognitive functions, while other negative effects remain unchanged [57]. When compared to occasional cannabis users, the acute effects of THC on divided attention, learning, and memory are blunted in frequent users, whereas impairments on reaction time do not seem to diminish [103]. Compared to infrequent users, regular users were also more accurate in their measure of the passage of time [7, 49].

Cannabis is also known to produce transient psychotic-like reactions and anxiety symptoms which are commonly encountered in cannabis-naive individuals who have not yet mastered the concept of initial dosage and titration. Accidental overdoses in experienced users may also occur, particularly when using unregulated edible products containing an undetermined amount of THC. However, anecdotal accounts of seasoned users being able to "come down" from cannabis-induced psychotic reactions have been reported since the mid-nineteenth century [102]. Recent studies have shown that even moderate previous exposure to cannabis may modulate these acute effects. In a recent double-blind randomized controlled trial comparing abstinent subjects having either low (less than 5 lifetime joints smoked) or modest (±9 lifetime joints smoked) cannabis exposure, participants with modest prior exposure demonstrated a blunted effect of THC on attentional salience and fear processing compared with those with low exposure. Attentional salience and emotional (or fear) processing refer to neural mechanisms that have been proposed to be involved in psychotic experiences and will be discussed in more detail in a separate section below.

This study suggests that individuals having even a modest experience with cannabis psychoactivity present less THC-induced psychotic symptoms than those with fewer cannabis experiences and also seem to recruit different brain areas to process attentional salient and emotional stimuli [31]. Written accounts dating back to the 1850s were indeed reporting that individuals more familiar with cannabis were thought to somehow "learn" to better manage some of the negative subjective effects such as paranoia and anxiety and also exhibit the ability to "come down" from states of marked intoxication [119]. These recent findings may therefore finally provide a neurophysiological basis explaining why the response in cannabis-naive subjects appears to be more variable and unpredictable than in experienced users.

For this reason, early introduction of cannabis in cancer and palliative care patients may be preferable in order to develop tolerance to mild psychoactive effects before global functioning and health status begin to decline. Consequently, it may also help to reduce the risk of future adverse reactions in patients whishing to explore higher dose psychoactivity.

8.4 Basic Precautions

Cannabis is not for everyone. Like with other types of medications, such as antidepressants, certain individuals do not develop a tolerance to even low doses of THC. However, risks of developing an initial undesirable adverse reaction can be reduced significantly by ruling out major contraindications, addressing trauma-sensitive individuals, and reviewing possible drug interactions (see Chaps. 5 and 6). Patients deemed to be appropriate candidates for a trial of cannabis can still present unforeseeable reactions, as seen with many other drugs such as opioids. However, this is considered a rare occurrence in the medical cannabis community, as long as the initial dosage remains low. A rich history of clinical experience dating back nearly 200 years coupled with recent and ongoing research has provided us with many valuable clues which can help in further reducing the probability of experiencing serious or unpleasant reactions [12, 87, 96, 102].

8.4.1 Introducing Cannabis Early in the Course of Life-Limiting Illnesses

Needless to say, it may take some time for cannabis-naive individuals to understand and manage the precarious emotional state which is produced by higher-dose cannabis psychoactivity. In some cases, it may require weeks or months to master the necessary elements of dose, set, and setting which will impact the overall benefit which can be drawn from these experiences. Hence, early introduction of cannabis-based medicines may provide cancer patients a window of opportunity to acclimatize themselves with psychoactivity.

Tolerance to increasing doses of cannabis can be described as having two phases. The initial tolerance phase involves physical and cognitive symptoms such as headache, dry mouth, dizziness, fatigue, and nausea. Most individuals will notice a gradual reduction of these symptoms over a few days or weeks.

As we will see later in this chapter, higher THC dosages produce an increase in the disruption of connectivity in the limbic system, the triad of default mode, salience and executive networks, the prefrontal cortex, and other brain regions.

Beyond a certain threshold dose, individuals will begin to gradually perceive a variety of subjective psychoactive effects that are unique to cannabis. These effects result in a partial loss of conscious control over attentional, emotional, and cognitive processing, which many may find difficult to endure, at least initially. Cannabis psychoactivity is considered by many to be a journey of exploration into the inner workings of human consciousness, and it may take several attempts before becoming acquainted with the feeling of having a reduced capacity to control the influx of unconscious material into the field of awareness.

With experience and counseling, most individuals eventually begin to understand the benefits of this shift in perspective. Considering the often unpredictable trajectory of cancer patients, who may exhibit a prolonged period of relative stability in their health status followed by a short period of evident decline (Fig. 8.3), introducing cannabis early in the course of the illness provides for a greater length of time to adjust to the particularities of cannabis psychoactivity.

8.4.2 Preventing Involuntary Intoxications

Preventing cannabis-related toxicity begins with the same approach as one would take with any other pharmaceutical, beginning with an appropriate knowledge of clinical pharmacology, dosing, and drug interactions. A detailed examination of all these topics can be found in previous chapters. In order to highlight the complex nature of cannabis, and THC in particular, it is important to remember that the unique dose-dependent neurocognitive effects share many similarities with the effects of traditional psychedelic compounds, such as LSD and psilocybin. For this reason, management of cannabis-based medicines containing any significant amount of THC requires mastering an additional skill set which stems from psychedelic research and their related treatment protocols. Fortunately, a resurgence of interest in the clinical applications of psychedelics has provided us with a fresh reiteration of guidelines initially developed in the early 1960s [72, 78]. Recent studies have indeed confirmed many of the earlier observations which emphasized the need to apply certain precautions when dealing with compounds that reduce conscious control over higher-order cognitive processes. Psychedelics have been shown to produce states of increased suggestibility and psychological vulnerability, which can be extremely destabilizing in unprepared individuals. For this reason, exploring psychoactivity with the use of any psychedelic compound, including cannabis, requires sufficient preparation and integration. This section will review the basic precautions for higher-dose cannabis use and introduce the personal and environmental factors that need to be taken into consideration in order to provide a safe exploration of cannabis psychoactivity, particularly in frail patients.

A thorough understanding of the overall cognitive effects of high-dose THC and other psychedelics requires a basic conceptual knowledge of progressive *ego dissolution*. Also known as *ego loss* or *ego death*, these are terms derived from Jungian psychoanalysis that describe the "loss of subjective identity" [85]. Recently, however, a better understanding and a more precise terminology have emerged which help describe the inner workings of both normal waking consciousness and the resulting *ego dissolution* which occurs as a result of high doses of THC and the use of other psychedelics [6, 63, 101]. In other words, the uncoupling of attentional processes from emotional and executive functions creates an experience during which the very notion of *self* gradually shifts from the unconscious realm and enters the conscious field of awareness and can thus become a subject for metaphysical contemplation.

8.4.3 Low Initial THC Dosing: The Cornerstone of Harm Reduction

A large enough dose of THC can produce a pronounced psychotic reaction in any healthy individual, even with an optimal set and setting. The early written accounts of Charles Baudelaire and Jacques Joseph Moreau in the mid-nineteenth century describe individuals presenting auditory and visual hallucinations in a waking state. This suggests that these early cannabis experimenters were taking very large doses of THC, since extremely high doses of THC are required to produce these effects *without* sensory deprivation. It's also well known that the dosage threshold of THC which produces psychedelic effects can vary widely from one individual to the next. Many of these higher-risk patients can be identified during patient evaluation, however (see Chap. 6).

Unlike LSD and psilocybin, however, THC-induced psychedelic experiences can often be accompanied by significant cardiovascular side effects such as hypotension and reflex tachycardia. With the exception of accidental overdoses [30, 109, 130], which are still commonly seen with unregulated products or inexperienced cannabis consumers, avoiding psychedelic dosage ranges is generally straightforward by using a low starting dose of THC and slow titration. Once patients reach levels of mild psychoactivity, they can be reassessed in order to determine the overall tolerability and can then be counseled if they wish to pursue higher dosage ranges. Patients unfamiliar with cannabis should be discouraged from using cannabis for psychedelic purposes and should be reminded that cannabis is not the drug of choice for psychedelic-assisted psychotherapy (PAP).

8.4.4 Route of Administration: Oral Versus Inhaled

Most medical cannabis patients treated for persistent symptoms are more likely to derive benefits from orally administered products which provide a longer duration of action [71]. Even with slow titration, mild psychoactivity is almost inevitable with doses of THC between 5 and 10 mg in most cannabis-naive individuals [79]. Patients should be regularly assessed in order to determine the dosage range that produces mild psychoactivity. At this point, and if these effects are well tolerated, patients who may wish to explore further ego dissolution might prefer to try a vaporized method, at least initially. The reasons are twofold. Firstly, vaporized cannabis is easier to titrate, as the effects appear more rapidly. One or two inhalations of low-to-medium potency strains will ensure modest THC plasma levels. After 5 or 10 min, a further inhalation may be attempted. This reduces the risk of accidental overdose. Furthermore, if anxiety or paranoia should manifest themselves, the effects will be of much shorter duration than with the oral route, lasting 2–4 h instead of 6–12 h. This subject is discussed in more detail in Chap. 6.

This completes the pharmacological precautions for exploring higher-dose cannabis psychoactivity. Once proper dosing, titration, and route of administration issues have been well assimilated, counseling on the non-drug parameters that influence psychedelic experiences as well as ensuring access to post-experience integration will provide additional safeguards in preventing distressing psychological adverse events.

8.5 Preparing Patients for Cannabis Psychoactivity

The reemergence of psychedelic medicine is in full swing, and researchers have dusted off and updated early study protocols. It has now become clear that psychedelic experiences require a series of precautions and interventions in order to reduce adverse events and increase potential benefits. This applies to higher-dose cannabis use as well. However, it is recommended that patients first understand the effects of altered brain connectivity and ensuing shift in awareness before proceeding (see Section 5 of this chapter for a more detailed description).

Fortunately, most cannabis-naive individuals do not exhibit distressing reactions to cannabis. Regular inquiry on the subjective experience following mild psychoactivity can provide further reassurance and open the possibility for titrating to higher doses. Frail patients can be particularly sensitive to these effects and require frequent monitoring while becoming acclimatized to the effects of low-dose THC effects before titrating upwards.

As mentioned earlier, the most important factor to assimilate remains the initial dose of THC and slow titration towards higher dose exposure. Once this crucial information is well understood, the further concepts of *set*, *setting*, and *integration* can be broached. These notions are now considered fundamental principles of psychedelic-assisted psychotherapy (PAP) and are among the most important harm reduction strategies which will determine how psychedelic experience will unfold [52]. However, they have not yet been fully integrated in the field of psychopharmacology, where the pharmacological actions of drugs such as antidepressants are still considered fully responsible for the objective and subjective effects. Appropriate set and setting play a vital role in providing a safe environment for the psychoactive or psychedelic experience. The additional concept of *integration* can also contribute to a positive outcome.

8.5.1 Set and Setting

Set and setting refer to the psychological, social, and cultural factors which influence the subjective experience of psychedelic drugs and other psychoactive compounds. Early psychedelic experimenters quickly recognized that using compounds which increased suggestibility and psychological vulnerability required more than simply determining a safe and appropriate dose. The terms *set* and *setting* were originally coined by Timothy Leary during the early days of psychedelic research in the 1960s [72].

The *set* is generally described as the internal state of the individual, which includes personality traits, the level of preparation, and the intention for having the experience, as well as "mood, expectations, fears, wishes" [72]. Leary divided the *set* into two subcategories: *long-range* and *immediate*. "*Long-range*" *set* factors refer to past experiences and established personality traits, including unconscious fears and recent conflicts and trauma, while the "*immediate*" *set* factors relating to set refer to the expectations about the experience itself.

Preparing the "setting" is more straightforward and refers to the physical and social environment in which the experience is taking place, the cultural background, and, if other individuals are present, the quality of those personal relationships. The setting should be a safe and supportive environment, and all those present should be made aware of the heightened state of suggestibility and vulnerability of the subject.

The notion of integrating these non-drug parameters goes back much further than the 1960s, however. Ancient shamanic healing rituals were carefully orchestrated events intended to better manipulate and enhance the healing process. Later, when hashish arrived in Europe in the nineteenth century and introduced Western society to the first psychedelic compound, early drug explorers and notable luminaries were quick to realize the influence of the surroundings and the state of mind of the individual on the quality of the overall experience. As mentioned earlier, psychiatrist Jacques Joseph Moreau, who also supplied the drug to the *Club des Hashischins*, observed that identical doses would produce different outcomes in the same individual and that the effects were highly suggestible to external stimuli, noting that "everything that strikes [the user's] eyes and his ears. A word, a gesture, a look, a sound or the slightest noise, by demanding his attention, will confer a special character on his illusions" [12]. Charles Baudelaire, another famous member of the *Club des Hashischins*, observed that cannabis can "exaggerate not only the individual but any and all surroundings and circumstances in their life" and that "those who were burdened with family worries or a broken heart should be careful" since their tribulations would "sound like a death knell through their drunkenness and poison their pleasure." Theophile Gautier, another member of the *Club des Hashischins*, recalled the necessity of adequate preparation before consuming cannabis. He suggested a "tranquil frame of mind and body," which would predict "ineffable pleasure" to those who followed this advice but "terror" and "suffering" for those who would disregard it.

8.5.2 Integration

The concept of *integration* is a more recent addition to the theory of non-drug influences of psychedelic-assisted therapy and refers to the pre- and post-experience environment that assists in the assimilation of subjectively relevant impressions which arise during the experience. This new dimension, developed by Betty Eisner in 1997, drew attention to factors occurring before and after a psychedelic experience that influence the outcome of psychedelic use and are now being recognized as an integral part of psychedelic-assisted psychotherapy [53].

In psychedelic-assisted psychotherapy, *integration* refers to the environment and therapeutic interventions that are generally undertaken, usually over a three-day period. The first day is dedicated to preparing for the drug session, which is carried out the following day usually with one or two *guides* or sitters. On the third day, an inquiry and integration session completes the assessment of the subjective experience and possible meaningful interpretations which may have arisen during or following the drug session. Although a detailed discussion on this subject is beyond the scope of this text, it is worth mentioning that pre- and post-session interventions are necessary in helping with psychedelic integration since these types of *peak* experiences can exhibit mystical qualities – aka "shaking the snow globe," which may prompt philosophical cogitations or impulsive lifestyle choices and therefore require the need for "a soft landing" through post-session inquiry and appropriate interpretation and guidance.

For these reasons, pre- and post-integration have been designed to establish a favorable environment into which patients can "return to" after mystical or *numinous* (having a strong religious or spiritual quality; indicating or suggesting the presence of a divinity) experiences. Although these inquiry techniques have been mostly studied with therapeutic LSD or psilocybin sessions, they may also be applicable in preparing inexperienced cannabis patients who may voluntarily or accidentally discover higher doses of THC bordering or crossing into the psychedelic realm.

8.5.3 Trauma Sensitivity

As with all related compounds, cannabis-induced psychedelic experiences can unearth unconscious memories. Reduced conscious control over memory and emotional processing places trauma-sensitive patients at greater risk of recalling intolerable memories. Cannabis-inexperienced individuals should be encouraged to seek counseling if they suspect this could become problematic for them. While reliving past memories may help in processing challenging life situations, trauma-sensitive individuals may be flooded with emotionally charged and unprocessed unconscious material. One study showed that up to 34% of children have experienced at least one trauma and exhibit evidence of post-traumatic stress without having a current diagnosis [46]. Since many survivors of trauma are unaware of their own personal history of childhood trauma, the use of high doses of THC can trigger spontaneous abreactions or flashbacks in these individuals.

This presents a serious dilemma. While these types of serious reactions have been encountered with the use of psychedelics, they are also encountered in other circumstances which lower ego identification, such as in mindfulness practices. Approaches such as these which use meditation techniques have been shown to be effective in relieving symptoms related to depression and anxiety. However, they can also produce adverse events in trauma survivors [47]. While there is actually no definitive method to accurately predict or prevent these types of reactions in this high-risk population, research is helping to provide certain clues. For example, many mindfulness-based approaches screen for trauma sensitivity and suggest using a slow "titration," beginning with shorter, well-structured meditations and allowing to interrupt the process at any time should the participant feel overwhelmed [121]. See Chap. 6 for information on screening and counseling trauma-sensitive individuals.

After evaluating for high-risk situations and if patients are considered having a low probability of reliving past trauma (*long-range set*), a careful review of recent stressors (*immediate set*) should then be undertaken, since emotional processing can quickly become overwhelming in an unprepared individual, particularly if they feel resistance in facing certain difficult emotional situations.

Moderate-dose cannabis psychoactivity, which may border on psychedelic experiences in certain individuals, does not necessarily require such an extensive monitoring framework. However, in advanced cancer and palliative care settings, neglecting to advise patients on the possible outcomes of higher-dose psychoactivity unnecessarily puts patients at higher risk of adverse events, particularly in cannabis-naive patients.

8.6 Dealing with an Involuntary Intoxication (Bad Trip)

Cannabis-naive individuals often find themselves unprepared for the gradual loss of conscious control over their mental processes which occurs with increasing doses of THC. Consequently, introducing certain safeguards can be helpful when facing challenging emotional reactions. Explaining the unique features of cannabis psychoactivity beforehand can be a very useful intervention in laying the groundwork for the experience of ego loss and reduced capacity to guide the focus of attention (see Section 5 below). It is also important to reassure future *psychonauts* that the events they encounter during the experience, whether cognitive, emotional, sensory, or hallucinatory, are transient creations generated by their own minds and do not necessarily reflect the reality they will return to once the drug wears off. The shape that their experience will take, and the relevance which will be attributed to its content, is an amalgamation of their own history, personality traits, and the influence of their immediate surroundings. If emotional processing becomes overwhelmed with anxiety or fear, it is important to recognize these events as transient mental constructs as well. By identifying and addressing them early, it is possible to avoid plunging further into a full-blown panic attack or delusional thinking.

Luckily, reduced control over attentional processing permits individuals subjected to this state of psychological vulnerability to be more easily distracted and amenable to gentle persuasion. Several principles stemming from psychedelic-assisted psychotherapy research have been developed to deal with this:

- *Grounding*: focusing the attention and connecting with the body (slow deep breaths, body scanning techniques) or gentle physical contact with another person [108].
- *Surrendering*: relaxing into the experience and letting go of expectations.
- *Curiosity*: taking note of the thought patterns, emotions, and imagery that arise. Prior experience with meditation techniques has been shown to provide a cushion for the experience of ego loss, since this concept is an intrinsic part of the meditative process [72].
- *Intention*: establishing a goal-oriented anchor prior to the experience can provide an emotional foundation to return to (understanding the nature of a difficult life situation, finding a creative way around an interference preventing play, fun, or joy).

Websites dedicated to recreational cannabis abound with advice on how to assist a victim in the throes of a "bad trip." Examples include listening to calm music or taking a walk in nature, both of which can be highly effective in reshaping the overall emotional experience. Some suggest watching online videos noted for their calming or positive content (Joy of Painting with Bob Ross, Alan Watts lectures, etc.). Several celebrities and cannabis advocates have also shared useful tips, such as chewing peppercorns to divert the attention towards an intense sensory stimulation.

When preparation, dose, set, and setting are not optimal, things may go temporarily awry. THC-induced paranoia and panic attacks share many similarities with non-drug-induced clinical syndromes, and this has led many to believe that abstinence is the only effective method to prevent these adverse events from reoccurring. This is indeed a prudent approach, since these reactions may be initial manifestations of a subclinical mental health problem. In many cases, these unpleasant effects do not dissuade many cannabis users from repeating the experience, which may lead to a clinical diagnosis requiring eventual treatment. However, the majority of healthy individuals who inadvertently find themselves *non compos mentis* due to cannabis intoxication eventually learn to anticipate these reactions and ascertain if their "set" is appropriate and if they find themselves in a safe and friendly *setting* where they can enjoy the full scope of the experience.

In some cases, these adverse reactions may act as an inner safety valve, releasing charged emotional "baggage" which can be an opportunity for exploring psychological conflicts leading to meaningful insights. However, offering psychodynamic interpretations while someone is dealing with an acute paranoid reaction or anxiety attack is generally not recommended and should be ideally dealt with during a post-experience integration session.

8.7 Overview of the Specific Neurocognitive Effects Associated with Cannabis Psychoactivity

With experience, individuals gradually become aware of the subtle differences in the neurocognitive effects of cannabis. In time, many grow to appreciate the benefits of certain psychoactive effects and also learn to mitigate other less desirable reactions. For some, the sought after effects remain limited to low-moderate dosage ranges which permit them to relax, unwind, or experience mild euphoria and help disconnect from their daily troubles. In this case, the sense of self is usually preserved, and psychotomimetic reactions are uncommon. Beyond a certain dosage threshold, more profound changes in connectivity occur, which can be a destabilizing experience for unprepared individuals. This section will examine this set of unique effects which often leads to a temporary state of psychological vulnerability.

The following information is intended to inform cannabis-naive individuals who wish to determine if higher-dose psychoactivity may be beneficial for them. We will review the specific neurocognitive effects and neuroimaging correlates associated with the use of high doses of THC, which are likely due to the agonistic effects on the CB1 receptor and further CB1-5HT2A receptor dimerization.

8.7.1 Slowed Down Perception of Time

One of the most prevalent and distinctive features of cannabis psychoactivity is a subjective feeling that the passage of time is slowing down, which can also vary from one experience to the next. While this effect is frequent, the underlying mechanisms which explain it are not completely understood. However, we can still draw certain preliminary conclusions based on the known effects of THC on brain circuitry.

There are multiple brain regions which regulate time perception, including the frontal cortex, basal ganglia, parietal cortex, cerebellum, and hippocampus. These regions are further influenced by sensory channels, emotional states, attention, memory, and even diseases [43]. Recent advancements in fMRI techniques have given us a glimpse of the neurological processes underlying cannabis psychoactivity and may also help to explain this phenomenon. THC-induced changes in brain function follow a pattern of increased connectivity in certain brain areas and reduced connectivity in others [132], which correlates with specific behavioral effects, including time perception. However, the results are still conflicting and are possibly due to small sample sizes, variable cannabis pre-exposure and study dosage within subjects.

The effects of THC on time perception may in fact be multifactorial, involving altered connectivity in brain regions associated with time perception and in other brain regions responsible for the attribution of attentional resources (salience attribution). By diverting the focus of awareness towards regions involved in memory and emotional processing, insight, metacognition, and self-referential processing, this global impact may provide a more comprehensive explanation for the subjective effects of time perception.

The effects of THC on attentional processes, including divided attention, have been well documented [17, 19, 94]. By disrupting the normal patterns of *attentional salience*, or the ability to "focus on what's important", THC may prevent other mental processes from obtaining the necessary attentional resources required to deal "normally" with content presented to the prefrontal cortex for higher order processing. Consequently, as time perception itself becomes less present in the field of awareness, brain activity shifts to other functional nodes and networks, thereby "amplifying" their content.

Thus, increased activity in the hippocampus, amygdala, and other regions may lift other stimuli or unconscious content into the field of awareness, bypassing the normal triaging of information which occurs during the normal waking state. This weakened ability to avoid focusing on peripheral stimuli and other background "noise" may in some cases restore memories that have been obscured by time or unconsciously denied for further emotional processing.

Cannabis-naive individuals are often stunned by the rapid flow of previously overlooked details in their surroundings and in their own thoughts. The simultaneous reattribution of brain activity which presents the field of awareness with unprocessed intrapsychic material can also generate spontaneous creative associations. In some individuals, this can be felt as a deconstruction of normal rigid thought patterns, producing a sense of balancing or equanimity in perception. Some may even recognize this as a useful, and sometimes necessary, exercise in order to "shake the snow globe" and find inspiration. The allocation of some of this processing activity to the central executive network (CEN) for higher-order cognitive management permits the unearthing of psychological conflicts as well (see Sect. 8.7.1.7). Many cannabis users learn to harness these effects in order to process and find creative options to help deal with difficult life situations. For this reason, advanced cancer patients are often ideal candidates for cannabis psychoactivity.

The awareness of the passage of time can be a dreadful experience for a newly diagnosed cancer patient. End-of-life distress and anticipatory grief can lead to an overwhelming sense of despair and many who find themselves in situations of life-threatening illnesses might find that cannabis-induced effects on time perception, and the ensuing awareness of the value of time, may provide greater benefits than symptom management alone. Furthermore, when a slowed down sense of time is accompanied by mild euphoria, an increased sensory awareness, subdued ruminations and reduced divided attention, several higher-order prefrontal activities such as metacognition and insight begin to focus their activity on the moment-to-moment content which is being presented in the field of awareness. The resulting overall experience may reestablish contact with simple pleasures and provide a higher appreciation of a more modest goal: having the permission to do the small things, deliberately, even purposefully, and see these tasks as a welcome reprieve from the tyrannical grips of apprehension.

8.7.2 Metacognition: Thinking About Thinking

> *"...along the track of the experience, the other sat looking down, observing, reasoning, and serenely weighing all the phenomena. This "calmer being", suffering with the other by sympathy, but did not lose its self possession."* – Fitz Hugh Ludlow, Confessions of a Hasheesh Eater

Metacognition, from the root word "meta" meaning "beyond" or "on top of," is defined as the ability to become self-aware of our thought processes and consequently reflect upon, understand, and control the thinking patterns that shape our belief system and influence our learning. Metacognition can also be defined more simply as a mental exercise by which people reflect on their memories and use that knowledge to regulate their reactions [69]. Hence, metacognition allows for evaluations of our decisions and permits us to avoid making "the same mistake twice" [84].

Some consider that metacognition sits at the top of a hierarchy of control over cognitive processes and allows for greater flexibility in planning and reacting to changing circumstances. Metacognition also helps in mental representations, such as anticipated regret, a uniquely human feature: we choose option A to avoid the regret we might feel if we choose option B [40]. Metacognition also helps us share our experiences with others by enabling us to paint a more accurate picture of the world. This allows for collaborative decision-making that can potentially lead to better outcomes in cognitive achievements and subjective well-being. Metacognitive abilities have also been shown to vary from one individual to the next. Research on students has demonstrated that individuals with higher metacognitive awareness are more strategic and perform better, possibly because metacognitive awareness allows individuals to plan, sequence, and monitor their learning more effectively [40].

Metacognitive functions have been shown to originate in the prefrontal cortex, along with other "higher brain functions" such as empathy, emotional regulation, morality, and intuition [114]. Studies with functional MRI have shown a positive correlation between the volume of gray matter in the most anterior region of the prefrontal cortex and metacognitive ability, and it has been suggested that this is the brain region which has undergone the most significant changes in connectivity during the course of hominid evolution [42]. This specific brain area, described anatomically as Brodmann's area 10, has also been associated with other higher cognitive functions, including prospective memory and task switching, and may serve as the apex of a hierarchy of prefrontal processes. Some suggest that the function of this region is to exert control over other cognitive processes, especially in situations that require "deliberate concentration on one's thoughts" [24]. The density of CB1 receptors varies in these regions (Fig. 8.2), and it is speculated that the endocannabinoid system (ECS) exhibits a marked influence on these and other brain areas involved with higher cognitive functions such as concentration, orientation, abstract thought, working memory, judgment, and problem-solving [37, 120].

The effects of cannabis on metacognition have also been studied. Previous anecdotal reports suggested that cannabis was capable of provoking "journeys of self-examination"; and it has been described as "forcing a broadly critical examination of who one is, where one is going and why" and thus creating a gateway into a mindset "freed from arbitrary and repressive constraints" – Doug Rushkoff [58]. Some authors go even further and propose the existence of a life *before* and *after* prolonged cannabis-induced self-examination: "straight" life being defined by dualism and seeing the world as having winners and losers and "stoned" life where one becomes aware that none of this really matters. However, the impact of cannabis on metacognitive abilities is more complex and awaits further research [58].

8.7.3 Metacognition Versus Mind Wandering

Mind wandering, commonly described as "zoning out," is known to occur in many clinical situations, such as nicotine withdrawal and alcohol intoxication [110, 111]. The effects of THC on mind wandering have also been confirmed [1]. This effect is associated with a decreased metacognitive accuracy when trying to evaluate task performance. In other words, THC leads to a decreased capacity for error monitoring when carrying out a specific task, and this deficit seems to become more pronounced as task duration increases. Thus, an increase in metacognition induced by cannabis does not necessarily equate with benefits in all circumstances and may in fact be counterproductive when goal oriented tasks are required.

However, metacognitive functions are also at play on a more "macro" level. It has been suggested that the ability to socialize is one of the outstanding features of humans and would depend critically on this metacognitive ability. It is considered a process of self-monitoring, beginning by the age of three, and it has been shown to be a teachable skill [84]. Meditative states have also been shown to improve metacognition and are a key feature of mindfulness-based treatment strategies [60, 62]. Consequently, while higher doses of THC may increase mind wandering and reduce metacognitive functioning in goal-directed tasks, the opposite may be true for insight catalysis and higher-order problem-solving.

In the normal waking state, access to the underlying process of metacognition varies from one person to the next, and self-reporting on our own and other's intentions is often inaccurate [44]. Although metacognition grants a temporary access into the larger inventory of our internalized perceptions and beliefs, this also includes our misconceptions and biases. In which case, metacognition may be laced with judgments or feelings involved with negative projections or self-evaluation. In these circumstances, metacognition could in fact detract from psychological well-being, as can be the case in depression. Consequently, insights which result from meditative practices or drug-induced metacognitive enhancements often require fact checking and inquiry in order to ascertain whether a balanced view of reality is taking place [95].

8.7.4 Metacognition Versus Insight

Metacognition requires a deliberate mental effort, whereas insight is considered more of a spontaneous understanding of the specific causes and effects of a given context. It is considered to occur relatively suddenly and described in terms such as "epiphany" or "eureka" moments. In psychiatric illness, it is considered the awareness of one's own mental health, its consequences, and need for treatment. Psychological insight refers to finding a spontaneous solution to a problem and has been attributed to increased activity in the temporal lobes and mid-frontal cortex [70].

Insight is also associated with spiritual development. The Pali word for "insight" is *vipassana*, which is now used to describe a type of Buddhist meditation practice. Recent research indicates that mindfulness meditation does facilitate insightful problem solving [106].

Several theories have been proposed to explain psychological insight mechanisms and include: suddenly seeing the problem in a new way, connecting the problem to another relevant problem, releasing cognitive bias from past experiences that are blocking the solution, or seeing the problem in a larger, more coherent context [34]. Solutions derived from insight have also been shown to be more accurate than those from non-insight conditions. The link between metacognition and insight is not well understood, but may depend on the capacity of certain neural circuits to synchronize [74].

Furthermore, low levels of insightfulness have been determined to be an important predictor in mental health outcomes [104], and research has begun to examine the insight-generating effects of psychedelics. In one study, the degree of insightfulness produced by a psilocybin session was significantly associated with a reduction in neuroticism, one of the five higher-order personality traits more likely associated with moodiness, anxiety, worry, fear, anger, frustration, jealousy, envy, guilt, depressed mood, and loneliness [39, 122]. Cannabis users often consider insight catalysis as a sought after feature of psychoactivity, and although cannabis use is associated with higher levels of psychological distress in highly introspective individuals [39], using cannabis psychoactivity in end-of-life settings in the pursuit of insight and self-examination shares little in common with youthful nihilistic self-explorations. As opposed to the long-term neuropsychiatric outcomes in young or otherwise healthy and functional individuals, the repeated use of cannabis in cancer or palliative care patients has a much greater probability of providing subjective benefits [113], but the possibility of dysphoria and depression must always be entertained if long-term survival is expected.

8.7.5 Introspective and Mystical/Spiritual Reflections

Cannabis experiences can occasionally have spiritual qualities. These are often perceived as very meaningful subjective experiences and described as being revelatory in nature. In many cases, they are considered as *ineffable*, meaning they cannot be described in words, and also possess a *noetic* quality, which William James described as "states of insight into depths of truth unplumbed by the discursive intellect." This is also accompanied by an impression that one is led passively through the experience.

Mystical experiences have been known to occur spontaneously in certain individuals without the need for external drugs. For example, Abraham Maslow was reported to experience these states by "simply resting in a lawn chair," according to his colleague William Richards. The explanation for this rare phenomenon is unclear. However, one theory suggests that DMT, the psychedelic compound found in Ayahuasca, is also present in brain tissue, although in minute quantities. Thus, certain individuals may exhibit transient elevations in their levels of DMT.

Spiritual issues are particularly relevant in oncology and palliative care, but the ability for patients to contemplate on such introspective subjects and generate insightful interpretations can vary from one individual to the other [123]. Although brain regions involved in higher cognitive functions such as metacognition and insight have been studied [34, 70, 123], the specific effects of THC on these regions and comparative effects between individuals with either low or high introspective abilities are still lacking [131]. However, cannabis users frequently report subjectively increased insight, introspection, and even mystical experiences. Subjects also often report feeling disconnected from their personal experience and exhibit feelings of *oceanic boundlessness*, or oneness with the external world, effects considered similar to when using other psychedelic compounds such as LSD or psilocybin.

When these experiences are explored on an occasional basis, the transient nature of cannabis psychoactivity allows these subjective psychic events to be reexamined after a return to normal brain functioning. Thus, inquiry into the psychological impact of these types of experiences should be routinely carried out in order to elicit any troublesome ruminations or delusional thinking which may require prompt counseling. Remaining in these states on a daily basis for extended periods of time can undoubtedly lead to reduced functioning and increased risks of more serious mental health problems.

Cannabis and other psychedelics may, in some cases, increase access to self-awareness, introspection, and spiritual insights. Recognizing these as clinically relevant situations requiring further evaluation, pharmacological intervention, and monitoring may eventually become standard medical knowledge. For now, it remains in the artistic realm of the profession.

8.7.6 Reduced Working Memory and Divided Attention

While certain higher brain networks remain relatively functional with high-dose THC, disruption in connectivity may be more pronounced in other brain regions displaying a higher density of CB1 receptors. In regions such as the amygdala, the hub of emotional processing, and the hippocampus, which is a key player in memory storage and retrieval, profound CB1 receptor activation disrupts communication between these nodes and higher cortical regions. The impact on working memory is particularly important to consider [61].

Working memory is the ability to temporarily hold information in mind, enabling a "workspace" to perform daily activities and for complex problem-solving. Working memory also plays a major role in the normal processing of the rapid flow of information which is essential for dealing with rapidly evolving situations, like driving a car. Disrupted working memory can be the result of disease processes, such as in schizophrenia [73], where it is hypothesized to be related to disruptions of the ECS in the dorsolateral prefrontal cortex (DLPFC) [28], another area rich in CB1 receptors [9, 33, 118]. The effect of THC on working memory may also be dose related [1] and increases with higher doses.

THC also affects the attentional network (parietal lobe, frontal lobe, and thalamus). When the effect of reduced working memory combines with a poorly controlled focus of attention, a reduced capacity for divided attention, and a highly suggestible salience network, the resulting disruption impairs the ability to access prior experiences in order to respond predictably to events as they are unfolding. This can be a particularly frustrating experience for many cannabis-naive individuals who often struggle to "regain control of one's senses," particularly if they are trying to engage in a complex goal oriented activity. Preparing inexperienced patients for the impact of disrupted connectivity and reduced functional capacity to control their "train of thought" is an important item to discuss in counseling before introducing cannabis. The negative impacts that result from this combined impairment require little explanation, which is why it is recommended to avoid safety sensitive tasks while under the influence of THC. However, as brain connectivity becomes disrupted and the normal cognitive patterns responsible for linear thinking spontaneously erode, this may in fact be beneficial in certain clinical situations since it may also prevent the mind from pursuing and overanalyzing undesirable ruminations.

One of the primary circuits implicated in obsessive thoughts and ruminations is the cortico-striatal-thalamo-cortical loop. This neural network can become particularly strong and active and is characteristic of obsessive-compulsive disorder (OCD). The trigger seems to arise from the dorsolateral prefrontal cortex (dlPFC), and a self-activating loop begins between these two regions. In one study, high doses of THC have been shown to reduce compulsions and intrusive thoughts in OCD patients [83]. If the effects of THC on ruminations and obsessive thoughts are indeed well founded, this surely warrants further investigation.

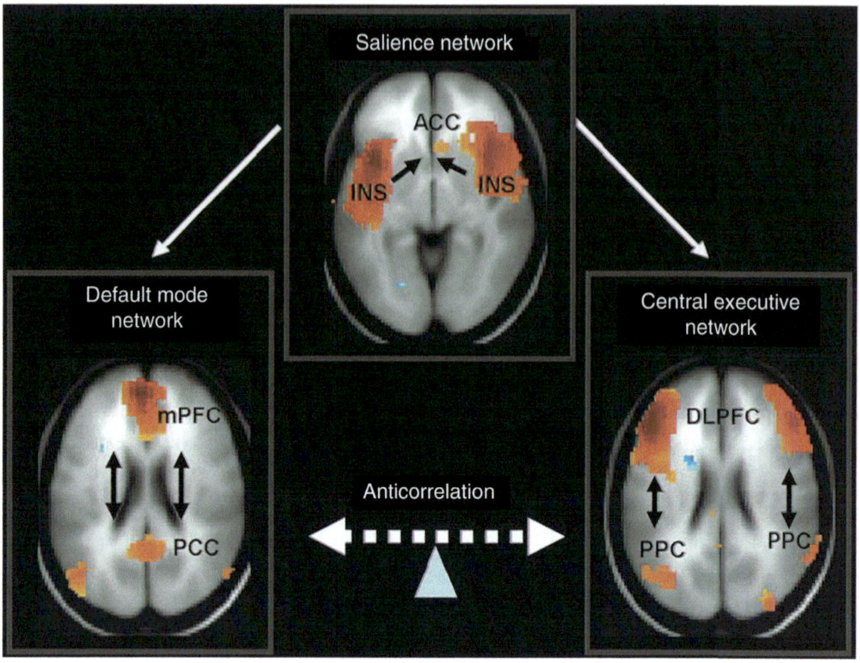

Fig. 8.1 This is an open-access article distributed under the terms of the Creative Commons Attribution License (CC-BY). The use, distribution, or reproduction in other forums is permitted, provided the original author(s) or licensor is credited and that the original publication in this journal is cited, in accordance with accepted academic practice. No use, distribution, or reproduction is permitted which does not comply with these terms. *Schematic figure of the triple network model consisting of the default mode network (DMN), salience network (SN), and central executive network (CEN).* According to this model, the anterior insula (belonging to the salience network) activates the CEN and deactivates the DMN in response to the salient stimuli. Legend: *ACC* anterior cingulate cortex, *DLPFC* dorsolateral prefrontal cortex, *PPC* posterior parietal cortex, *mPFC* medial prefrontal cortex, *PPC* posterior cingulate cortex, *INS* anterior insula [92]. In healthy humans, the SN efficiently allocates attentional resources to either the DMN or CEN. This anticorrelation (i.e., negative relationship) is necessary for optimal functioning

However, cannabis use has also been reported to *induce* ruminations in some individuals. These events may either manifest themselves as emotionally neutral “mind wanderings” and being “lost in thought” or contemplating philosophical musings. They may also deepen into brooding negative self-explorations, where the experimenter will have a tendency to overanalyze and “cling” to an idea. Many cannabis users acknowledge this phenomenon. However, like experienced meditators, most learn to eventually recognize the pointless nature of falling down these rabbit holes and learn to “let go” of their ruminations and let the salience of attention float downstream and focus on whatever “it” wants to focus on. With experience and increased metacognitive awareness, individuals often become accustomed to this process, and further exploration of cannabis psychoactivity often shifts into a journey of heightened curiosity.

8.7.7 *Heightened Sense of Awareness and Nonspecific Amplification: The Effects of THC on the Triad Network – Default Mode, Salience, and Central Executive*

Over the last few years, neuroimaging studies have provided us with an increased understanding of fundamental brain functions. While it was known that certain brain regions were responsible for specific tasks (memory, emotions, etc.), recent data has now shown that the organization of our major thought processes may in fact be orchestrated by three large neural networks. Hence, our minds are able to effectively process and analyze information, generate abstractions, and organize complex tasks thanks in great part to this triad of networks involved in determining:

1. What is important (salience network - SN)
2. Carrying out specific tasks (central executive network - CEN)
3. Monitoring ourselves and our reactions (default mode network - DMN)

The salience network (SN) seems to play a pivotal role in determining the activity of both the default mode network (DMN) and the central executive network (CEN). In essence, the salience network (SN) influences "anticorrelated" activation of the DMN or the CEN, thus alternately enabling one network and deactivating the other depending on "what's the most important thing to do right now." By doing so, the SN optimizes the attentional resources on either self-reflection (DMN) or performing a task (CEN) in order for either to function optimally (Fig. 8.1). In healthy individuals, the SN effectively switches activity between the DMN and the CEN, ensuring an optimal level of overall functionality [126].

It is now also widely believed that aberrant orchestration or switching between these networks explains many of the features of various psychiatric disorders such as schizophrenia and depression. It may also explain many of the effects of THC: when attentional processing becomes uncoupled from the memory and emotional processing hubs (hippocampus and amygdala), the remaining focus of attention becomes a "free agent," and higher cognitive control loses the ability to maintain its habitual level of awareness on what the salience network considers *important.* Cultural and social cues, as well as learned behavior, play a role in attentional processes and higher-order learning as well [45]. In disease states, a disruption in attentional processing may lead to aberrant perceptions or behaviours. However, in otherwise healthy individuals, overactive attentional processing may explain patterns of rigid thinking. Hence, the loosening of this system by way of the neuromodulatory effects of CB1 receptor activation in certain brain areas may provide a different perspective to an individual's take on reality. This has been described as "seeing things with a fresh pair of eyes," "returning to a state of childlike wonder," or "dishabituation" [58]. Regular cannabis users often become aware of this distinctive cognitive pattern which, when left to its own devices, can provide an opportunity for self-examination and a "heightened state of awareness"

Repeated experience of this kind have been known to lead to behavioral changes [77]. For example, individuals who let their hair naturally form into dreads, when asked to explain the reason why they chose not to groom their hair, often answer that they gradually became convinced, after being exposed to THC-induced increased awareness of social constructs, of the futility for much of "hair care." Thus, the subjective importance, or salience, given to time perception may dictate much of attentional salience resources and influence behaviors. The effect on the ECS seems to play a major role in reallocating attentional resources to consciously suppressed networks in most individuals who tolerate this level of psychoactivity.

These three interconnected neurocognitive networks have been determined to be essential in supporting efficient cognition and play a major role in cannabis psychoactivity. The default mode network (DMN), salience network (SN), and central executive network (CEN) have been identified based on their level of activity during specific brain functions:

8.7.7.1 The Default Mode Network (DMN)

Recent fMRI research looking at the "background noise" in resting brain activity revealed low-frequency signal fluctuations which correlated with functional anatomical systems [115]. This led to an entirely new brain mapping paradigm that is shedding light on the neural mechanisms explaining many cognitive functions and communications between brain regions in the corticolimbic system, including many of the effects of cannabis psychoactivity. These brain regions are now being described as communications "networks," "hubs," or "nodes" which, when activated, correlate with specific brain activities such as self-awareness, daydreaming, insight, recognizing social boundaries, empathy, attention, and task performance. The DMN is the largest of the three and consists of brain regions that increase in activity during resting state, when an individual is not focused on the outside world. The major nodes include the ventromedial prefrontal cortex (vmPFC), the dorsomedial prefrontal cortex (DMPFC), and the posterior cingulate cortex (PCC), and it is considered the backbone of cortical integration [6]. The DMN is involved in emotional processing, self-referential mental activity, and the recollection of prior experiences [101]. For many researchers, activity in the DMN is correlated with a corresponding level of *self-awareness* and is an area of great interest which may explain the pathophysiology of several neuropsychiatric disorders [86]. As such, DMN activity has been shown to be increased in mood disorders such as depression, which is typically accompanied by increased negative self-ruminations. Maintaining activity in the salience network may also become more difficult in depression as DMN hyperactivation seizes a larger portion of the brain's activity, preventing other brain networks from getting access to the amount of attentional salience that is required to function normally. This tug-of-war between a hyperactive DMN and other brain regions could explain why depressed patients often exhibit impaired concentration, attention, emotional control over negative thoughts, working memory, and other cognitive functions which all require a minimum level of brain activity in order to function properly. In contrast to depression, the DMN appears to be decreased in illnesses characterized by a fragmented sense of self-awareness, such as schizophrenia. This could explain why these patients report having a reduced sense of self and have difficulty to discriminate information which may or may not pertain to them. It has been demonstrated that the DMN can also be deactivated *voluntarily* in experienced meditators [23]. This observation has led some to propose that the DMN is the neuroanatomical site responsible for generating the *ego* or sense of self. THC has been shown to increase DMN activation, which may impair task performance by diminishing effective activation of the central executive network (CEN) [21].

8.7.7.2 The Central Executive Network (CEN)

The central executive network (CEN) is composed of the dorsolateral PFC and the lateral posterior parietal cortex and is involved in maintaining and manipulating working memory, executive function, and cognitive control processes. It is also responsible for decision-making and problem-solving and goal-directed behavior. In other words, the CEN becomes active while performing a task, resulting in a decreased activation of the DMN (i.e., losing oneself in one's work). CEN hypoactivity has been associated in depression, which would explain decreased levels of cognitive functioning. This may result from hyperactivity in the DMN in depressed patients, allocating more attentional resources to negative self-referential processes. In which case, an increased effort is required to overcome the effects of ruminations [20].

8.7.7.3 The Salience Network (SN)

The salience network (SN) is composed primarily of the dorsal anterior cingulate cortex (daCC) and the anterior insula (AI). Unsurprisingly, the function of the SN relies greatly on components of the r*eward system*, which is composed of the amygdala, ventral striatum, and substantia nigra/ventral tegmental area, brain regions which are particularly rich in both dopamine and CB1 receptors [127]. The salience network is responsible for *salience attribution*, whereby a stimulus that is more prominent or noticeable than others is allocated a larger portion of the available attention resources (i.e., it becomes *salient*). These regions function as an information processing loop which represents and then responds to relevant internal or external stimuli by instilling these stimuli with emotional weight [115]. In other words, the SN filters out irrelevant information and assigns memory, attentional, and other cognitive resources on stimuli considered to be more *important*. It is also thought to participate in shifting brain activity back and forth between self-referential thinking (DMN) to goal-oriented tasks (CEN). There are clinical examples of salience network dysfunction. Disorders of social-emotional regulation, such as frontotemporal dementia, schizophrenia, bipolar disorder, major depression, attention deficit hyperactivity, anxiety states, autism spectrum, and substance abuse have been linked to volume loss or altered connectivity in salience networks. This could explain some of the symptoms encountered in these conditions, such as

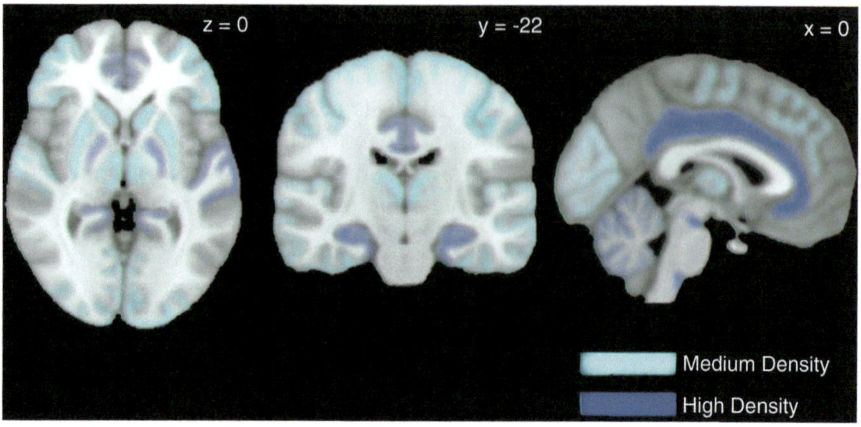

Fig. 8.2 This is an open-access article distributed under the terms of the Creative Commons CC-BY license, which permits unrestricted use, distribution, and reproduction in any medium, provided the original work is properly cited. *The distribution of CB1Rs across the human brain.* Regions with high CB1R concentration include the amygdala (not in view) and substantia nigra (related to salience network), cerebellum, cingulate gyrus, dorsal motor nucleus of the vagus, entorhinal cortex, globus pallidus, hippocampal formation, middle frontal gyrus, and Wernicke's area. Regions with medium CB1R concentration include the auditory cortex (right), caudate nucleus, mediodorsal nucleus of the thalamus, motor cortex, occipitotemporal gyrus, putamen, somatosensory cortex, and visual cortex. Montreal Neurological Institute coordinates (x, y, z) are shown above [18]

difficulties in orchestrating and maintaining the focus of attention on objectively relevant tasks. However, when functioning normally, the DMN and the CEN exchange the bulk of attentional salience on demand which permits focusing most of the available attentional resources on either self-reflection and analysis or performing a task. Focused attention to these two activities, which are influenced by emotions and memory, makes up for most of daily consciousness. With the possible exception of meditative states which produce a unique pattern in connectivity, most functional adults find it difficult to envision any other possible way of experiencing consciousness, which may possibly explain why cannabis produces such intense reactions in some individuals.

These three important networks (DMN, SN, CEN) are densely populated with CB1 receptors (Fig. 8.2), producing significant disruptions in connectivity when exposed to THC. This may explain several negative side effects of cannabis such as reduced capacity for effective executive functioning (i.e., carrying out complex tasks) and delusional thinking. Despite this growing body of research, the full impact of THC on these networks is not completely understood. Brain mapping studies looking into the effects of THC have focused mostly on the negative mental health and cognitive outcomes. This has attracted much interest since comparable disruptions have been found to exist in other mental health conditions and psychosis in particular. In trauma-sensitive individuals, meditation has been shown to produce, possibly by way of default mode deactivation (DMN), severe psychiatric reactions such as panic attacks [47]. THC psychoactivity can produce a similar deactivation pattern in the DMN, which can expose trauma-sensitive individuals to repressed and emotionally charged memories. This makes for a very unstable *set*. For this reason, it is crucial to reiterate the importance of introducing cannabis with very low doses and slow titration. However, repressed memories that do not carry much weight can be more easily metabolized and won't flood emotional regulation nodes. Emotional processing is also disrupted in THC-induced psychosis, and this can prevent an individual from controlling their emotional reactions to stimuli and thoughts.

Cannabis has long been described as a "nonspecific amplifier," producing a "heightened sense of awareness" [49, 132]. These popular terms have been used to express the subjective experience of becoming aware that our "natural" tendency to guide our focus of attention to external or internal stimuli and events no longer follows routine cues. Details that would have otherwise gone unnoticed become more salient and grab attentional resources. This effect fits the general description of aberrant attentional and salience network attribution. Aberrant salience attribution is a theoretical framework developed in 2003 by Dr Shitij Kapur in order to unify the biological, phenomenological, and pharmacological mechanisms that are responsible for the development of psychotic disorders [64]. While the role of a hyperactive dopaminergic state has been generally accepted as having a significant role in "reward" and "reinforcement," he and others proposed that dopamine also plays a role in *motivational salience*. According to this hypothesis, the mesolimbic dopamine system mediates the conversion of emotionally "neutral" information into an "attractive" entity. This process, whereby benign thoughts or external stimuli come to "grab our attention," is termed *salience attribution*. In a normally functioning brain, relevant information is processed and actions taken according to the importance or *salience* which has been attributed to this information. In psychotic states, as well as under the influence of THC, the normal pathways governing the attribution of salience are disrupted, leading to an increased "amplification" or "heightened awareness" of information previously regarded as irrelevant.

DMN disruption by THC has also been associated with several psychotic-like symptoms. Normally, the DMN and resulting self-referential processing is "quieted," while activity in the central executive network (CEN) increases in order to effectively perform a goal oriented task. However, patients with schizophrenia exhibit an inability to deactivate their DMN when doing so, which may explain certain cognitive deficits found in this illness. THC also suppresses DMN deactivation when asked to perform a task [21]. When this occurs, both the DMN and the CEN are only partially active.

Taken together, these neurological "events" come with great risks of misinterpretations and delusions. They can, however, when combined with reduced ego control over psychological defense mechanisms, present the field of awareness with overlooked conscious or even pre-conscious material that warrant further contemplation. When examined from this perspective, the same neurocognitive effects of THC which can produce paranoid ideations or delusional thinking can also create an altered state of consciousness more favorable for insight catalysis and creative problem-solving. It then becomes a matter of determining the clinical situations that could benefit from these effects and applying the appropriate harm reduction measures in carefully selected patients.

8.7.7.4 Psychotomimetic Properties of THC: The Aberrant Salience Model

The psychoactive effects of THC by way of CB1 receptor activation are well known. However, THC effects on neurocognitive functions may also be related to its agonistic effects on the 5HT2A receptor as well. Agonism of 5HT2A has been clearly associated with the psycholytic and psychedelic effects of LSD and psilocybin [59].

Hence, the "psychoactive effects" of cannabis are more complex than previously thought. They are also involved in impairment and functional changes in brain regions responsible for anxiety, learning/memory, reward processing/motivation, euphoria, and psychosis. The acute subjective effects of CB1 receptor activation have been associated with disrupted connectivity in the amygdala, hippocampus, striatum, and prefrontal cortex, respectively [41]. Chronic cannabis use has also been associated with unique features, including disrupted activation in brain regions associated with behavioral control, learning, memory, reward and pain processing, social judgments, attention, and inhibition control [18]. Persistent structural changes in the hippocampus have also been identified in some but not all studies. A recent meta-analysis suggests that cognitive performance seems to return to the level of controls after 25 days of abstinence, at least in adult cannabis consumers. The same may not be true for adolescents, however [16].

Cannabis is considered as having psychotomimetic properties, which is defined as any drug capable of producing psychotic-like effects. THC does not only mimic the subjective experience of psychosis; recent neuroimaging data has shown that it also reduces functional connectivity in the same brain regions involved in the pathogenesis of schizophrenia [14, 18, 32]. As seen previously, one of these key areas is collectively known as the *salience network* (SN), and are responsible for the processing of information from various inputs, filtering out irrelevant stimuli and determining what is most important for the focus of attention which leads to further judgments and actions. The successive neural connections which permit our attention to selectively grab and eventually manage relevant information are known as *salience attribution*. When functioning normally, the salience network filters the constant stream of sensory inputs and correctly identifies relevant events which help guide our attention and behavior. It therefore plays an important role in learning and survival.

Aberrant salience, or the misattribution of the importance or meaning of sensory information, is a core feature of psychosis and is involved in the genesis of delusional thinking and hallucinations. As such, aberrant salience provides an interesting theoretical framework for understanding the development of psychotic disorders [64] [65]. Disrupted salience attribution is also a core feature of cannabis psychoactivity [127]. The aberrant salience model suggests that the onset of positive symptoms can occur gradually across a pre-psychotic period of heightened awareness, characterized by increasing assignment of marked and deviant importance to internal and external stimuli [65]. THC-induced disrupted salience can indeed produce very traumatic psychotic reactions. However, these same disruptions, when experienced in a prepared and controlled environment and with a clear intent, can take a completely different path and produce some rather unusual benefits. The conditions which help determine the overall tolerability and possible usefulness of these psychotic-like states have been observed and documented for nearly 200 years.

Psychosis has been largely considered a symptom associated with a disease state. This is understandable, since there are few accounts of positive outcomes that happen as a result of an unpredictable and disruptive psychotic episode. Psychotic illnesses are associated with significant distress, both acute and chronic, and are accompanied by reduced levels of functioning due to their chronic and relapsing nature. However, it is important to point out that a psychotic experience in itself does not necessarily herald negative long-term outcomes. In fact, brief psychotic episodes are common, and most individuals do not progress to chronic illness and reduced functional status [17]. They are a hallmark of type 1 bipolar disease during manic phases and have been associated with increased creativity in these circumstances [2].

Psychedelic compounds, including cannabis, can produce transient psychotic-like states that are virtually indistinguishable from acute disease states and may even increase the risk of triggering or accelerating the onset of a true psychotic illness. However, the outcome for the vast majority of individuals is a return to their baseline level of cognition and functioning [68]. Furthermore, the subjective qualities of the experiences, whether pleasant or distressing, do not depend solely on individual or idiosyncratic factors, as we have been led to believe. Although a moderate dose of THC can indeed provoke a psychotic reaction, this seems to occur largely in unprepared, predisposed, or trauma-sensitive individuals or when experienced in a particularly inhospitable surroundings or unfavorable mindset. The vast majority of cannabis experiences have not been shown to produce unpleasant long term psychological effects in well-informed, low-risk individuals and in an appropriate set and setting [49]. Later inquiry can also be helpful by reminding the subject to carefully examine and question the impact of subjectively meaningful introspections that may have arisen during the experience. In some individuals, these can take the form of profound revelations that can lead to premature conclusions and impulsive actions. In which case, subjects should be advised to pursue their reflections during a prolonged period of abstinence. Prompt referral for counseling is also advisable in some cases. In most instances, however, these states provide a fertile environment for insight catalysis and creative problem-solving that withstand the test of time.

8.7.8 Aversive Memory Extinction

"*Memory is the enemy of wonder*" – Julie Holland, The Pot Book

The devastating impact of dementia and other neurodegenerative diseases has led many to consider that reduced functional memory is synonymous with impairment. However, this may not always be the case. Post-traumatic stress disorder, a very common condition affecting nearly 10% of the population with varying degrees, may in fact be a clinical setting where an increased memory capacity is not generally considered beneficial. Moreover, cancer patients, much like survivors of myocardial infarction and stroke, often experience feelings related to post-traumatic stress disorder, including anger, anxiety, fear, hopelessness, and intrusive illness-related thoughts [129].

Acquiring and storing aversive memories is considered a basic neurological function intended to reinforce behavioral changes. Brain regions involved include the amygdala, infralimbic and prelimbic subregions of the medial prefrontal cortex (mPFC), and dorsal anterior cingulate (dACC) cortices. In the case of PTSD, this function, which was initially designed for survival in the animal kingdom, will more likely produce detrimental effects. The ECS has been shown to be involved in memory formation and retrieval and also plays a role in processing traumatic memories [82].

On the other hand, *aversive memory extinction* is a form of unlearning which inhibits or suppresses the expression of the original traumatic memory and acts as a counterweight to aversive memory formation and storage. This balancing function has been proposed as being essential to cope with stressful events which occur in an ever-changing environment. Data has also shown that the ECS also plays a central role in modulating aversive memory processing [82]. Patients with PTSD display a hypoactive vmPFC, a hyperactive dACC and amygdala, and a hypofunctional hippocampus. They also seem to have a dysregulated ECS, with low levels of circulating endocannabinoids and upregulated CB1 receptors in the hippocampus, dACC, and amygdala [8]. CB1 receptors in the mPFC have been shown to be involved not only in the extinction of conditioned fear but also in the adaptation to aversive situations in rat models [8, 75, 76]. Activation of CB1 receptors around the formation of traumatic memories has been shown to improve memory extinction of these events [76]. In a recent review, smaller doses of THC with added CBD have been shown to produce the most benefit in patients with PTSD. This review also noted that CBD may exert anxiolytic effects on higher-dose THC-induced anxiety and particularly when the dose of CBD is at least equal or higher than the dose of THC [105].

Acute medical situations such as myocardial infarction and certain medical or surgical treatments have been known to increase the risk of PTSD in patients and is associated with a lower quality of life [117]. Oncology patients are often exposed to multiple stresses, discomfort, and unpredictable escalations in symptoms occasionally requiring aggressive treatments. This is the type of clinical situation where the use of cannabis may be helpful by altering two separate memory functions: initially, by inhibiting memory formation, as a result of disrupted working memory and storage of traumatic events such as chemo or radiation therapy. After the trauma, it may also help relieve the ensuing hyperarousal states.

8.8 Other Benefits of Cannabis Use in End of Life Situations

8.8.1 *Cannabis and Creativity*

"If you're going to write stoned, edit sober" – Allen Ginsberg

The effect on creativity has been a central theme in cannabis lore and literature. In 1795, French botanist M. Marcendier observed that cannabis seemed to be useful for the "arts as well as medicine" [81]. Some even claim that jazz would not have existed without cannabis, and it is suspected that much of the music and art of the later half of the twentieth century was influenced to varying degrees by cannabis. However, the artistic process involved in producing jazz music is not necessarily applicable to other forms of art. Many artistic endeavors often require a more structured approach to produce a polished result. Ginsberg's observation was indeed perspicacious. While it is true that cannabis experiences may occasionally produce subjectively meaningful creative insights, these may not necessarily retain their relevance and stand up to scrutiny in a non-intoxicated mindset. The editing process, a crucial part of many artistic endeavors, is difficult to achieve without a fully functional prefrontal cortex, as Ginsberg intuitively pointed out. Hence, those who wish to enhance their creativity with cannabis may need to do so sparingly if they intend to complete their work.

8.8.2 *Higher-Order Problem-Solving*

Cannabis use is often directed to problem-solving or metaphysical musings, particularly in teenagers and young adults. Patients who are not faced with a life-threatening illness who present with a possible cannabis use disorder (CUD) might be advised to prioritize their high-dose cannabis use as an occasional problem-solving strategy. This can be a non-judgmental way to remind patients that the true value of "connecting with oneself" by getting high is the opportunity it presents to find ways of better connecting with others. In advanced cancer and palliative care, patients commonly face difficult personal or existential life situations that may benefit from a shift in perspective. Regular inquiry and monitoring of cannabis use as a

Table 8.1 Clinical indications for palliative sedation

Indications for palliative sedation
Refractory physical symptoms (pain, dyspnea, vomiting)
Refractory neuropsychiatric symptoms (seizures, delirium, agitation, anxiety, depression)
Severe social problems (discrimination, rejection, existential distress)

Adapted from the Oxford Textbook of Palliative Medicine. 5th ed. Edited by Nathan Cherny, Marie Fallon, Stein Kaasa, Russell K. Portenoy, and David C. Currow. Oxford University Press, 2015

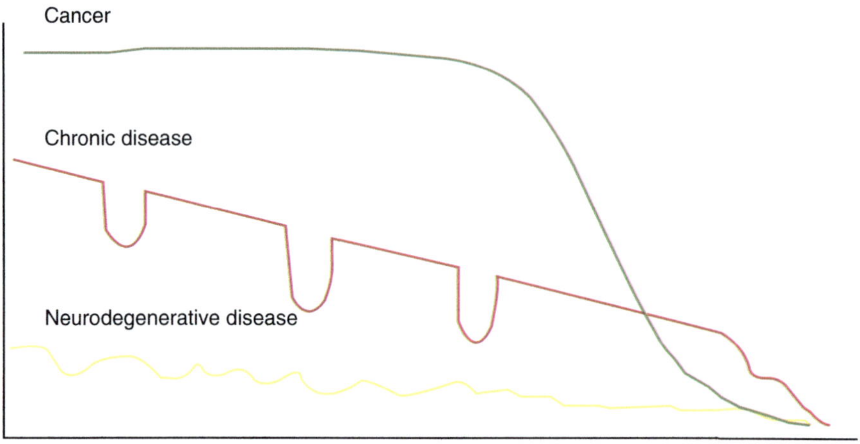

Fig. 8.3 Illness trajectories in palliative care. (Adapted from: Murray et al. [90])

problem-solving strategy for these purposes is an important harm reduction principle of cannabis medicine.

8.8.3 Delaying Palliative Sedation

Advanced cancer and palliative care often present clinicians with difficult challenges. Even with the best intentions, patients may not be able to find a momentary escape from the torments of their ordeals. The tools at our disposition have certainly improved in the last decades and we can certainly reduce much of the physical pain and anxiety. When the situation becomes truly intolerable, there is always the option of inducing palliative sedation as a last resort. Palliative sedation is defined as a controlled induction of sedation, sometimes to the point of unconsciousness, which is intended to relieve severe refractory suffering of a terminally ill patient, despite aggressive efforts to determine and treat the underlying cause. Choosing to initiate a palliative sedation protocol is often the final decision a cancer patient takes. In which case, patients spend the remaining hours or days of their lives in an unconscious or semi-conscious state and communication with others is generally no longer possible. There are many reasons why palliative sedation may be indicated, which include physical as well as neuropsychiatric or even social/existential reasons (Table 8.1). The need for palliative sedation in existential distress evidently remains an option only in certain extraordinary circumstances. Intensive "dignity therapy" by way of psychological counseling and spiritual guidance is often of benefit in these situations [29]. The consideration for palliative sedation in these clinical settings may be ethically challenging to manage. It's possible that the future integration of psychedelics may offer an alternative for these patients.

As opposed to other life-limiting diseases, cancer patients do not typically follow a steady and progressive trajectory during their illness [97]. For example, neurodegenerative diseases tend to follow a steady and gradual decline. In cancer patients, the level of functioning can remain stable after remission and usually tends to drop rapidly during the final stages of the disease (Fig. 8.3).

Very high dose cannabis psychoactivity can lead to dissociative states and may provide an additional alternative to address physical, psychological, and existential suffering during the final hours and days of life and may, in selected individuals, temporarily postpone the need for palliative sedation. Tolerance to high dose cannabis use, as discussed earlier, can take some time for cannabis-naive patients. Hence, introducing these very high dosage regimens near the end of life may not be tolerable for many patients and produce significant altered states of perception and pronounced motor incoordination or sedation. Although tolerance may build very quickly, this approach is probably better suited for patients with established tolerability to moderate-high doses of THC or with considerable prior cannabis experience.

Daily doses of THC surpassing 2000 mg or more are not uncommon, and, other than sedation and extreme forgetfulness, individuals may display few noticeable signs of impairment. Although patients may feel noticeably dissociated, they often maintain the ability to articulate thoughts and communicate coherently, which is usually not the case with high-dose opioids.

8.8.4 Coping with Forced Confinement

As a footnote to the benefits of cannabis psychoactivity, it is worth reviewing the potential impacts of cannabis use during the forced confinement set forth by the worldwide COVID-19 pandemic. This global disruption has been emotionally destabilizing for many individuals. This did not spare palliative care patients and seniors who presented with significant anxiety, depression, and other mental health issues [48], and who, in many tragic cases, were forced to die alone.

Cannabis sales in Canada have been increasing steadily since legalization for recreational use in October 2018. At the beginning of the COVID pandemic in March 2020, cannabis sales spiked in Canada and then pursued their previous upward trend, while sales of alcohol and potato chips also increased [99, 100]. This situation has also created an opportunity to compare the eventual outcomes of large-scale increases in higher-risk coping strategies.

The effects of THC on working memory and divided attention have portrayed cannabis as an imprudent recreational intoxicant for individuals working in safety-sensitive occupations (i.e., pilot, air traffic controller, bus driver, etc.) or who are responsible for the safety of infants or small children. Chronic cannabis use has also been anecdotally reported to increase tolerance to solitude and may indeed be a causal factor of social isolation in certain mental health conditions such as social anxiety disorder [10, 93] – Although the mental health outcomes of using cannabis as a coping mechanism in times of confinement are not yet known [10], in situations with few alternatives to interact with loved ones, it may provide some reprieve from the suffering brought on by forced isolation.

8.9 Conclusion

Multidisciplinary and holistic approaches to cancer care are progressively being embraced by oncologists. Learning how to harness and manage the potential benefits of altered connectivity in neural networks by way of mindfulness-based cancer recovery [26, 27, 112], psychedelic-assisted psychotherapy [50], and moderate- to high-dose cannabis psychoactivity is also gaining ground [3]. These approaches all share common therapeutic objectives, centered on providing a safe environment for self-exploration and moment to moment awareness and acceptance.

The pharmacological effects of high-doses of THC borrow some of the same receptor pathways as other psychedelics like LSD or psilocybin and the altered connectivity in the various nodes and networks involved can induce a similar dose-dependent state of heightened psychological vulnerability and suggestibility. The resulting effects can either enable higher-order problem-solving or derail into a terrifying psychotic reaction. Fortunately, most adverse events can be prevented by implementing the supportive frameworks developed in psychedelic-assisted psychotherapy, which are centered on appropriate dosage, set, setting, and integration.

As opposed to mindfulness-based techniques and structured psychedelic-assisted therapy sessions, the boundary between the necessary and excessive use of cannabis remains unclear at the present time. The risks of abuse and other potential adverse events are legitimate issues in cancer and palliative care, particularly if long-term survival is expected. However, many of these harms can be effectively mitigated, and the knowledge required to safely integrate and manage psychedelic experiences in cancer patients is being validated. Though the science is still evolving, the available data strongly suggests that these concerns should not preclude its use in most cancer and palliative care patients.

In essence, the psychoactive experience induced by cannabis requires special attention to several factors which will greatly influence the overall benefits. This knowledge is important to acquire in order to provide counseling which increases the likelihood of a more deserving outcome: the chance to leave life's torments aside, even for a brief moment, and have a bit more fun with the time that is left to live.

References

1. Adam KCS, Doss MK, Pabon E, Vogel EK, de Wit H. Δ9-Tetrahydrocannabinol (THC) impairs visual working memory performance: a randomized crossover trial. Neuropsychopharmacology. 2020;45:1807–16. https://doi.org/10.1038/s41386-020-0690-3.
2. Addington J, Farris M, Devoe D, Metzak P. Progression from being at-risk to psychosis: next steps. NPJ Schizophr. 2020;6:1–7. https://doi.org/10.1038/s41537-020-00117-0.
3. Aggarwal SK. Use of cannabinoids in cancer care: palliative care. Curr Oncol. 2016;23:S33–6. https://doi.org/10.3747/co.23.2962.
4. Ahmed AIA, van den Elsen GAH, Colbers A, Kramers C, Burger DM, van der Marck MA, Olde Rikkert MGM. Safety, pharmacodynamics, and pharmacokinetics of multiple oral

doses of delta-9-tetrahydrocannabinol in older persons with dementia. Psychopharmacology. 2015;232:2587–95. https://doi.org/10.1007/s00213-015-3889-y.
5. Almog S, Aharon-Peretz J, Vulfsons S, Ogintz M, Abalia H, Lupo T, Hayon Y, Eisenberg E. The pharmacokinetics, efficacy, and safety of a novel selective-dose cannabis inhaler in patients with chronic pain: a randomized, double-blinded, placebo-controlled trial. Eur J Pain. 2020; https://doi.org/10.1002/ejp.1605.
6. Alves PN, Foulon C, Karolis V, Bzdok D, Margulies DS, Volle E, Thiebaut de Schotten M. An improved neuroanatomical model of the default-mode network reconciles previous neuroimaging and neuropathological findings. Commun Biol. 2019;2:1–14. https://doi.org/10.1038/s42003-019-0611-3.
7. Atakan Z, Morrison P, Bossong MG, Martin-Santos R, Crippa JA. The effect of cannabis on perception of time: a critical review. Curr Pharm Des. 2012;18:4915–22. https://doi.org/10.2174/138161212802884852.
8. Barad M, Gean P-W, Lutz B. The role of the amygdala in the extinction of conditioned fear. Biol Psychiatry. 2006;60:322–8. https://doi.org/10.1016/j.biopsych.2006.05.029.
9. Barbey AK, Koenigs M, Grafman J. Dorsolateral prefrontal contributions to human working memory. Cortex. 2013;49:1195–205. https://doi.org/10.1016/j.cortex.2012.05.022.
10. Bartel SJ, Sherry SB, Stewart SH. Self-isolation: a significant contributor to cannabis use during the COVID-19 pandemic. Subst Abus. 2020;41:409–12. https://doi.org/10.1080/08897077.2020.1823550.
11. Battistella G, Fornari E, Annoni J-M, Chtioui H, Dao K, Fabritius M, Favrat B, Mall J-F, Maeder P, Giroud C. Long-term effects of cannabis on brain structure. Neuropsychopharmacology. 2014;39:2041–8. https://doi.org/10.1038/npp.2014.67.
12. Baudelaire C. Les Paradis artificiels. Paris: Auguste Poulet-Malassis; 1860.
13. Bhaskar A, Bell A, Boivin M, Briques W, Brown M, Clarke H, Cyr C, Eisenberg E, de Oliveira Silva RF, Frohlich E, Georgius P, Hogg M, Horsted TI, MacCallum CA, Müller-Vahl KR, O'Connell C, Sealey R, Seibolt M, Sihota A, Smith BK, Sulak D, Vigano A, Moulin DE. Consensus recommendations on dosing and administration of medical cannabis to treat chronic pain: results of a modified Delphi process. J Cannabis Res. 2021;3:22. https://doi.org/10.1186/s42238-021-00073-1.
14. Bhattacharyya S, Fusar-Poli P, Borgwardt S, Martin-Santos R, Nosarti C, O'Carroll C, Allen P, Seal ML, Fletcher PC, Crippa JA, Giampietro V, Mechelli A, Atakan Z, McGuire P. Modulation of mediotemporal and ventrostriatal function in humans by Delta9-tetrahydrocannabinol: a neural basis for the effects of Cannabis sativa on learning and psychosis. Arch Gen Psychiatry. 2009;66:442–51. https://doi.org/10.1001/archgenpsychiatry.2009.17.
15. Black N, Stockings E, Campbell G, Tran LT, Zagic D, Hall WD, Farrell M, Degenhardt L. Cannabinoids for the treatment of mental disorders and symptoms of mental disorders: a systematic review and meta-analysis. Lancet Psychiatry. 2019; https://doi.org/10.1016/S2215-0366(19)30401-8.
16. Blest-Hopley G, Giampietro V, Bhattacharyya S. Regular cannabis use is associated with altered activation of central executive and default mode networks even after prolonged abstinence in adolescent users: results from a complementary meta-analysis. Neurosci Biobehav Rev. 2019;96:45–55. https://doi.org/10.1016/j.neubiorev.2018.10.026.
17. Bloomfield MAP, Mouchlianitis E, Morgan CJA, Freeman TP, Curran HV, Roiser JP, Howes OD. Salience attribution and its relationship to cannabis-induced psychotic symptoms. Psychol Med. 2016;46:3383–95. https://doi.org/10.1017/S0033291716002051.
18. Bloomfield MAP, Hindocha C, Green SF, Wall MB, Lees R, Petrilli K, Costello H, Ogunbiyi MO, Bossong MG, Freeman TP. The neuropsychopharmacology of cannabis: a review of human imaging studies. Pharmacol Ther. 2019;195:132–61. https://doi.org/10.1016/j.pharmthera.2018.10.006.
19. Böcker KBE, Gerritsen J, Hunault CC, Kruidenier M, Mensinga TT, Kenemans JL. Cannabis with high δ9-THC contents affects perception and visual selective attention acutely: an event-related potential study. Pharmacol Biochem Behav. 2010;96:67–74. https://doi.org/10.1016/j.pbb.2010.04.008.

20. Borders A. Rumination and related constructs 2020.
21. Bossong MG, Jansma JM, van Hell HH, Jager G, Kahn RS, Ramsey NF. Default mode network in the effects of Δ9-tetrahydrocannabinol (THC) on human executive function. PLoS One. 2013;8 https://doi.org/10.1371/journal.pone.0070074.
22. Breitbart W, Gibson C, Chochinov HM. Textbook of Psychosomatic Medicine. (American Psychiatric Publishing, Inc., 2005).
23. Brewer JA, Worhunsky PD, Gray JR, Tang Y-Y, Weber J, Kober H. Meditation experience is associated with differences in default mode network activity and connectivity. PNAS. 2011;108:20254–9. https://doi.org/10.1073/pnas.1112029108.
24. Burgess PW, Dumontheil I, Gilbert SJ. The gateway hypothesis of rostral prefrontal cortex (area 10) function. Trends Cogn Sci. 2007;11:290–8. https://doi.org/10.1016/j.tics.2007.05.004.
25. Carlini BH, Garrett SB, Carter GT. Medicinal cannabis: a survey among health care providers in Washington state. Am J Hosp Palliat Care. 2017;34:85–91. https://doi.org/10.1177/1049909115604669.
26. Carlson LE, Doll R, Stephen J, Faris P, Tamagawa R, Drysdale E, Speca M. Randomized controlled trial of Mindfulness-based cancer recovery versus supportive expressive group therapy for distressed survivors of breast cancer. J Clin Oncol. 2013;31:3119–26. https://doi.org/10.1200/JCO.2012.47.5210.
27. Carlson LE, Beattie TL, Giese-Davis J, Faris P, Tamagawa R, Fick LJ, Degelman ES, Speca M. Mindfulness-based cancer recovery and supportive-expressive therapy maintain telomere length relative to controls in distressed breast cancer survivors. Cancer. 2015;121:476–84. https://doi.org/10.1002/cncr.29063.
28. Carter E, Wang X-J. Cannabinoid-mediated disinhibition and working memory: dynamical interplay of multiple feedback mechanisms in a continuous attractor model of prefrontal cortex. Cereb Cortex. 2007;17(Suppl 1):i16–26. https://doi.org/10.1093/cercor/bhm103.
29. Cherny N. Oxford textbook of palliative medicine, Oxford textbook of palliative medicine. Oxford University Press; 2015.
30. Choi NG, Marti CN, DiNitto DM, Choi BY. Older adults' marijuana use, injuries, and emergency department visits. Am J Drug Alcohol Abuse. 2018;44:215–23. https://doi.org/10.1080/00952990.2017.1318891.
31. Colizzi M, McGuire P, Giampietro V, Williams S, Brammer M, Bhattacharyya S. Previous cannabis exposure modulates the acute effects of delta-9-tetrahydrocannabinol on attentional salience and fear processing. Exp Clin Psychopharmacol. 2018;26:582–98. https://doi.org/10.1037/pha0000221.
32. Colizzi M, Ruggeri M, Bhattacharyya S. Unraveling the intoxicating and therapeutic effects of cannabis ingredients on psychosis and cognition. Front Psychol. 2020;11:833. https://doi.org/10.3389/fpsyg.2020.00833.
33. D'Esposito M, Postle BR. The cognitive neuroscience of working memory. Annu Rev Psychol. 2015;66:115–42. https://doi.org/10.1146/annurev-psych-010814-015031.
34. Davidson JE, Sternberg RJ, editors. The nature of insight. Cambridge: A Bradford Book; 1994.
35. Dyck E. Psychedelics and dying care: a historical look at the relationship between psychedelics and palliative care. J Psychoactive Drugs. 2019;51:102–7. https://doi.org/10.1080/02791072.2019.1581308.
36. Earleywine M, Ueno LF, Mian MN, Altman BR. Cannabis-induced oceanic boundlessness. J Psychopharmacol. 2021;35:841–7. https://doi.org/10.1177/0269881121997099.
37. Eggan SM, Lewis DA. Immunocytochemical distribution of the cannabinoid CB1 receptor in the primate neocortex: a regional and laminar analysis. Cereb Cortex. 2007;17:175–91. https://doi.org/10.1093/cercor/bhj136.
38. Ermel JA, Moran EK, Culbreth AJ, Barch DM. Psychotic like experiences as part of a continuum of psychosis: associations with effort-based decision-making and reward responsivity. Schizophr Res. 2019;206:307–12. https://doi.org/10.1016/j.schres.2018.10.026.
39. Erritzoe D, Roseman L, Nour MM, MacLean K, Kaelen M, Nutt DJ, Carhart-Harris RL. Effects of psilocybin therapy on personality structure. Acta Psychiatr Scand. 2018;138:368–78. https://doi.org/10.1111/acps.12904.

40. Filiz-Ozbay E, Ozbay EY. Auctions with anticipated regret: theory and experiment. Am Econ Rev. 2007;97:1407–18. https://doi.org/10.1257/aer.97.4.1407.
41. Finn K, editor. Cannabis in medicine: an evidence-based approach. Springer International Publishing; 2020. https://doi.org/10.1007/978-3-030-45968-0.
42. Fleming SM, Weil RS, Nagy Z, Dolan RJ, Rees G. Relating introspective accuracy to individual differences in brain structure. Science. 2010;329:1541–3. https://doi.org/10.1126/science.1191883.
43. Fontes R, Ribeiro J, Gupta DS, Machado D, Lopes-Júnior F, Magalhães F, Bastos VH, Rocha K, Marinho V, Lima G, Velasques B, Ribeiro P, Orsini M, Pessoa B, Leite MAA, Teixeira S. Time perception mechanisms at central nervous system. Neurol Int. 2016;8 https://doi.org/10.4081/ni.2016.5939.
44. Frith CD. The role of metacognition in human social interactions. Philos Trans R Soc Lond Ser B Biol Sci. 2012;367:2213–23. https://doi.org/10.1098/rstb.2012.0123.
45. Gariépy J-F, Watson KK, Du E, Xie DL, Erb J, Amasino D, Platt ML. Social learning in humans and other animals. Front Neurosci. 2014;8:58. https://doi.org/10.3389/fnins.2014.00058.
46. Gonzalez A, Monzon N, Solis D, Jaycox L, Langley AK. Trauma exposure in elementary school children: description of screening procedures, level of exposure, and post-traumatic stress symptoms. School Ment Health. 2016;8:77–88. https://doi.org/10.1007/s12310-015-9167-7.
47. Goodman A, Sommers-Flanagan J. David A. Treleaven, trauma-sensitive mindfulness: practices for safe and transformative healing. J Contemp Psychother. 2019;49:127–8. https://doi.org/10.1007/s10879-018-9407-x.
48. Gorenko JA, Moran C, Flynn M, Dobson K, Konnert C. Social isolation and psychological distress among older adults related to COVID-19: a narrative review of remotely-delivered interventions and recommendations. J Appl Gerontol. 2021;40:3–13. https://doi.org/10.1177/0733464820958550.
49. Government of Canada. Final report of the Commission of Inquiry into the Non-medical Use of Drugs/Gerald Le Dain, chairman: H21-5370/2E-PDF – Government of Canada Publications – Canada.ca [WWW Document]. URL https://publications.gc.ca/site/eng/9.699765/publication.html 2002. Accessed 19 Jul 2021.
50. Griffiths RR, Johnson MW, Carducci MA, Umbricht A, Richards WA, Richards BD, Cosimano MP, Klinedinst MA. Psilocybin produces substantial and sustained decreases in depression and anxiety in patients with life-threatening cancer: a randomized double-blind trial. J Psychopharmacol. 2016;30:1181–97. https://doi.org/10.1177/0269881116675513.
51. Grinspoon L, Bakalar J. The psychedelic drug therapies, psychedelic drugs reconsidered. A drug policy classic reprint from the lindesmith center. New York: Lindesmith; 1997.
52. Hartogsohn I. Constructing drug effects: a history of set and setting. Drug Sci Policy Law. 2017;3:2050324516683325. https://doi.org/10.1177/2050324516683325.
53. Hartogsohn I. American trip: set, setting, and the psychedelic experience in the twentieth century. Cambridge: MIT Press; 2020.
54. Hasin DS. US epidemiology of cannabis use and associated problems. Neuropsychopharmacology. 2018;43:195–212. https://doi.org/10.1038/npp.2017.198.
55. Health Canada. For health care professionals: Cannabis and cannabinoids – Canada.ca [WWW Document]. URL https://www.canada.ca/en/health-canada/services/drugs-medication/cannabis/information-medical-practitioners/information-health-care-professionals-cannabis-cannabinoids.html 2018. Accessed 19 Jul 2021
56. Health Canada. Canadian cannabis survey 2020: summary [WWW document]. URL https://www.canada.ca/en/health-canada/services/drugs-medication/cannabis/research-data/canadian-cannabis-survey-2020-summary.html 2020. Accessed 19 Jul 2021.
57. Hirvonen J, Goodwin R, Li C-T, Terry G, Zoghbi S, Morse C, Pike V, Volkow N, Huestis M, Innis R. Reversible and regionally selective downregulation of brain cannabinoid CB1 receptors in chronic daily cannabis smokers. Mol Psychiatry. 2012;17:642–9. https://doi.org/10.1038/mp.2011.82.
58. Holland J, editor. The pot book: a complete guide to cannabis: its role in medicine, politics, science, and culture. Rochester: Park Street Press; 2010.

59. Ibarra-Lecue I, Mollinedo-Gajate I, Meana JJ, Callado LF, Diez-Alarcia R, Urigüen L. Chronic cannabis promotes pro-hallucinogenic signaling of 5-HT2A receptors through Akt/mTOR pathway. Neuropsychopharmacology. 2018;43:2028–35. https://doi.org/10.1038/s41386-018-0076-y.
60. Isbel B, Summers MJ. Distinguishing the cognitive processes of mindfulness: developing a standardised mindfulness technique for use in longitudinal randomised control trials. Conscious Cogn. 2017;52:75–92. https://doi.org/10.1016/j.concog.2017.04.019.
61. Jacobus J, Tapert SF. Effects of cannabis on the adolescent brain. Curr Pharm Des. 2014;20:2186–93.
62. Jankowski T, Holas P. Metacognitive model of mindfulness. Conscious Cogn. 2014;28:64–80. https://doi.org/10.1016/j.concog.2014.06.005.
63. Johnson M, Richards W, Griffiths R. Human hallucinogen research: guidelines for safety. J Psychopharmacol. 2008;22:603–20. https://doi.org/10.1177/0269881108093587.
64. Kapur S. Psychosis as a state of aberrant salience: a framework linking biology, phenomenology, and pharmacology in schizophrenia. AJP. 2003;160:13–23. https://doi.org/10.1176/appi.ajp.160.1.13.
65. Kapur S, Mizrahi R, Li M. From dopamine to salience to psychosis—linking biology, pharmacology and phenomenology of psychosis. Schizophr Res. 2005;79:59–68. https://doi.org/10.1016/j.schres.2005.01.003.
66. Kast E. LSD and the dying patient. Chic Med Sch Q. 1966;26:80–7.
67. Kast E. A concept of death. In: Psychedelics: the uses and implications of hallucinogenic drugs. Garden City: Anchor Books; 1970.
68. Kim HS, Monte AA. Colorado cannabis legalization and its effect on emergency care. Ann Emerg Med. 2016;68:71–5. https://doi.org/10.1016/j.annemergmed.2016.01.004.
69. Koriat A. Metacognition and consciousness, in: the Cambridge handbook of consciousness. New York: Cambridge University Press; 2007. p. 289–325. https://doi.org/10.1017/CBO9780511816789.012.
70. Kounios J, Beeman M. The Aha! Moment: the cognitive neuroscience of insight. Curr Dir Psychol Sci. 2009;18:210–6. https://doi.org/10.1111/j.1467-8721.2009.01638.x.
71. Kruger DJ, Korach NJ, Kruger JS. Requirements for cannabis product labeling by U.S. state. Cannabis Cannabinoid Res. 2021; https://doi.org/10.1089/can.2020.0079.
72. Leary T. The psychedelic experience: a manual based on the Tibetan book of the dead. New York: University Books; 1964.
73. Lee J, Park S. Working memory impairments in schizophrenia: a meta-analysis. J Abnorm Psychol. 2005;114:599–611. https://doi.org/10.1037/0021-843X.114.4.599.
74. Leonhardt BL, Vohs JL, Bartolomeo LA, Visco A, Hetrick WP, Bolbecker AR, Breier A, Lysaker PH, O'Donnell BF. Relationship of metacognition and insight to neural synchronization and cognitive function in early phase psychosis. Clin EEG Neurosci. 2019; https://doi.org/10.1177/1550059419857971.
75. Lin H-C, Mao S-C, Su C-L, Gean P-W. The role of prefrontal cortex CB1 receptors in the modulation of fear memory. Cereb Cortex. 2009;19:165–75. https://doi.org/10.1093/cercor/bhn075.
76. Lisboa SF, Vila-Verde C, Rosa J, Uliana DL, Stern C, et al. Tempering aversive/traumatic memories with cannabinoids: a review of evidence from animal and human studies. Psychopharmacology. 2019;236:201–26. https://doi.org/10.1007/s00213-018-5127-x.
77. Lorenzetti V, Alonso-Lana S, J Youssef G, Verdejo-Garcia A, Suo C, Cousijn J, Takagi M, Yucel M, Solowij N. Adolescent cannabis use: what is the evidence for functional brain alteration? Curr Pharm Des. 2016;22:6353–65.
78. Ludlow FH. The hasheesh eater: being passages from the life of a pythagorean. New York: Harper; 1857.
79. MacCallum CA, Russo EB. Practical considerations in medical cannabis administration and dosing. Eur J Intern Med. 2018;49:12–9. https://doi.org/10.1016/j.ejim.2018.01.004.
80. Mahvan TD, Hilaire ML, Mann A, Brown A, Linn B, Gardner T, Lai B. Marijuana use in the elderly: implications and considerations. Consult Pharm. 2017;32:341–51. https://doi.org/10.4140/TCP.n.2017.341.

81. Marcandier M. Traité du Chanvre. Paris, Chez André [et] Debray, An troisieme [i.e. 1795]. Paris: Chez André [et] Debray; 1795.
82. Marsicano G, Wotjak CT, Azad SC, Bisogno T, Rammes G, Cascio MG, Hermann H, Tang J, Hofmann C, Zieglgänsberger W, Di Marzo V, Lutz B. The endogenous cannabinoid system controls extinction of aversive memories. Nature. 2002;418:530–4. https://doi.org/10.1038/nature00839.
83. Mauzay D, LaFrance EM, Cuttler C. Acute effects of cannabis on symptoms of obsessive-compulsive disorder. J Affect Disord. 2021;279:158–63. https://doi.org/10.1016/j.jad.2020.09.124.
84. Medina MS, Castleberry AN, Persky AM. Strategies for improving learner metacognition in health professional education. Am J Pharm Educ. 2017;81 https://doi.org/10.5688/ajpe81478.
85. Metzner R, Leary T. On programming psychedelic experiences. Psychedelic Rev. 1967;9:5–19.
86. Mohan A, Roberto AJ, Mohan A, Lorenzo A, Jones K, Carney MJ, Liogier-Weyback L, Hwang S, Lapidus KAB. The significance of the default mode network (DMN) in neurological and neuropsychiatric disorders: a review. Yale J Biol Med. 2016;89:49–57.
87. Moreau J-J. Du Haschich et de l'aliénation Mentale: études psychologiques. Paris: Fortin-Masson; 1845.
88. Murillo-Rodriguez E, Pastrana-Trejo JC, Salas-Crisóstomo M, de-la-Cruz M. The endocannabinoid system modulating levels of consciousness, emotions and likely dream contents. CNS Neurol Disord Drug Targets. 2017;16:370–9. https://doi.org/10.2174/1871527316666170223161908.
89. Murillo-Rodriguez E, Pandi-Perumal SR, Monti JM, editors. Cannabinoids and neuropsychiatric disorders, advances in experimental medicine and biology. Springer International Publishing; 2021. https://doi.org/10.1007/978-3-030-57369-0.
90. Murray SA, Kendall M, Boyd K, Sheikh A. Illness trajectories and palliative care. BMJ. 2005;330:1007–11.
91. National Academies of Sciences, Engineering, and Medicine. The health effects of cannabis and cannabinoids: the current state of evidence and recommendations for research. National Academies Press; 2017.
92. Nekovarova T, Fajnerova I, Horacek J, Spaniel F. Bridging disparate symptoms of schizophrenia: a triple network dysfunction theory. Front Behav Neurosci. 2014;8 https://doi.org/10.3389/fnbeh.2014.00171.
93. Nelemans SA, Hale WW, Raaijmakers QAW, Branje SJT, van Lier PAC, Meeus WHJ. Longitudinal associations between social anxiety symptoms and cannabis use throughout adolescence: the role of peer involvement. Eur Child Adolesc Psychiatry. 2016;25:483–92. https://doi.org/10.1007/s00787-015-0747-8.
94. Newmeyer MN, Swortwood MJ, Taylor ME, Abulseoud OA, Woodward TH, Huestis MA. Evaluation of divided attention psychophysical task performance and effects on pupil sizes following smoked, vaporized and oral cannabis administration. J Appl Toxicol. 2017;37:922–32. https://doi.org/10.1002/jat.3440.
95. Norman E. Why metacognition is not always helpful. Front Psychol. 2020;11:1537. https://doi.org/10.3389/fpsyg.2020.01537.
96. O'Shaughnessy WB. On the preparations of the Indian Hemp, or Gunjah. Prov Med J Retrosp Med Sci. 1843;5:363–9.
97. Oxford Textbook of Palliative Medicine. Oxford textbook of palliative medicine. Oxford University Press; n.d.
98. Phillips JR, Hewedi DH, Eissa AM, Moustafa AA. The cerebellum and psychiatric disorders. Front Public Health. 2015;3:66. https://doi.org/10.3389/fpubh.2015.00066.
99. Pollard MS, Tucker JS, Green HD. Changes in adult alcohol use and consequences during the COVID-19 pandemic in the US. JAMA Netw Open. 2020;3:e2022942. https://doi.org/10.1001/jamanetworkopen.2020.22942.
100. Potatoes USA. Marketing year 2020 – total potato sales. Potatoes USA. URL https://potatoesusa.com/research-reports/marketing-year-2020-total-potato-sales/ 2020. Accessed 19 Jul 2021.

101. Raichle ME. The Brain's default mode network. Annu Rev Neurosci. 2015;38:433–47. https://doi.org/10.1146/annurev-neuro-071013-014030.
102. Ramaekers JG, Kauert G, Theunissen EL, Toennes SW, Moeller MR. Neurocognitive performance during acute THC intoxication in heavy and occasional cannabis users. J Psychopharmacol. 2009;23:266–77. https://doi.org/10.1177/0269881108092393.
103. Ramaekers JG, Theunissen EL, de Brouwer M, Toennes SW, Moeller MR, Kauert G. Tolerance and cross-tolerance to neurocognitive effects of THC and alcohol in heavy cannabis users. Psychopharmacology. 2011;214:391–401. https://doi.org/10.1007/s00213-010-2042-1.
104. Ramu N, Kolliakou A, Sanyal J, Patel R, Stewart R. Recorded poor insight as a predictor of service use outcomes: cohort study of patients with first-episode psychosis in a large mental healthcare database. BMJ Open. 2019;9:e028929. https://doi.org/10.1136/bmjopen-2019-028929.
105. Raymundi AM, Da Silva TR, Sohn J, Bertoglio LJ, Stern CA. Effects of Δ 9 -tetrahydrocannabinol on aversive memories and anxiety: a review from human studies. BMC Psychiatry. 2020;20:1–17. https://doi.org/10.1186/s12888-020-02813-8.
106. Ren J, Huang Z, Luo J, Wei G, Ying X, Ding Z, Wu Y, Luo F. Meditation promotes insightful problem-solving by keeping people in a mindful and alert conscious state. Sci China Life Sci. 2011;54:961–5. https://doi.org/10.1007/s11427-011-4233-3.
107. Russo EB. Clinical endocannabinoid deficiency reconsidered: current research supports the theory in migraine, fibromyalgia, irritable bowel, and other treatment-resistant syndromes. Cannabis Cannabinoid Res. 2016;1:154–65. https://doi.org/10.1089/can.2016.0009.
108. Sahi RS, Dieffenbach MC, Gan S, Lee M, Hazlett LI, Burns SM, Lieberman MD, Shamay-Tsoory SG, Eisenberger NI. The comfort in touch: immediate and lasting effects of handholding on emotional pain. PLoS One. 2021;16:e0246753. https://doi.org/10.1371/journal.pone.0246753.
109. Saltz G. The power of different. The link between disorder and genius. Little, Brown Book Group; 2017.
110. Sayette MA, Reichle ED, Schooler JW. Lost in the sauce the effects of alcohol on mind wandering? Psychol Sci. 2009;20:747–52. https://doi.org/10.1111/j.1467-9280.2009.02351.x.
111. Sayette MA, Schooler JW, Reichle ED. Out for a smoke: the impact of cigarette craving on zoning out during reading. Psychol Sci. 2010;21:26–30. https://doi.org/10.1177/0956797609354059.
112. Schellekens MP, Tamagawa R, Labelle LE, Speca M, Stephen J, Drysdale E, Sample S, Pickering B, Dirkse D, Savage LL, Carlson LE. Mindfulness-Based Cancer Recovery (MBCR) versus Supportive Expressive Group Therapy (SET) for distressed breast cancer survivors: evaluating mindfulness and social support as mediators. J Behav Med. 2017;40:414–22. https://doi.org/10.1007/s10865-016-9799-6.
113. Schleider LB-L, Mechoulam R, Lederman V, Hilou M, Lencovsky O, Betzalel O, Shbiro L, Novack V. Prospective analysis of safety and efficacy of medical cannabis in large unselected population of patients with cancer. Eur J Intern Med. 2018;49:37–43. https://doi.org/10.1016/j.ejim.2018.01.023.
114. Schraw G, Dennison RS. Assessing metacognitive awareness. Contemp Educ Psychol. 1994;19:460–75. https://doi.org/10.1006/ceps.1994.1033.
115. Seeley WW. The salience network: a neural system for perceiving and responding to homeostatic demands. J Neurosci. 2019;39:9878–82. https://doi.org/10.1523/JNEUROSCI.1138-17.2019.
116. Sewell RA, Schnakenberg A, Elander J, Radhakrishnan R, Williams A, Skosnik PD, Pittman B, Ranganathan M, D'Souza DC. Acute effects of THC on time perception in frequent and infrequent cannabis users. Psychopharmacology. 2013;226:401–13. https://doi.org/10.1007/s00213-012-2915-6.
117. Singh A, Agrawal S, Gargya S, Saluja S, Kumar A, Kumar A, Kalra K, Thind M, Saluja S, Stone LE, Ali F, Duarte-Chavez R, Marchionni C, Sholevar F, Shirani J, Nanda S. Posttraumatic stress disorder after myocardial infarction and coronary artery bypass grafting. Int J Crit Illn Inj Sci. 2017;7:84–90. https://doi.org/10.4103/IJCIIS.IJCIIS_27_17.

118. Smith EE, Jonides J. Storage and executive processes in the frontal lobes. Science. 1999;283:1657–61. https://doi.org/10.1126/science.283.5408.1657.
119. Striley SLL, Catherine W. Marijuana use among adults 50 years or older in the 21st century. Gerontol Geriatr Med. 2018; https://doi.org/10.1177/2333721418781668.
120. Tao R, Li C, Jaffe AE, Shin JH, Deep-Soboslay A, Yamin R, Weinberger DR, Hyde TM, Kleinman JE. Cannabinoid receptor CNR1 expression and DNA methylation in human prefrontal cortex, hippocampus and caudate in brain development and schizophrenia. Transl Psychiatry. 2020;10:158. https://doi.org/10.1038/s41398-020-0832-8.
121. Tarrant J. Trauma-informed mindfulness|psychology today Canada [WWW Document]. URL https://www.psychologytoday.com/ca/blog/choosing-your-meditation-style/202006/trauma-informed-mindfulness 2020. Accessed 19 Jul 2021.
122. Thompson ER. Development and validation of an international English big-five mini-markers. Personal Individ Differ. 2008;45:542–8. https://doi.org/10.1016/j.paid.2008.06.013.
123. Tik M, Sladky R, Luft CDB, Willinger D, Hoffmann A, Banissy MJ, Bhattacharya J, Windischberger C. Ultra-high-field fMRI insights on insight: neural correlates of the aha!-moment. Hum Brain Mapp. 2018;39:3241–52. https://doi.org/10.1002/hbm.24073.
124. Turna J, Balodis I, Munn C, Van Ameringen M, Busse J, MacKillop J. Overlapping patterns of recreational and medical cannabis use in a large community sample of cannabis users. Compr Psychiatry. 2020;102:152188. https://doi.org/10.1016/j.comppsych.2020.152188.
125. van den Elsen GAH, Ahmed AIA, Verkes R-J, Feuth T, van der Marck MA, Olde Rikkert MGM. Tetrahydrocannabinol in behavioral disturbances in dementia: a crossover randomized controlled trial. Am J Geriatr Psychiatry. 2015;23:1214–24. https://doi.org/10.1016/j.jagp.2015.07.011.
126. Wang X, Öngür D, Auerbach RP, Yao S. Cognitive vulnerability to major depression: view from the intrinsic network and cross-network interactions. Harv Rev Psychiatry. 2016;24:188–201. https://doi.org/10.1097/HRP.0000000000000081.
127. Wijayendran SB, O'Neill A, Bhattacharyya S. The effects of cannabis use on salience attribution: a systematic review. Acta Neuropsychiatr. 2018;30:43–57. https://doi.org/10.1017/neu.2016.58.
128. Wilkinson ST, Radhakrishnan R, D'Souza DC. Impact of cannabis use on the development of psychotic disorders. Curr Addict Rep. 2014;1:115–28. https://doi.org/10.1007/s40429-014-0018-7.
129. Wolfson PE, Andries J, Feduccia AA, Jerome L, Wang JB, Williams E, Carlin SC, Sola E, Hamilton S, Yazar-Klosinski B, Emerson A, Mithoefer MC, Doblin R. MDMA-assisted psychotherapy for treatment of anxiety and other psychological distress related to life-threatening illnesses: a randomized pilot study. Sci Rep. 2020;10:20442. https://doi.org/10.1038/s41598-020-75706-1.
130. Yeung MEM, Weaver CG, Janz K, Haines-Saah R, Lang E. Clearing the air: a study of cannabis-related presentations to urban Alberta emergency departments following legalization. CJEM. 2020;1–8 https://doi.org/10.1017/cem.2020.384.
131. Zablocki B, Aidala A, Hansell S, White HR. Marijuana use, introspectiveness, and mental health. J Health Soc Behav. 1991;32:65–79.
132. Zaytseva Y, Horáček J, Hlinka J, Fajnerová I, Androvičová R, Tintěra J, Salvi V, Balíková M, Hložek T, Španiel F, Páleníček T. Cannabis-induced altered states of consciousness are associated with specific dynamic brain connectivity states. J Psychopharmacol. 2019;33:811–21. https://doi.org/10.1177/0269881119849814.
133. Zeisser C, Thompson K, Stockwell T, Duff C, Chow C, Vallance K, Ivsins A, Michelow W, Marsh D, Lucas P. A 'standard joint'? The role of quantity in predicting cannabis-related problems. Addict Res Theory. 2012;20:82–92. https://doi.org/10.3109/16066359.2011.569101.

Summary of Recommendations

- Encourage the use of regulated and accurately labeled products.
- Proceed with caution when starting or transitioning to any product of unknown potency.
- Avoid smoking cannabis.
- Avoid mixing cannabis with tobacco.
- Avoid THC in patients at clinical high risk of psychosis or with unstable cardiovascular disease.
- Avoid all cannabis products containing either THC or CBD during pregnancy and breastfeeding.
- There are few absolute contraindications for low-range THC dosing regimens in advanced cancer and palliative care patients.
- There are even fewer absolute contraindications for mid- to high-range CBD dosing regimens.
- Setting-specific *SMART* goals may be more helpful than general pain scales in order to determine efficacy.
- Doses of cannabinoids (and THC in particular) are calculated in milligrams, not drops, bites, or puffs.
- Titration is the key to avoiding *serious* adverse events with THC.
- A starting dose of THC of less than 1 mg is safe in *nearly* every patient.
- Tolerance to *minor* adverse events occurs rapidly.
- Patients who have developed a tolerance to high doses of THC may require harm reduction counseling if long-term survival is expected.
- Paying attention to *set*, *setting*, and *integration* can reduce the severity of anxiety and paranoid reactions encountered with higher THC dosages.
- Anxiety and paranoid reactions can occur at very high doses of THC even in experienced cannabis users.
- Remain available to assess and inquire on any psychological adverse events or persisting distress related to psychoactivity, particularly in trauma-sensitive patients.

C. Cyr et al., *Cannabis and Cannabinoid-Based Medicines in Cancer Care*,
https://doi.org/10.1007/978-3-030-89918-9

- In patients who are expecting long-term survival, monitor for near-daily use of high psychoactive doses of THC, which may lead to tolerance, lower levels of functioning, and social isolation.
- Monitoring for tolerance and euphoria-seeking behavior may be less relevant near end-of-life settings.
- Very high THC dosing produces psychedelic effects similar to LSD and psilocybin by way of CB1-5HT2A dimerization but often with more adverse physiological effects.
- Patients wishing to maximize benefits and reduce the harms of psychedelic experiences should be referred for psychedelic-assisted psychotherapy (PAP).
- The use of extremely high doses of cannabinoids as anti-tumor agents has not been clinically proven and may in fact increase tumor progression in some cases.
- Clinically relevant CYP450 drug interactions can occur but usually with *high* doses of THC or CBD.
- Cannabis use can reduce the effectiveness of certain immunomodulatory drugs (i.e., checkpoint inhibitors).

Suggestions for Which Evidence is Still Lacking

- Only rough dosing guidelines are available: initial dose, titration, maintenance doses, and frequency of use are highly individualized.
- Cannabis may be more effective for treating multiple rather than single symptoms.
- The benefits of using high-CBD products to treat cancer symptoms have not yet been evaluated.
- The optimal CBD/THC ratio for treating various conditions or symptoms is unknown.
- The optimal CBD/THC ratio or threshold dose of CBD intended to reduce THC psychotropic effects is unknown but probably much higher than previously thought.
- Encourage the use of orally administered products for persistent symptoms.
- Reserve inhalation (vaporization) for breakthrough symptoms requiring short duration of effects or when first exploring higher dose psychoactivity.
- Inquire regularly on the daily dose of THC taken by the patient.
- Inquire regularly on the frequency and impact of using higher-dose THC for psychoactive or recreational purposes
- Low bid or tid THC dosing is often effective (1–10 mg/dose) if the desired goal is symptom management.
- The therapeutic range of THC for symptom management is usually below 30–40 mg per day.
- Less is more: occasional use of higher THC dosing requires close monitoring and should be reserved for experienced patients who report no serious adverse effects with mild psychoactivity

- If patients do not retain low dosage ranges for symptom management, monitor for reduced functioning and early clues of cannabis use disorder (CUD).
- Dealing with overdoses and adverse psychological reactions can often be managed with techniques such as *grounding, surrendering*, *curiosity*, and *intent.*
- Providing gentle distractions can also be effective for panic attacks and paranoid reactions.
- Psychoactivity can provide a space for creative problem-solving.
- Psychoactivity can also facilitate healing.
- Healing often requires spiritual guidance.
- Other benefits of psychoactivity include a sense of distancing from ruminations; a heightened awareness and appreciation of food, music, and art; and increased attention and reflection on overlooked details or unconscious psychic material.
- Psychoactivity may induce reinterpretations of personal opinions and cultural beliefs (dishabituation).

Cannabis in Cancer Index 2021

Number of natural cannabinoids found in the cannabis plant as of 2016: 144 [1]
Number of natural cannabinoids that have undergone human clinical trials: 2
Number of synthetic cannabinoids according to EMCDDA as of 2016: 169 [2]
Number of synthetic cannabinoids (or endocannabinoid system modulators) that have undergone human clinical trials: 5 [3]
Number of synthetic cannabinoids that are presently available for clinical use: 2
Number of synthetic cannabinoids detectable with routine drug tests: 0 [4]
Remaining number of orphan human G-protein-coupled receptors which have yet to be paired with an endogenous ligand: 100 [5]
Current number of orphan human G-protein-coupled receptors recently found to interact with cannabinoids: 10 [6]
Number of human G-protein-coupled receptors/cannabinoid interactions associated with subjective psychoactive effects and intoxication: 1
Year when morphine, cocaine, CBD, and THC were isolated, respectively: 1805, 1855, 1942, and 1964
Estimated median lethal dose (LD50) of THC in humans: 4000 mg [7]
Estimated increased CB1 receptor affinity ratio of newly isolated tetrahydrocannabiphorol (Δ9-THCP) vs Δ9-THC: 30:1 [8]
Estimated number of known cannabis strain names: 2300 [9]
Number of strains that contain significant amounts of the newly discovered tetrahydrocannabiphorol (Δ9-THCP): 1 [8]
Number of medical associations which have recognized cannabis as a *primary* treatment for any condition or symptom: 0
Percentage of cancer patients who have started using cannabis for the first time *after* learning about their diagnosis: 36% [10]
Frequency of cancer-related pain, nausea, or other cancer symptoms as reasons given for using cannabis in these patients, respectively: 46%, 34%, and 31%
Frequency of "non-cancer related reasons" given for using cannabis in these patients: 56%

C. Cyr et al., *Cannabis and Cannabinoid-Based Medicines in Cancer Care*,
https://doi.org/10.1007/978-3-030-89918-9

Percentage of oncologists who consider cannabis as a helpful adjunct to standard care: 67% [11]
Percentage of oncologists who feel equipped to make clinical recommendations regarding medical cannabis: 30%
Maximum amount of THC found in hemp flowers: 0.3%
Amount of cannabinoids found in hemp seeds: 0

References

1. Aizpurua-Olaizola O, Soydaner U, Öztürk E, Schibano D, Simsir Y, Navarro P, Etxebarria N, Usobiaga A. Evolution of the cannabinoid and Terpene content during the growth of cannabis sativa plants from different chemotypes. J Nat Products. 2016.
2. https://www.emcdda.europa.eu/system/files/publications/2753/POD_Synthetic%20cannabinoids_0.pdf
3. https://www.clinicaltherapeutics.com/article/S0149-2918(18)30332-1/pdf1.1
4. Barnes AJ, Spinelli E, Young S, Martin TM, Klette KL, Huestis MA. Validation of an ELISA synthetic cannabinoids urine assay. Ther Drug Monit. 2015;37(5):661–9. https://doi.org/10.1097/FTD.0000000000000201
5. Irving A, Abdulrazzaq G, Chan SLF, Penman J, Harvey J, Alexander SPH. Cannabinoid receptor-related orphan G protein-coupled receptors. Adv Pharmacol. 2017;80:223–47. https://doi.org/10.1016/bs.apha.2017.04.004
6. Morales P, Reggio PH. An update on non-CB1, non-CB2 cannabinoid related G-protein-coupled receptors. Cannabis Cannabinoid Res. 2017;2(1):265–73. https://doi.org/10.1089/can.2017.00361.
7. https://www.who.int/medicines/access/controlled-substances/Section3-thc-Toxicology.pdf?ua=11.
8. Citti C, Linciano P, Russo F, et al. A novel phytocannabinoid isolated from Cannabis sativa L. with an in vivo cannabimimetic activity higher than Δ 9 -tetrahydrocannabinol: Δ 9 -Tetrahydrocannabiphorol. Sci Rep. 2019;9(1):20335. https://doi.org/10.1038/s41598-019-56785-1
9. Schleuss, Jon. Medical marijuana name game. Los Angeles Times.1, 2017.
10. Martell K, Fairchild A, LeGerrier B, Sinha R, Baker S, Liu H, Ghose A, Olivotto IA, Kerba M. Rates of cannabis use in patients with cancer. Curr Oncol. 2018;25:219–2251.
11. Braun IM, Wright A, Peteet J, et al. Medical oncologists' beliefs, practices, and knowledge regarding Marijuana used therapeutically: a nationally representative survey study. J Clin Oncol. 2018;36:1957–196

Patient Evaluation and Monitoring Checklist

Checklist for the Medical Assessment of the Patient Asking about Medical Cannabis

- ☐ Date of visit
- ☐ Date of Birth
- ☐ Female ☐ Male

Patient Identifier

- ☐ Primary Symptom :
- ☐ Location
- ☐ Onset/cause
- ☐ Quality
- ☐ Duration
- ☐ Intens ity
- ☐ Aggravating/Alleviating factors
- ☐ Other Symptoms:

Quantitative measures

NRS Scales

BPI Inference Scale Score

ADL / IADL

☐ Prior Treatments Pharmacological	☐ Reason for discontinuation	☐ Prior Treatments Non - Pharmacological	☐ Reason for discontinuation

☐ Current Pharmacological Treatments	☐ Dose/duration	☐ Effect

☐ Current non-pharmacological treatments	☐ Frequency	☐ Effect

Disclaimer: **This checklist is intended to be a reference tool for the evaluation of a patient for medical cannabis by a health professional.** This is not intended for use as a screening questionnaire. This is not a validated clinical guideline. It is intended to provide a basis for a thorough assessment of the patient, their health status, risk factors, contraindications and expectations, to guide specific examination strategies, and to establish goals for medical cannabis use and monitoring. Version Date: 22-Apr-2014.

C. Cyr et al., *Cannabis and Cannabinoid-Based Medicines in Cancer Care*,
https://doi.org/10.1007/978-3-030-89918-9

Checklist for the Medical Assessment of the Patient Asking about Medical Cannabis

Past Medical History

- ☐ **Psychosis (personal)***
- ☐ **Psychosis (family)**
- ☐ **Schizophrenia***
- ☐ Anxiety
- ☐ Bipolar disorder
- ☐ Paranoia
- ☐ **Unstable heart disease***
- ☐ Ischemic heart disease
- ☐ Arrhythmias
- ☐ Cerebrovascular disease
- ☐ Liver disease
- ☐ Hypertension
- ☐ COPD
- ☐ Emphysema
- ☐ Pregnancy
- ☐ Breastfeeding

***Contra-indications for cannabinoids**

Notes:

Substance Use

- ☐ Alcohol ____ Amount / week ____ Duration ____
- ☐ Cigarettes ____ Pack years ____
- ☐ Other recreational drugs ____
- ☐ Recreational Cannabis Frequency Amount Duration ____

Notes:

Cessation attempts

Treatments, if any

- ☐ Medical Cannabis Use Frequency ____ Amount ____ Duration ____
- ☐ Dose, current (g/day) ____ Dose change over time ____
- ☐ Mode of administration ____ Self-titration ____
- ☐ Onset/how started ____
- ☐ Prescription Cannabinoids tried/used ☐ Nabilone ☐ Dronabinol ☐ Nabiximols
- ☐ Self-reported impact of cannabis on:
- ☐ Primary symptom: ____
- ☐ Other symptom(s): ____
- ☐ Function
- ☐ Mood
- ☐ Quality of life
- ☐ Sleep
- ☐ Driving ability
- ☐ Cognitive function

Social History

- ☐ Police issues Past / Ongoing ____
- ☐ Spousal / partner cannabis use ____
- ☐ Occupational Status:
  - ☐ FT employed
  - ☐ PT employed
  - ☐ Stay at home
  - ☐ Retired
  - ☐ Student
  - ☐ Temporary disability
  - ☐ Permanent disability
  - ☐ Unemployed
  - ☐ Other

Notes: *Legal issues*

Disclaimer: **This checklist is intended to be a reference tool for the evaluation of a patient for medical cannabis by a health professional.** This is not intended for use as a screening questionnaire. This is not a validated clinical guideline. It is intended to provide a basis for a thorough assessment of the patient, their health status, risk factors, contraindications and expectations, to guide specific examination strategies, and to establish goals for medical cannabis use and monitoring. Version Date: 22-Apr-2014.

Checklist for the Medical Assessment of the Patient Asking about Medical Cannabis

Physical Examination

The patient seeking medical cannabis use may present with a wide range of medical conditions, and since the effects of cannabis may affect multiple symptoms, a full physical examination is recommended to establish baseline health status and confirm diagnosis.

- [ ] Pulse
- [ ] Blood pressure
- [ ] Mood
- [ ] Mental status
- [ ] Speech content
- [ ] Speech quality

Notes:

- [ ] Jaundice
- [ ] Cyanosis
- [ ] Lymphadenopathy
- [ ] Edema
- [ ] Needle marks/scars
- [ ] Respiratory exam
- [ ] Cardiovascular exam
- [ ] Musculoskeletal exam
- [ ] Other exams

Notes:

Assessment / Diagnosis:

- [ ] **DSM V Cannabis use Disorder**

- [ ] Referring diagnosis (if applicable)
- [ ] Information from other physicians/sources
- [ ] Other treating physicians acknowledge that cannabis is being used or considered

- [ ] Describe what the patient expects to gain from medical cannabis prescription
- [ ] Specific functional goals for cannabis treatment
- [ ] Other alternatives have been discussed and considered

Disclaimer: **This checklist is intended to be a reference tool for the evaluation of a patient for medical cannabis by a health professional.** This is not intended for use as a screening questionnaire. This is not a validated clinical guideline. It is intended to provide a basis for a thorough assessment of the patient, their health status, risk factors, contraindications and expectations, to guide specific examination strategies, and to establish goals for medical cannabis use and monitoring. Version Date: 22-Apr-2014.

Checklist for the Medical Assessment of the Patient Asking about Medical Cannabis

Treatment Plan:

- [ ] **Medical cannabis will be part of the treatment plan:** [ ] **Yes** [ ] **No** [ ] **Deferred**
- [ ] Consideration of prescription cannabinoids and alternative treatment options

Document reasons why alternatives not considered

- [ ] Consideration of patient concerns and questions

Resources provided

- [ ] Objectives of cannabis treatment

Primary symptom, other symptom(s), function, mood, sleep, quality of life

- [ ] Cannabis dose authorized g/day Duration

1 cigarette = 0.5 g
Typical analgesic dose <1-3 g/day
Watchful dose 5g/day

Mode of administration
- [ ] Smoking
- [ ] Vaporization
- [ ] Other

- [ ] Specific precautions [ ] Safety [ ] Storage [ ] Aberrant behaviours

- [ ] If cannabis is prescribed: THC (%) CBD (%)
- [ ] Cannabis Brand or Identifier Licensed Producer Name

Monitoring Targets

- [ ] Scheduled Follow up [ ] 1 month [ ] 3 months [ ] 6 months [ ] 1 year [ ] Other
- [ ] Follow up with whom
- [ ] Effect on Specified Objectives

NRS Scales
BPI Inference Scale Score
Pain Function scales
Canadian Occupational Performance Measure

- [ ] Adverse events to be monitored

Supporting Documentation

- [ ] Medical history [ ] Referring diagnosis [ ] Urine drug screen [ ] Treatment contract
- [ ] Functional goal setting [ ] Informed consent [ ] Opioid agreement
- [ ] Other

Disclaimer: **This checklist is intended to be a reference tool for the evaluation of a patient for medical cannabis by a health professional.** This is not intended for use as a screening questionnaire. This is not a validated clinical guideline. It is intended to provide a basis for a thorough assessment of the patient, their health status, risk factors, contraindications and expectations, to guide specific examination strategies, and to establish goals for medical cannabis use and monitoring. Version Date: 22-Apr-2014

Checklist for the Medical Assessment of the Patient Asking about Medical Cannabis

Follow up

- ☐ *Complete at next appointment*
- ☐ Date of visit
- ☐ Months since last visit ☐ 1 ☐ 3 ☐ 6 ☐ 12 ☐ other

Patient Identifier

- ☐ Effects of Medical cannabis on treatment objectives
- ☐ Change in
  - ☐ Primary symptom
  - ☐ Other symptom
  - ☐ Function
  - ☐ Mood
  - ☐ Sleep
  - ☐ Quality of life

NRS Scales
BPI Inference Scale Score
ADL / IADL
Canadian Occupational Performance Measure

- ☐ Treatments added ☐ Dose/duration/frequency
- ☐ Treatments discontinued ☐ Reason

- ☐ **Decision to continue with medical cannabis as part of the treatment plan** ☐ **Yes, continue** ☐ **No, do not continue** ☐ **Deferred**
- ☐ Reason for continuation or discontinuation
- ☐ Consideration of patient concerns and questions

If continuing

- ☐ Review / revise objectives of cannabis treatment
- ☐ Cannabis dose authorized g/day duration Mode of administration

1 cigarette = 0.5 g *Typical analgesic dose is<1-3 g/day* *Watchful dose = 5g/day*

THC (%) CBD (%) Cannabis Brand or Identifier Licensed Producer Name

- ☐ Specific precautions
- ☐ Safety / Storage reminders and concerns
- ☐ Monitoring targets
- ☐ Scheduled Follow up ☐ 1 month ☐ 3 months ☐ 6 months ☐ 1 year ☐ Other

Disclaimer: **This checklist is intended to be a reference tool for the evaluation of a patient for medical cannabis by a health professional.** This is not intended for use as a screening questionnaire. This is not a validated clinical guideline. It is intended to provide a basis for a thorough assessment of the patient, their health status, risk factors, contraindications and expectations, to guide specific examination strategies, and to establish goals for medical cannabis use and monitoring. Version Date: 22-Apr-2014.

Clinical High Risk for Psychosis Checklist

Patients without a history of psychotic illness but who present with predisposing factors or prodromal symptoms are at higher risk of developing more severe THC-induced psychotic symptoms. These include:

1. Early life stress:
   (a) Obstetric complications
   (b) Prenatal/postnatal infection
   (c) Maternal malnutrition/stress
2. Childhood stress:
   (a) Abuse
   (b) Head injury
3. Later life stress:
   (a) Drug use (particularly <15 years)
   (b) Migration/ethnicity
   (c) Urbanization
   (d) Social adversity
   (e) Life events
4. First-degree family history of psychosis
5. Schizotypal personality disorder
6. Presence of attenuated psychotic symptoms (APS) *particularly* if accompanied by poor functioning, long duration of symptoms, high levels of depression and reduced attention:
   (a) Derealization
   (b) Overvalued beliefs
   (c) Auditory hallucinations
   (d) Mild delusions
   (e) Having increased levels of suspiciousness

C. Cyr et al., *Cannabis and Cannabinoid-Based Medicines in Cancer Care*,
https://doi.org/10.1007/978-3-030-89918-9

(f) Disorganized speech

7. Other risk factors encountered in cancer and palliative care

(a) Brain metastasis
(b) Hypercalcemia
(c) Electrolyte and metabolic abnormalities
(d) Thyroid disorders
(e) Strokes (particularly right sided)
(f) Steroids
(g) Opioids and anticholinergics (in the elderly)
(h) Benzodiazepine and alcohol withdrawal
(i) Malnutrition (vitamin B)
(j) Specific cancers: ovarian teratoma, small cell lung cancer
(k) Neurological conditions (dementia, Parkinsons, epilepsy,...)
(l) Chemotherapy (capecitabine)

Trauma Sensitive Screening

Intended to reduce the risk of certain adverse events such as panic attacks and dissociative states which may occur with higher psychoactive doses of THC. Similar adverse events are also encountered in these individuals during meditative states [1].

High risk patients may disclose any of the following information during history taking:

- Has a diagnosis of PTSD or describes PTSD symptoms
- Divulges a trauma history or history of traumatic events, regardless of chronology
- Becomes lost in a traumatic "story"; and
- Is having traumatic stress symptoms such as panic attacks, nightmares, flashbacks, and dissociation.

If patients divulge any of the preceding items, further questioning should include:

1. "What are your current stressors?" "Your sources of stress?"
2. "Are there any past events that are still stressful for you?"
3. "What are your current stress symptoms?"
4. "Do you have a history of trauma?"
5. "Are you actively experiencing symptoms that feel connected to this trauma? Examples include flashbacks, nightmares, and having difficulty with attention
6. "Are you currently seeing a therapist?"
7. "Who else is helping you with any of the above?"
8. "Have you ever attempted to take your life and if so, can you tell me about it?"

Reference

1. Treleaven DA. Trauma-sensitive mindfulness: Practices for safe and transformative healing. W W Norton & Co. 2018.

C. Cyr et al., *Cannabis and Cannabinoid-Based Medicines in Cancer Care*,
https://doi.org/10.1007/978-3-030-89918-9

Glossary of Terms

Cannabinoid-Based Medicines in Cancer Care

Readers have surely noticed that the medical and recreational cannabis landscape uses several and often overlapping terms which are commonly used interchangeably to describe the many functions, characteristics, and products arising from this emerging field of science. While the authors of this textbook do not have the authority to formally establish which of these terms should be used preferentially, they have chosen to limit the use of certain vernacular or otherwise vague expressions in order to avoid possible confusion. The more specifically used terms chosen among the following list are mentioned at the beginning of each chapter.

1. *Endocannabinoid system (ECS)*: The ECS is a biological system composed of endocannabinoids, which are endogenous lipid-based retrograde neurotransmitters, the metabolic enzymes responsible for the synthesis and degradation of endocannabinoids and the cannabinoid receptor proteins that are expressed throughout the central nervous system (including the brain), peripheral nervous system and other organs.
2. *Endocannabinoidome (eCBome)*: The eCBome is an expanded view of the ECS, proposed to include several endocannabinoid-like lipid mediators, their metabolic enzymes, and their molecular targets that encompass several non-endocannabinoid long-chain fatty acid amides and esters, including (i) the congeners of anandamide (the N-acylethanolamines, NAEs) and 2-AG (the 2-acylglycerols, 2-AcGs); (ii) the N-acyl-amino acids; (iii) acylated neurotransmitters such as the N-acyl-dopamines and N-acyl-serotonins; and (iv) the primary fatty acid amides. These lipid mediators often share metabolic enzymes with anandamide and 2-AG but not necessarily their receptors, which include orphan GPCRs, ligand-activated ion channels, and peroxisome proliferator-activated nuclear receptors (PPARs). Strictly speaking, these molecules may not be considered endocannabinoids, but instead endocannabinoid-like mediators (or modulators). This expanded endocannabinoid system, which includes

C. Cyr et al., *Cannabis and Cannabinoid-Based Medicines in Cancer Care*,
https://doi.org/10.1007/978-3-030-89918-9

more than 100 lipid mediators, 20 enzymes, and 20 receptors, is now known as the endocannabinoidome [2].

3. *Cannabis (taxonomic definition)*: There is actually no consensus on the taxonomic classification system for the cannabis family (Cannabaceae), and some authors suggest an overhaul of the current botanical terminology [8]. The original sixteenth-century classification system categorized cannabis as a single species *Cannabis sativa* L., which was later divided into various subcategories based on morphology or usefulness as fiber, oil, seed, or drug [14]. Recently, genetic evidence has suggested three major group accessions: Sativa (fiber/seed landraces), Indica (fiber/seed landraces and drug strains), and Ruderalis [13]. The vernacular classification system, which has evolved independent of science, is still commonly used by the illicit and medical cannabis markets. It consists of numerous cultivars or strains with names such as White Widow, Northern Lights, AK-47, etc. [7]. Vernacular classification is based mostly on plant morphology (shape, height, color, smell) and subjective effects and is usually accompanied by the further descriptives Sativa, Indica, or Hybrid subcategories. Chemical analyses of available strains from the medical market have consistently shown that the vernacular product name was not a reliable indicator of cannabinoid or terpenoid content [9, 10]. Medical use of the cannabis plant minimally requires an accurate knowledge of THC and CBD potency. However, the absence of industry standards combined with outdated botanical classification systems and unreliable labeling information continue to plague the clinical integration of these products. In response to this, the US Pharmacopeia (USP) outlined a plan in 2020 to support the quality of cannabis for medical use [12]. Another prominent figure in the movement to raise industry standards is Americans for Safe Access (ASA). This not-for-profit organization has become the first cannabis organization to receive ISO 17605 accreditation by the American Association for Laboratory Accreditation (A2LA) for their Patient Focused Certification (PFC) program [11]. This allows ASA to deliver PFC certifications to medical cannabis businesses and services and ensure reliability of medical cannabis products as to strength, composition, purity, and identity (https://patientfocusedcertification.org/).
4. *Hemp*: Term used to describe fiber-/seed-producing plants of the Cannabaceae family, often containing significant amounts of CBD. The FDA states that hemp must also produce no more than 0.3 percent of THC on a dry weight basis. However, certain cannabis drug strains, which are genetically dissimilar to hemp, can also contain low THC levels and appreciable amounts of CBD.
5. *Cannabis cultivar*: A cultivar is any cultivated plant according to the International Code of Nomenclature for Cultivated Plants (ICNCP). It is the most basic and general classification category for a cultivated plant variety, uniform and stable in its characteristics [4]. Generally, these characteristics include form, color, size and yield, flavor, resistance to disease, etc. More than 700 different cannabis cul-

tivars have already been described, though it is unclear whether this type of classification reflects any relevant differences in chemical composition [5].

6. *Cannabis landrace*: Term used to describe cultivars that had evolved genetically in an ecogeographical location either naturally or using breeding techniques [6].
7. *Cannabis chemovar*: Proposed mapping system of cannabis varieties based on chemical composition [7].
8. *Cannabis clone*: Type of asexual propagation producing genetically identical plants, usually cultivated with a cutting from a stable mother plant and commonly used as a preferred method in the production of cannabis for therapeutic purposes.
9. *Cannabis extract*: Oily resin containing most of the active and nonactive chemical constituents of the cannabis plant extracted through several methods, including mechanical compression (hashish), ice (kief), heat (rosin), edible fats (oil, butter), petroleum solvents (butane, naphtha), isopropyl or ethyl alcohol, and supercritical CO_2.
10. *Cannabis distillate*: Purified cannabis extract containing higher levels of cannabinoids and trace amounts of secondary compounds (terpenes, flavonoids, etc.). Petroleum solvents are most often used to obtain these products.
11. *Endocannabinoid system modulators (ESM)*: Any chemical compound, either naturally occurring (endogenous and plant based) or synthetic, which interacts with or modulates the endocannabinoid system or endocannabinoidome. These include:

    (a) *Cannabinoids*: Any biologically active chemical compound that is functionally similar to cannabinoids derived from cannabis or hemp. There are three types of cannabinoids:

        (i) *Endocannabinoids* (classical or canonical) are produced by the human body (anandamide, 2-AG).
        (ii) *Phytocannabinoids* are derived from cannabis but also found in other plants or produced by genetically modified organisms (yeast).
        (iii) *Synthetic cannabinoids* are manufactured artificially. They encompass a variety of distinct chemical classes: the classical cannabinoids structurally related to THC; the nonclassical cannabinoids (cannabimimetics) including the aminoalkylindoles, 1,5-diarylpyrazoles, quinolines, and arylsulfonamides; and eicosanoids related to endocannabinoids. Some have demonstrated increased potency as compared with natural THC and are being studied for potential clinical use, while others are used recreationally.

    (b) *Endocannabinoid-like mediators* (e.g., PEA, OEA, SEA)
    (c) *MAGL, FAAH inhibitors*

(d) *FABP competitors*
(e) *Other*

12. *Cannabinoid-Based Medicine (CBM)*: CBM is a general term intended to describe pharmaceutical grade plant-derived or synthetic cannabinoids products which have been studied in human trials and are presently available for clinical use. These include:

    (a) *Synthetic medical cannabinoids (nabilone, dronabinol)*: These medications are available in several jurisdictions where they fall under the regulations governing the use of approved pharmaceuticals. These compounds require a *prescription* from an authorized HCP.
    (b) *Medical cannabis/Cannabis-Based Medicines (CBM)*: These terms are meant to describe the properly monitored use of pharmaceutical grade, plant-derived Cannabinoid-Based Medicines (CBM), which includes approved cannabis extracts such as Sativex™ and Epidiolex™. The latter requires a *prescription*, whereas the former is usually acquired using a *medical document* allowing patients to obtain the legal authorization to purchase cannabis products intended for medical use. These compounds require a *prescription* from a HCP and, at present, represent a minority of patients using cannabis. Criteria include:

        (i) For a recognized clinical condition or as off-label use
        (ii) Under the supervision of a HCP with an appropriate level of cannabinoid medicine experience
        (iii) With a valid medical authorization

13. *Medical marij(h)uana (MM)/cannabis (cannabinoids) for therapeutic purposes (CTP)*: Terms intended to distinguish between proper and improper use of CBM and are meant to describe the use of cannabis products or unapproved synthetic cannabinoids in either an unsupervised or inadequately structured clinical environment. This presently represents the majority of patients who have limited access to adequate resources and support. Criteria for defining MM/CTP include:

    (a) Use as self-medication without clinical supervision
    (b) Use without authorization or consent from the HCP (harm reduction strategy)
    (c) Use without guidance as to product choice and dosage
    (d) Use for an undiagnosed or inappropriate clinical condition
    (e) Use of unregulated natural or synthetic cannabinoid products

    Using the terms MM/CTP versus CBM helps to discern between two vastly different practices, one using non-standardized products in a non-existent or loosely structured setting and the other using safe and predictable products in a properly supervised clinical practice. When possible, patients should be encouraged to migrate their MM/CTP use to either CBM or CBM.

14. *High-CBD products/CBD-rich products/CBD-dominant products*:
    (a) *Full-spectrum CBD/broad-spectrum CBD*: CBD derived from cannabis sativa and not hemp.
    (b) *CBD isolate*: Purified CBD from a natural source containing trace amounts of other cannabis plant compounds. This term has been known to appear on labels containing in fact "full" or "broad" spectrum CBD products.
    (c) *Hemp-derived CBD*: Derived from the hemp plant, which is genetically similar to cannabis. Maximum THC concentration of 0.3% by dry weight.
    (d) *Synthetic CBD*
15. *Psychoactivity*: Psychoactive substances are substances that, when taken in or administered into one's system, affect mental processes, e.g., cognition or affect. This term and its equivalent, psychotropic drug, are the most neutral and descriptive term for the whole class of substances, licit (antidepressants, neuroleptics, etc.) and illicit, of interest to drug policy. "Psychoactive" does not necessarily imply dependence-producing, and in common parlance, the term is often left unstated, as in "drug use" or "substance abuse" (WHO). Does not mean impairment or intoxication.
16. *Impairment*: It is an absence of or significant difference in a person's body structure or mental functioning (CDC).
17. *Intoxication*: Intoxication is a condition that follows the administration of a psychoactive substance and results in disturbances in the level of consciousness, cognition, perception, judgment, affect, or behavior or other psychophysiological functions and responses (WHO).
18. *Peak experience*: Peak experiences are multifaceted transcendental and ecstatic states of extreme happiness, fulfillment, and loss of self in a mystical and transpersonal dimension. They represent crucial components of healthy human functioning which characterize self-actualizing individuals [3]. These experiences have been known to occur spontaneously in some individuals and in other circumstances, such as religious experiences, high-level sporting events, and with the use of certain drugs.

References

1. Ramer R, Schwarz R, Hinz B. Modulation of the endocannabinoid system as a potential anticancer strategy. Front Pharmacol. 2019. https://doi.org/10.3389/fphar.2019.004301.

2. Di Marzo V. The endocannabinoidome as a substrate for noneuphoric phytocannabinoid action and gut microbiome dysfunction in neuropsychiatric disorders. Dialogues Clin Neurosci. 2020;22(3):259–69.
3. Bassi M, Delle Fave A. Peak experiences vs. everyday feelings. In: Michalos A.C. (eds) Encyclopedia of quality of life and well-being research. Springer, Dordrecht, 2014. https://doi.org/10.1007/978-94-007-0753-5_2109.
4. Pollio A. The name of cannabis: a short guide for nonbotanists. Cannabis Cannabinoid Res. 2016;1:234–238.1.
5. Hazekamp A, Fischedick JT. Cannabis - from cultivar to chemovar. Drug Test Anal. 2012;4:660–667.1.
6. Casañas F, Simó J, Casals J, Prohens J. Toward an evolved concept of landrace. Front Plant Sci. 2017;8.1.
7. Hazekamp A, Tejkalová K, Papadimitriou S. Cannabis: From Cultivar to Chemovar II—A metabolomics approach to cannabis classification. Cannabis Cannabinoid Res. 2016;1(1):202–15. Available from: https://www.liebertpub.com/doi/full/10.1089/can.2016.0017.
8. McPartland J, Guy G. Correct (ed) vernacular nomenclature of Cannabis. O'Shaugnessy's Online Journal. Edition 4, January 2015.
9. Lynch RL, Vergara D, Tittes S, et al. Genomic and chemical diversity in cannabis. BioRxiv, 2015.
10. Hillig KW. Genetic evidence for speciation in Cannabis (cannabaceae). Genet Resour Crop Evol. 2005;52:161–180.
11. https://cannabisindustryjournal.com/news_article/americans-for-safe-access-accredited-to-iso-17065/.
12. Sarma ND, Waye A, ElSohly MA, Brown PN, Elzinga S, Johnson HE, et al. Cannabis inflorescence for medical purposes: USP considerations for quality attributes. J Nat Prod. 2020;83(4):1334–51.1.
13. Small E. Evolution and Classification of Cannabis sativa (Marijuana, Hemp) in Relation to Human Utilization. Bot Rev. 2015;81:189–294.
14. Small E, Cronquist A. A Practical and Natural Taxonomy for Cannabis. TAXON. 1976;25:405–35.

Index

A
Addiction issues, 177
Allosteric modulators, 8, 9
Anandamide (AEA), 3, 15, 43
Anti-cancer agents
  antineoplastic activity, 119–122
  breast cancer, 118
  CB1 and CB2 receptors, 117
  effects of THC, 121
  gliomas, 118
  GvHD, 122, 123
  high dose cannabinoids, 124
  immune checkpoint inhibitors, 123
  melanoma, 118
  oncologists, 118
  pancreatic cancer, 118
  preclinical evidence of, 120
Anticoagulants, 65
Antidepressants, 48
Anxiety, 213
Arachidonic acid, 3
2-Arachidonoyl glycerol (2-AG), 16–18, 43
Aversive memory extinction, 270

B
Benzodiazepines, 64
Bipolar disease, 176

C
Cachexia, 136
Caco-2, 102
Cancer-related cachexia anorexia syndrome (CACS), 136
Cancer symptom management
  appetite stimulation, 136–137
  cancer-related pain, 129
  dose-response curve, 131
  drug-sparing effects, 141–142
  higher-dose THC, 132
  multimodal symptom treatment, 143–144
  nausea and vomiting, 129, 133–135
  noncancer-related reasons, 129
  observational investigations, 130
  pain, 137–140
  randomized clinical trials, 131
  reproducibility, 131
  standardized formulations, 132
  wound healing and analgesia, 142–143
Cannabichromene (CBC), 119
Cannabidiol (CBD), 43, 57–59, 197
Cannabigerol (CBG), 119
Cannabinoid-based medicine (CBM), 131, 134, 136, 143, 302
Cannabinoid ligands, 14
Cannabinoid-opioid interactions, 47
Cannabinoid receptor-interacting protein 1a (CRIP-1a), 6
Cannabinol (CBN), 43
Cannabis, 154, 155, 180, 181, 236, 237, 239–241
  addiction issues, 177
  anxiety, 176, 213
  appetite stimulation, 212
  basic precautions, 247–250
  bipolar disease, 176
  cardiovascular effects, 162, 170, 171
  CBD, 197
  chemovar, 301

C. Cyr et al., *Cannabis and Cannabinoid-Based Medicines in Cancer Care*,
https://doi.org/10.1007/978-3-030-89918-9

Cannabis (*cont.*)
clinical high risk for psychosis, 174
clinical setting, 209, 210
clone, 301
contraindications, 160, 161
cultivar, 300
default mode network, 241
dementia patients, 157
depression, 176, 214
diagnostic criteria, 227
distillate, 301
endocannabinoidome, 155
extract, 301
financial, 167
formulation, 206–208
gastrointestinal effects, 172
general considerations, 194–196
history, 180
5HT2A receptor, 239
immune system modulatory effects, 173
increased cancer risk, 159, 160
inhalation, 201, 202, 204
initial interview, 165–168
intra-rectal, 205
involuntary intoxication, 253, 254
landrace, 301
managing patient expectations, 163, 164
managing physician expectations, 162, 163
medication history, 179
metabolism, 209
mild cognitive impairment, 178
mystical experience, 260
neurocognitive effects, 255–259, 264, 273
neurological effects, 168–170
neuropathic pain, 211
official guidelines, 155, 156
oral ingestion, 200
oromucosal ingestion, 201
patent trolling, 192
patient evaluation, 164, 165
peak experience, 240
pharmaceutical, 205, 206
post-traumatic stress disorder, 177
precautions, 162
precise dosing recommendations, 217, 218, 221–225
preparing patients, 250–252
principal active ingredients, 196, 197
prior experience, 157
psychiatric history, 174
psychoactivity, 241–246
PTSD, 215, 216
pulmonary effects, 172
risks, 157–159
salience network, 261
sleep disturbances, 216
smoke, 202, 203
THC, 175, 192, 197
THCA, 198
timing, 156
topical salves, 205
trauma-sensitive patients, 178, 179
travel, 166
Cannabis use disorder (CUD), 180, 226, 285
Cannabis withdrawal syndrome (CWS), 226
Cardiovascular effects, 170, 171
Central executive network (CEN), 256, 265, 267
Cerebral ischemia, 10
Chemotherapy, 66
Chemotherapy induced nausea and vomiting (CINV), 134, 212
Chronic morphine, 46
Chronic pain, 210
Clinical toxicity, 104
Clopidogrel, 65
Clozapine, 52
Constitutive activity, 8
Corticosteroids, 48, 62
COVID pandemic, 130

D

Default mode network (DMN), 264, 265
9-delta-tetrahydrocannabinol (THC), 4
Delta 1-THC-7-oic acid, 19
Depression, 214
Detailed psychiatric history, 173, 174
Dexamethasone, 62
Diacylglycerol lipase-alpha and-beta (DAGLs), 2
Diet, 42
Dorsolateral prefrontal cortex (DLPFC), 261
Dravet syndrome, 64
Dronabinol, 60, 92, 135, 206

E

Eicosanoid system, 19–20
Endocannabinoid system (ECS), 118, 155, 193, 238, 240, 299
AEA, 15
allosteric modulators, 8, 9
2-arachidonoyl glycerol (2-AG), 16–18
astrocytes and microglia, 9
cannabinoid ligands, 14

constitutive activity, 8
endogenous opioid systems, 13
heterodimers and membrane influences, 7–8
intracellular binding proteins, 20
NAEs, 21–23
neurophysiology of, 10–11
NMDA receptor, 14
orphan receptor, 11, 12
P-glycoprotein 1 (Pgp or P-gp), 20, 21
receptor locations, 9–10
tetrahydrocannabinol, 19–20
THC, 18
TRP channels, 12
Endocannabinoid system modulators (ESM), 301
Endocannabinoid tone, 49, 50
Endocannabinoidome (eCBome), 2, 4, 43, 93, 118, 132, 155, 193, 240, 299
Endocannabinoids, 301
Endogenous cannabinoids, 43
Endogenous opioid systems, 13
Epidiolex ™, 62, 64
Ethanol, 65

F
Fatty acid binding proteins (FABPs), 20

G
Gamma aminobutyric acid (GABA), 9
Gastrointestinal effects, 172
Glutamate receptors, 11
GPR3 modulates, 12
G-protein interactions, 2, 6
G-protein receptor 55 (GPR55), 117
Graft-versus-host disease (GvHD), 122

H
Habitual cannabis, 242
Hemp, 300
High-CBD products, 303
HIV medications, 65–66
5-hydroxytryptamine (5HT3) receptor antagonists, 134

I
Inhalation, 201
Integration, 252

L
Lennox-Gastaut syndrome, 64
Ligands, 9

M
Morphine equivalent daily dose (MEDD), 141
Mystical experience, 260

N
N-(2-acylethanolamine)-hexadecanamide, 100
Nabilone, 60, 92, 100, 135
Nabiximols, 135, 206
N-acylethanolamines (NAEs), 3, 21–23
Naproxen, 63
Neuropathic pain, 211
Nivolumab, 123
NMDA receptor, 14
Nonspecific amplifier, 267

O
Obsessive-compulsive disorder (OCD), 261
Oceanic boundlessness, 238
Oleoylethanolamide (OEA), 23
Omega-3 fatty acids, 54, 55
Oncologists, 118
Opioid receptors, 46
Oral ingestion, 199
Oromucosal ingestion, 199, 201
Orphan receptor, 11, 12
Orthosteric ligands, 7

P
Palliative sedation, 272
Palmitoylethanolamide (PEA), 21, 93, 100–105
Peak experience, 240
P-glycoprotein 1 (Pgp or P-gp), 20, 21, 62
Pharmacodynamics, 101
Pharmacokinetics, 101–103
Pharmacology and drug interactions
absorption, 42
active aryl hydrocarbons, 61
anxiety and depression, 48–50
CBD ICD50, 61
clinical and animal studies of, 46–48
cyclooxygenase and, 44–45
cytochrome system, 60
endocannabinoid physiology, 43, 44

Pharmacology and drug interactions (*cont.*)
  endocannabinoid tone, 49, 50
  glucocorticoid receptors, 45
  omega-3 fatty acids, 54, 55
  and opioids, 46
  pharmacokinetic
    anticoagulants, 65
    anticonvulsants, 64
    antidepressants, 63
    antiplatelet medications, 65
    antipsychotics, 64
    benzodiazepines, 64
    chemotherapy, 66
    corticosteroids, 62
    ethanol, 65
    HIV medications, 65–66
    janus kinase inhibitors, 63
    naproxen, 63
    opioids, 63
    theophylline, 66
  PTSD, 51
  schedule of administration, 42
  THC IC50, 61
Phoenix tears, 124
Phytocannabinoids, 42, 99, 301
Piperidine, 59
Plasticity, 11
Polypharmacy, 154
Post-traumatic stress disorder (PTSD), 50, 51, 176, 215
Prostamides, 44
Psychoactive effects, 268
Psychoactivity, 237, 239, 303
Pulmonary effects, 172

R
Reproducibility, 131
Rick Simpson oil, 124
Rimonobant, 49
Roland-Morris disability questionnaire (RMDQ), 104

S
Safety-sensitive tasks, 168
Salience network (SN), 263, 265
Social anxiety disorder (SAD), 273
Stiripentol, 64
Substance abuse, 303
Synthetic cannabinoids (SC), 301
  anti-inflammatory responses, 92
  antinociception, 92
  anti-seizure activity, 92
  black mamba, 91
  dronabinol, 92
  nabilone, 92
  PEA, 100
  pharmacodynamics of, 94–97, 101
  pharmacokinetics, 101–103
  safety, 103–105
  spice, 91
  synthetic cannabinoid toxicity, 99–100
  use in community, 94
  weight loss, 92
  withdrawal symptoms, 100

T
Tetrahydrocannabinol (THC), 18, 43, 197
THC-induced psychotic symptoms, 295
Theophylline, 66
Tofacitinib, 63
Tolerance, 177
Topical salves, 204
Tramadol, 63
Transient receptor potential (TRP) channels, 12
Trauma sensitive screening, 297
Trauma sensitivity, 252, 253
Tropical Synergy, 92

V
Vanilloid receptors (TRPV1), 46

W
Withdrawal symptoms, 100

Y
Yucatan fire, 92

9783030899172